Antibody Engineering Protocols

Methods in Molecular Biology™ Series
John M. Walker, SERIES EDITOR

55. **Plant Cell Electroporation and Electrofusion Protocols,** edited by *Jac A. Nickoloff, 1995*

54. **YAC Protocols,** edited by *David Markie, 1995*

53. **Yeast Protocols:** *Methods in Cell and Molecular Biology,* edited by *Ivor H. Evans, 1995*

52. **Capillary Electrophoresis:** *Principles, Instrumentation, and Applications,* edited by *Kevin D. Altria, 1995*

51. **Antibody Engineering Protocols,** edited by *Sudhir Paul, 1995*

50. **Species Diagnostics Protocols:** *PCR and Other Nucleic Acid Methods,* edited by *Justin P. Clapp, 1995*

49. **Plant Gene Transfer and Expression Protocols,** edited by *Heddwyn Jones, 1995*

48. **Animal Cell Electroporation and Electrofusion Protocols,** edited by *Jac A. Nickoloff, 1995*

47. **Electroporation Protocols for Microorganisms,** edited by *Jac A. Nickoloff, 1995*

46. **Diagnostic Bacteriology Protocols,** edited by *Jenny Howard and David M. Whitcombe, 1995*

45. **Monoclonal Antibody Protocols,** edited by *William C. Davis, 1995*

44. **Agrobacterium Protocols,** edited by *Kevan M. A. Gartland and Michael R. Davey, 1995*

43. **In Vitro Toxicity Testing Protocols,** edited by *Sheila O'Hare and Chris K. Atterwill, 1995*

42. **ELISA:** *Theory and Practice,* by *John R. Crowther, 1995*

41. **Signal Transduction Protocols,** edited by *David A. Kendall and Stephen J. Hill, 1995*

40. **Protein Stability and Folding:** *Theory and Practice,* edited by *Bret A. Shirley, 1995*

39. **Baculovirus Expression Protocols,** edited by *Christopher D. Richardson, 1995*

38. **Cryopreservation and Freeze-Drying Protocols,** edited by *John G. Day and Mark R. McLellan, 1995*

37. **In Vitro Transcription and Translation Protocols,** edited by *Martin J. Tymms, 1995*

36. **Peptide Analysis Protocols,** edited by *Ben M. Dunn and Michael W. Pennington, 1994*

35. **Peptide Synthesis Protocols,** edited by *Michael W. Pennington and Ben M. Dunn, 1994*

34. **Immunocytochemical Methods and Protocols,** edited by *Lorette C. Javois, 1994*

33. **In Situ Hybridization Protocols,** edited by *K. H. Andy Choo, 1994*

32. **Basic Protein and Peptide Protocols,** edited by *John M. Walker, 1994*

31. **Protocols for Gene Analysis,** edited by *Adrian J. Harwood, 1994*

30. **DNA–Protein Interactions,** edited by *G. Geoff Kneale, 1994*

29. **Chromosome Analysis Protocols,** edited by *John R. Gosden, 1994*

28. **Protocols for Nucleic Acid Analysis by Nonradioactive Probes,** edited by *Peter G. Isaac, 1994*

27. **Biomembrane Protocols:** *II. Architecture and Function,* edited by *John M. Graham and Joan A. Higgins, 1994*

26. **Protocols for Oligonucleotide Conjugates:** *Synthesis and Analytical Techniques,* edited by *Sudhir Agrawal, 1994*

25. **Computer Analysis of Sequence Data:** *Part II,* edited by *Annette M. Griffin and Hugh G. Griffin, 1994*

24. **Computer Analysis of Sequence Data:** *Part I,* edited by *Annette M. Griffin and Hugh G. Griffin, 1994*

23. **DNA Sequencing Protocols,** edited by *Hugh G. Griffin and Annette M. Griffin, 1993*

22. **Microscopy, Optical Spectroscopy, and Macroscopic Techniques,** edited by *Christopher Jones, Barbara Mulloy, and Adrian H. Thomas, 1993*

21. **Protocols in Molecular Parasitology,** edited by *John E. Hyde, 1993*

20. **Protocols for Oligonucleotides and Analogs:** *Synthesis and Properties,* edited by *Sudhir Agrawal, 1993*

19. **Biomembrane Protocols:** *I. Isolation and Analysis,* edited by *John M. Graham and Joan A. Higgins, 1993*

18. **Transgenesis Techniques:** *Principles and Protocols,* edited by *David Murphy and David A. Carter, 1993*

17. **Spectroscopic Methods and Analyses:** *NMR, Mass Spectrometry, and Metalloprotein Techniques,* edited by *Christopher Jones, Barbara Mulloy, and Adrian H. Thomas, 1993*

16. **Enzymes of Molecular Biology,** edited by *Michael M. Burrell, 1993*

15. **PCR Protocols:** *Current Methods and Applications,* edited by *Bruce A. White, 1993*

14. **Glycoprotein Analysis in Biomedicine,** edited by *Elizabeth F. Hounsell, 1993*

13. **Protocols in Molecular Neurobiology,** edited by *Alan Longstaff and Patricia Revest, 1992*

12. **Pulsed-Field Gel Electrophoresis:** *Protocols, Methods, and Theories,* edited by *Margit Burmeister and Levy Ulanovsky, 1992*

11. **Practical Protein Chromatography,** edited by *Andrew Kenney and Susan Fowell, 1992*

10. **Immunochemical Protocols,** edited by *Margaret M. Manson, 1992*

9. **Protocols in Human Molecular Genetics,** edited by *Christopher G. Mathew, 1991*

8. **Practical Molecular Virology:** *Viral Vectors for Gene Expression,* edited by *Mary K. L. Collins, 1991*

7. **Gene Transfer and Expression Protocols,** edited by *Edward J. Murray, 1991*

6. **Plant Cell and Tissue Culture,** edited by *Jeffrey W. Pollard and John M. Walker, 1990*

5. **Animal Cell Culture,** edited by *Jeffrey W. Pollard and John M. Walker, 1990*

Methods in Molecular Biology™ • 51

Antibody Engineering Protocols

Edited by

Sudhir Paul

University of Nebraska Medical Center, Omaha, NE

Humana Press ✴ **Totowa, New Jersey**

Printed in the United States of America. 10 9 8 7 6 5 4 3 2 1

Library of Congress Cataloging in Publication Data

Main entry under title:

Methods in molecular biology™.

Antibody engineering protocols / edited by Sudhir Paul.
         p.   cm. -- (Methods in molecular biology™ ; 51)
      Includes index.
      ISBN 0-89603-275-2 (alk. paper)
      1. Immunoglobulins--Biotechnology. 2. Protein engineering.
   I. Paul, Sudhir. II. Series: Methods in molecular biology™ (Totowa,
   NJ) ; 51.
   TP248.65.I49A585 1995
   616.07'93--dc20   95-423
                                                                       CIP

Preface

Antibodies are the instruments of immune defense and attack. They can bind small atomic arrays as well as large epitopes with high affinity. *Antibody Engineering Protocols* presents advanced protocols in the field of antibody engineering, reviews of basic principles and methodology, and a historical perspective on the development of currently held beliefs about antibody structure–function relationships. The topics cover analysis of antibody sequences, three-dimensional structure, delineation of antibody characteristics in polyclonal mixtures, phage display of natural and synthetic antibodies, and antibody catalysis.

Ligand recognition by antibodies occurs primarily at a subset of amino acid residues located in the complementarity determining regions (CDRs) found in the light (L) and heavy (H) chain subunits. Specific antibodies are developed by immunization with molecules identical to or related in structure to the target ligand. The immune repertoire from nonimmunized individuals also contains pre-existing specificities that can be selected by screening libraries composed of hybridoma cells or phage particles displaying F_v domains or individual variable domains of the light (V_L) and heavy (V_H) chains. Random or site-directed mutagenesis in vitro can be used to refine the pre-existing specificities or produce new specificities *de novo*. Another level at which new specificities may be generated in vitro is V_L and V_H domain-swapping and CDR-swapping. The former procedure embodies a variation of natural mechanisms of generating antibody diversity. The latter procedure produces new intramolecular CDR combinations not found in nature. Application of anti-idiotypic imagery can also be utilized to replicate and modify the active site of antibodies and enzymes.

In the biological sciences, many conceptual advances have been driven by new methodology. In the case of antibody research, recent methodological developments make possible mechanistic study of the role of antibodies in immune defense and autoimmune disease, and encourage the belief that antibody fragments will find important uses in industry and medicine. In particular, the discovery of catalysis by natural antibodies offers simple means to derive new catalysts from the immune response. Immunization with transition-state and charged-substrate analogs has previously been observed to generate esterolytic and amidolytic antibodies. Combined with the natural propensity of the immune system to produce catalytic antibodies, the "nudge" toward catalysis by substrate and transition state analog immunizations may permit development of efficient catalysts.

     I thank each of the authors for painstaking descriptions of the nuts and bolts of their techniques. Donna Dutch and Angela Plendl typed many of the manuscripts, scanned them into the computer, and generally helped in generating a comprehensible text, for which I am in their debt. I thank John Walker for editorial guidance and Humana Press for producing this volume.

Sudhir Paul

Contents

Preface v

Contributors ix

Ch. 1. SEQHUNT: *A Program to Screen Aligned Nucleotide*
  and Amino Acid Sequences,
  George Johnson, Tai Te Wu, and Elvin A. Kabat 1

Ch. 2. Molecular Modeling of Antibody-Combining Sites,
  David M. Webster and Anthony R. Rees 17

Ch. 3. Structure and Properties of Human Immunoglobulin Light-Chain Dimers,
  Fred J. Stevens and Marianne Schiffer 51

Ch. 4. Crystallographic and Chromatographic Methods for Study
  of Antibody Light Chains and Other Proteins,
  Marianne Schiffer and Fred J. Stevens 83

Ch. 5. Detection of Human Variable Gene Family Expression
  at the Single-Cell Level,
  Moncef Zouali 99

Ch. 6. Purification of Reduced and Alkylated Antibody Subunits,
  Mei Sun and Sudhir Paul 111

Ch. 7. Murine Monoclonal Antibody Development,
  Donald R. Johnson 123

Ch. 8. Comparative Properties of Polyclonal and Monoclonal Antibodies,
  L. Scott Rodkey 139

Ch. 9. Evaluation of Antibody Clonality,
  L. Scott Rodkey 151

Ch. 10. Affinity Immunoblotting,
  Keith A. Knisley and L. Scott Rodkey 165

Ch. 11. Epitope and Idiotope Mapping Using Monoclonal Antibodies,
  Srinivas Kaveri 171

Ch. 12. Anti-Idiotypic Antibodies That Mimic Opioids,
  Jay A. Glasel and Dianne Agarwal 183

Ch. 13. Catalytic Antibodies: *Structure and Possible Applications,*
  Howard Amital, Ilan Tur-Kaspa, Zeev Tashma,
  Israel Hendler, and Yehuda Shoenfeld 203

Ch. 14. Preparation and Assay of Acetylcholinesterase Antibody,
  Alain Friboulet and Ladan Izadyar-Demichèle 211

Ch. 15. DNA Hydrolysis by Antibodies,
Alexander G. Gabibov and Oxana Makarevitch 223

Ch. 16. Screening Strategies for Catalytic Antitransition-State Analog Antibodies,
Alfonso Tramontano 237

Ch. 17. Expression of Chimeric Immunoglobulin Genes in Mammalian Cells,
Sergey M. Deyev and Oleg L. Polanovsky 251

Ch. 18. Single-Chain Anti-DNA F_v,
Michael Polymenis and B. David Stollar 265

Ch. 19. Molecular Cloning of Antiground-State Proteolytic Antibody Fragments,
Qing-Sheng Gao and Sudhir Paul 281

Ch. 20. Cloning and Bacterial Expression of an Esterolytic sF_v,
Rodger G. Smith, Mark T. Martin, Rosa Sanchez,
and John H. Kenten 297

Ch. 21. Site-Directed Mutagenesis of Antibody-Variable Regions,
Qing-Sheng Gao and Sudhir Paul 319

Ch. 22. Synthetic Antibody Gene Libraries for In Vitro Affinity Maturation,
Su-jun Deng, C. Roger MacKenzie, and Saran A. Narang 329

Ch. 23. Chaperonins in Phage Display of Antibody Fragments,
Eskil Söderlind, Marta Dueñas, and Carl A. K. Borrebaeck ... 343

Ch. 24. Phage-Display Libraries of Murine and Human Antibody Fab Fragments,
Jan Engberg, Peter Sejer Andersen, Leif Kofoed Nielsen,
Morten Dziegiel, Lene K. Johansen,
and Bjarne Albrechtsen 355

Ch. 25. Selection of Human Immunoglobulin Light Chains
from a Phage-Display Library,
Sonia Tyutyulkova, Qing-Sheng Gao, and Sudhir Paul 377

Ch. 26. Purification of Antibody Light Chains by Metal Affinity
and Protein L Chromatography,
Sonia Tyutyulkova and Sudhir Paul 395

Ch. 27 Rapid Purification of Recombinant Antibody Fragments
for Catalysis Screening,
Han Huang, Brian Fichter, Robert Dannenbring,
and Sudhir Paul 403

Ch. 28. Assay of Radiolabeled VIP Binding and Hydrolysis by Antibodies,
Han Huang and Sudhir Paul 409

Ch. 29 Methods of Measuring Thyroglobulin and Peptide-
Methylcoumarinamide Hydrolysis by Autoantibodies,
Lan Li, Ravishankar Kalaga, Srinivas Kaveri,
and Sudhir Paul 417

Ch. 30. Radiolabeling of Antibodies for Therapy and Diagnosis,
Janina Baranowska-Kortylewicz, Glenn V. Dalrymple,
Syed M. Quadri, and Katherine A. Harrison 423

Index 441

Contributors

DIANNE AGARWAL • Department of Biochemistry, University
of Connecticut Health Center, Farmington, CT

BJARNE ALBRECHTSEN • Department of Biology, Danmarks
Farmaceutiske Højskole, Copenhagen, Denmark

HOWARD AMITAL • Department of Medicine 'B' and Research Unit
of Autoimmune Diseases, Sheba Medical Center,
Tel-Hashomer, Sackler Faculty of Medicine, Tel-Aviv University

PETER SEJER ANDERSEN • Department of Biology, Royal Danish
School of Pharmacy, Copenhagen, Denmark

JANINA BARANOWSKA-KORTYLEWICZ • Department of Radiology,
University of Nebraska Medical Center, Omaha, NE

CARL A. K. BORREBAECK • Department of Immunotechnology,
Lund University, Lund, Sweden

GLENN V. DALRYMPLE • Department of Radiology, University
of Nebraska Medical Center, Omaha, NE

ROBERT DANNENBRING • Department of Anesthesiology, University
of Nebraska Medical Center, Omaha, NE

SU-JUN DENG • Institute for Biological Sciences, National Research
Council of Canada, Ottawa, Ontario, Canada

SERGEY M. DEYEV • Engelhardt Institute of Molecular Biology,
Russian Academy of Sciences, Moscow, Russia

MARTA DUEÑAS • Department of Immunotechnology, Lund University,
Lund, Sweden

MORTEN DZIEGIEL • Department of Biology, Royal Danish School
of Pharmacy, Copenhagen, Denmark

JAN ENGBERG • Department of Biology, Royal Danish School
of Pharmacy, Copenhagen, Denmark

BRIAN FICHTER • Department of Anesthesiology, University
of Nebraska Medical Center, Omaha, NE

ALAIN FRIBOULET • *Laboratoire de Technologie Enzymatique, Université de Technologie de Compiègne, France*

ALEXANDER G. GABIBOV • *Engelhardt Institute of Molecular Biology, Russian Academy of Sciences, Moscow, Russia*

QING-SHENG GAO • *Department of Anesthesiology, University of Nebraska Medical Center, Omaha, NE*

JAY A. GLASEL • *Department of Biochemistry, University of Connecticut Health Center, Farmington, CT*

KATHERINE A. HARRISON • *Department of Radiology, University of Nebraska Medical Center, Omaha, NE*

ISRAEL HENDLER • *Israeli Defense Forces–Medical Corps, Tel-Aviv, Israel*

HAN HUANG • *Department of Anesthesiology, University of Nebraska Medical Center, Omaha, NE*

LADAN IZADYAR-DEMICHÈLE • *Laboratoire de Technologie Enzymatique, Université de Technologie de Compiègne, France*

LENE K. JOHANSEN • *Department of Biology, Royal Danish School of Pharmacy, Copenhagen, Denmark*

DONALD R. JOHNSON • *Department of Pathology and Microbiology, University of Nebraska Medical Center, Omaha, NE*

GEORGE JOHNSON • *Department of Biochemistry and Molecular Cell Biology, Northwestern University, Evanston, IL*

ELVIN A. KABAT • *Department of Microbiology, Columbia University, New York, NY*

RAVISHANKAR KALAGA • *Department of Anesthesiology, University of Nebraska Medical Center, Omaha, NE*

SRINIVAS KAVERI • *INSERM U28, Hôpital Broussais, Paris, France*

JOHN H. KENTEN • *Proneuron, Inc., Rockville, MD*

KEITH A. KNISLEY • *Department of Cell Biology and Biochemistry, Texas Tech University Health Science Center, Lubbock, TX*

LAN LI • *Department of Anesthesiology, University of Nebraska Medical Center, Omaha, NE*

C. ROGER MACKENZIE • *Institute for Biological Sciences, National Research Council of Canada, Ottawa, Ontario, Canada*

OXANA MAKAREVITCH • *Engelhardt Institute of Molecular Biology, Russian Academy of Sciences, Moscow, Russia*

MARK T. MARTIN • *IGEN Inc., Rockville, MD*
SARAN A. NARANG • *Institute for Biological Sciences, National Research Council of Canada, Ottawa, Ontario, Canada*
LEIF KOFOED NIELSEN • *Department of Biology, Royal Danish School of Pharmacy, Copenhagen, Denmark*
SUDHIR PAUL • *Department of Anesthesiology, University of Nebraska Medical Center, Omaha, NE*
OLEG L. POLANOVSKY • *Engelhardt Institute of Molecular Biology, Russian Academy of Sciences, Moscow, Russia*
MICHAEL POLYMENIS • *Department of Biochemistry, Tufts University School of Medicine, Boston, MA*
SYED M. QUADRI • *Department of Radiology, University of Nebraska Medical Center, Omaha, NE*
ANTHONY R. REES • *School of Biology and Biochemistry, University of Bath, UK*
L. SCOTT RODKEY • *Department of Pathology, University of Texas-Houston Medical School, Houston, TX*
ROSA SANCHEZ • *IGEN Inc., Rockville, MD*
MARIANNE SCHIFFER • *Center for Mechanistic Biology and Biotechnology, Argonne National Laboratory, Argonne, IL*
YEHUDA SHOENFELD • *Department of Medicine 'B' and Research Unit of Autoimmune Diseases, Sheba Medical Center, Tel-Hashomer, Sackler Faculty of Medicine, Tel-Aviv University*
RODGER G. SMITH • *IGEN Inc., Rockville, MD*
ESKIL SÖDERLIND • *Department of Immunotechnology, Lund University, Lund, Sweden*
FRED J. STEVENS • *Center for Mechanistic Biology and Biotechnology, Argonne National Laboratory, Argonne, IL*
B. DAVID STOLLAR • *Department of Biochemistry, Tufts University School of Medicine, Boston, MA*
MEI SUN • *Department of Anesthesiology, University of Nebraska Medical Center, Omaha, NE*
ZEEV TASHMA • *Israeli Defense Forces–Medical Corps, Tel-Aviv, Israel*
ALFONSO TRAMONTANO • *IGEN Research Institute, Rockville, MD*
ILAN TUR-KASPA • *Israeli Defense Forces–Medical Corps, Tel-Aviv, Israel*

SONIA TYUTYULKOVA • *Department of Anesthesiology, University of Nebraska Medical Center, Omaha, NE*

DAVID M. WEBSTER • *School of Biology and Biochemistry, University of Bath, UK*

TAI TE WU • *Department of Biochemistry and Molecular Cell Biology, Northwestern University, Evanston, IL*

MONCEF ZOUALI • *Département d'Immunologie, Institut Pasteur, Paris, France*

CHAPTER 1

SEQHUNT

A Program to Screen Aligned Nucleotide and Amino Acid Sequences

George Johnson, Tai Te Wu, and Elvin A. Kabat

1. Introduction

We have been collecting nucleotide and amino acid sequences of proteins of immunological interest, and aligning them in order to understand the structure and function relations of these proteins *(1)*. To aid in organizing and analyzing this collection, a computer program, called SEQHUNT, was written.

The SEQHUNT program is written in PL/PROPHET *(2,3)*. SEQHUNT uses a preprocessed form of the database as its search data. SEQHUNT can pattern match nucleotide and amino acid sequences with the aligned data, pattern match phrases in the annotation fields of the sequences, and compare specified regions in similarly aligned sequences.

The SEQHUNT program can be used only on a machine with the PL/PROPHET environment present and with the PL/PROPHET table representation of the database present. To allow greater accessibility to the matching capabilities of the program, a partial implementation of SEQHUNT is available via electronic mail.

2. Materials

The variable and constant regions of immunoglobulins and T-cell receptors for antigen, and the various domains of MHC class I and class II molecules have been aligned *(1)*. These aligned sequences and

From: *Methods in Molecular Biology, Vol. 51: Antibody Engineering Protocols*
Edited by: S. Paul Humana Press Inc., Totowa, NJ

sequences of related proteins *(1)*, together with new sequences published recently, have been stored in the NIH-supported PROPHET computer system *(2,3)* in the form of PL/PROPHET data tables. SEQHUNT uses this Kabat database *(1)* for its searching and region analysis.

3. Methods

SEQHUNT is a computer program written in PL/PROPHET for use in the PL/PROPHET environment. The program performs three main types of analyses. The first is matching. Given a nucleotide or amino acid sequence and restrictions on the number of allowable mismatches and data tables to search through, SEQHUNT will return aligned matches of all sequences with mismatches equal to or less than the allowable number. The second function of SEQHUNT allows searching for specified patterns in the sequence annotations. Name, antibody specificity, T-cell receptor classification, and reference fields may be searched for the desired pattern. Moreover, the full implementation of SEQHUNT allows region analysis of any one or a number of sequence stretches in similarly aligned sequences, e.g., all immunoglobulin heavy (H) chains. The program queries for the given region, such as the entire light (L) chain variable region (positions 1–107) or a combination of several complementarity determining regions (CDRs), for example, CDRL1, CDRL2, and CDRL3 together. All sequences are called as search patterns, and the entire set of sequences is used as the search pool. Redundant matching is eliminated to reduce output. Any number of mismatches may be specified, although the output for mismatches above 1 or 2 is usually massive. These three types of searches may be performed on nucleotide or amino acid data, and matching and annotation searches also may be performed on unaligned data.

SEQHUNT, as written, must be called from the PL/PROPHET environment. To allow greater access to the program, an interface has been developed that allows specially formatted queries to be sent via electronic mail for processing. The interface supports all functions of the original SEQHUNT, except region analysis.

3.1. Sequence Pattern Match

The nucleotide sequence pattern-matching capabilities of SEQHUNT are shown in Fig. 1. In this example, the nucleotide sequence to match (TARGET SEQUENCE) is the H-chain variable region of the IgM

BALB/c murine monoclonal antibody (MAb) PR1 *(4)*, which has specificity for the PR1 antigen on human prostate cancer cells and normal human prostate cells. This SEQHUNT search was restricted to 12 or fewer mismatches among the sequences of all H-chain variable regions of all species currently in the database. In Fig. 1, several sequences with 6, 7, or 11 mismatches are shown. They are listed in order of increasing mismatches. An upper-case base is a mismatch, and all lower-case bases are matches. Dashes are for alignment *(1)*. To save space, several other sequences with fewer than 12 mismatches are not listed (*see* Notes 1 and 2 for other examples).

Figure 2 shows the results of a search of all H-chain variable regions for matches with a segment of the human D-minigene D2 *(5)*. Human D-minigenes sometimes match segments other than the third CDR of human H chains *(6)*. As shown in Fig. 2, a segment of 14 nucleotides from human D2 is found in the second CDR of human, mouse, and rabbit H chains (*see* Note 3). For nucleotide sequences in the human CDRH3 region, additional matches are found on both sides of the 14 nucleotides. RF-SJ2 matches human D2 for 24 bases, ttg*tagtggtggtagc*tgctactc, and L42 for 28 bases, ggatatt*gtagtggtggtagc*tgctact. The 14 matches in Fig. 2 are underlined. Usually, only short segments of human D-minigenes are incorporated into CDRH3s *(7)*. When some of these short segments of the human D-minigenes, e.g., aactgg, a segment of DHQ52 *(5)*, are searched, identical matches occur frequently over the entire H-chain variable region (Fig. 3).

3.2. Antibody Specificity Search

An example of antibody specificity searching is shown in Fig. 4 for a SEQHUNT search called with the specified pattern "HIV," the abbreviation for Human Immunodeficiency Virus. Only a few of the matches are shown. The search was restricted to all H-chain variable region sequences in the database. SEQHUNT scans the antibody specificities and looks for exact matches with the "HIV" pattern. This search, Fig. 4, found antibodies directed against p24, gp120, and gp41. Even for the same protein, the numbers of dashes in the last three lines of the sequences are different, indicating that the length of H-chain CDR3 can vary more extensively than those of CDR1 and CDR2 *(8)*. Most likely, the antibodies are directed toward different parts of one of the HIV proteins. Searches of the name and reference fields are also allowed.

Rowname	NAME	DIFFERENCES	SEQUENCE	SPECIES	BEGIN	END	SPECIFICITY	REFERENCE
1.	TARGET SEQUENCE	0	*(sequence illegible)*					
2.	M3	6	*(sequence illegible)*	MOUSE	1	94	ANTI-3-FUCOSYLLACTOSAMINE HYBRIDOMA	KIMURA,H.,BU-ESCHER,E.S./BALL,E.D.& MARCUS,D.M.(1989) EUR.J.IMMUNOL.,19-,1741-1746.
3.	W3129	7	*(sequence illegible)*	MOUSE	1	94	ANTI-ALPHA 1,6 DEXTRAN	BORDEN,E.A.(FABAT,E.A.(1990) PROC.N ATL.ACAD.SCI.USA,04,2440-2443.
4.	10L-126-7	7	*(sequence illegible)*	MOUSE	1	94	ANTI-AMINOFHENYL-BETA-N-ACETYLGLUCOS-AMINIDE,A/F R/8/34 INFLU-ENZA VIRUS	BONILLA,F.A.-ZAGHOUANI,H.-RUBIN,M.&-BONA,C.(19-90) J.IMMUNO-22,145,616-6

5.	3A9	11	g a G g t g A a g c t T C t C g a g t c t g g a g - g t g g c c t g g t g c a g c c t g g a g g a t c - c c t g a a a G t c t c c t g t g c a g c c t c a - g g a t t c g a t t t t a g t a g a t a c t g g a - t g a g t - - - - - - t g g g t c c g g c a g g c - t c c a g g g a a a g g g c t a g a a t g g a t t - g g a g a a a t t a a t c c a - - - - - - g a t a - g T a g t a c g C t a a a c t a t G c g c C a t c - t c t a a a g g a t a a a t t c a t c a t c t c c - a g A g a c a a c g c c a a a a a t a c A c t g t - a c c t g c a a a t g a g c a a a g t g a g a t c - t g a g g a c a c a g c c c t t t a t t a c t g t - g c a a g a	MOUSE	1	94	ANTI-GALACTO-SYLGLOBOSIDE	SNYDER, J.G., -WENG, N., YU-L-EE, L. & MARC-US, D.M. (199-0) EUR. J. IMM-UNOL., 20, 267-3-2677.
6.	mAb402-10	11	g a G g t g A a g c C T C t C g a g t c t g g a g - g t g g c c t g g t g c a g c c t g g a g g a t c - c c t g a a a c t c t c c t g t g c a g c c t c a - g g a t t c g a t t t t a g t a g a t a c t g g a - t g a g t - - - - - - t g g g t c c g g c a g g c - t c c a C g g a a a C g g c t a g a a t g g a t t - g g a g a a a t t a a t c c a - - - - - - g a t a - g c a g t a c g a t a a C c t a t a c g c c a t c - t c t a a a g g a t a a a t t c a t c a t c t c c - a g A g a c a a c g c c a a a a a t a c g c t g t - a c c t g c a a a t g a g c a a a g t g a g a t c - t g a g g a c a c a g c c c t t t a t t a c t g t - g c a a g T	MOUSE	1	94	ANTI-MORPHIN-E-6-HEMISUCC-INATE-BSA	KUSSIE, P.H., -ANCHIN, J.M., -SUBRAMANIAM, -S., GLASEL, J.-A. & LINTHIC-UM, D.S. (199-1) J. IMMUNOL-., 146, 4248-4-257.

Fig. 1. Matching a nucleotide sequence of a H-chain variable region, positions 1–94. The sequence, PR1, is shown in row 1 labeled as TARGET SEQUENCE. Some of the sequences in the database with 6, 7, or 11 mismatches are listed in the order of increasing mismatches as shown in column 2. Names of these sequences are given in column 1. Columns 4–8 indicate species, beginning position, ending position, antibody specificity, and reference, respectively.

0 Powname	1 NAME	2 DIFFER-ENCES	3 SEQUENCE	4 SPECIES	5 BEGIN	6 END	7 SPECIFICITY	8 REFERENCE
1.	TARGET SEQUENCE	0	g t a g t g g t a g c					
2.	914	0	g t - - - a g t g - / g t a g t a g c	MOUSE	52	56	UNKNOWN	LEVY,N.S.,MALIFIERO,U.V.,LEBEC-QUE,S.G. & GEARHART,P.J. (1989) J.EXP.MED.,169,2007-2019.
3.	RVH720	0	g t - - - a g t g - / g t g g t a g c	RABBIT	52	56	UNKNOWN	ROUX,K.H.,DHANARAJAN,P.,GOTTSC-HALK,V.,McCORMACK,W.T. & PENSH-AW,R.M. (1991) J.IMMUNOL.,146,2027-2036.
4.	19/9	0	g t - - - a g t g g t a g - / g t a g c	HUMAN	52A	56	ANTI-DNA AUT-OANTIBODY HY-BRIDOMA	DERSIMONIAN,H.,SCHWARTZ,R.S.,B-ARRETT,K.J. & STOLLAR,B.D. (19-87) J.IMMUNOL.,139,2496-2501.

5.	RF-SJ2	0	g t a g t g g t a g c	HUMAN	98	100B ANTI-IGG1, IG-G2,IGG4 RHEU-MATOID FACTOR	PASCUAL,V.,RANDEN,I.,THOMPSON,-K.,SIOUD,M.FORRE,O.,NATVIG,J.-& CAPRA,J.D. (1990) J.CLIN.INV-EST.,86,1320-1328; RANDEN I.,B-ROWN,D.,THOMPSON,K.M.,HUGHES-J-ONES,N.,PASCUAL,V.,VICTOR,K.,C-APRA,J.D.,FORRE,O. & NATVIG,J.-B. (1992) J.IMMUNOL.,148,3296--3301.
6.	L42	0	g t a g t g g t a g c	HUMAN	100	100D AUTOANTIBODY	KIPPS,T.J. & DUFFY,S.F. (1991)-J.CLIN.INVEST.,87,2087-2096.

Fig. 2. Matching segments of D-minigenes. The format of this figure is identical to that of Fig. 1. The TARGET SEQUENCE pattern consists of 14 bp from the human D2-minigene. It matches identically to nucleotide segments in the CDRH2 region of 914 (mouse), RVH720 (rabbit) and 18/9 (human) as shown in rows 2, 3, and 4 respectively. It also matches human CDRH3 segments of RF-SJ2 and L42 shown in rows 5 and 6. For details, *see* section 3.1.

0 Pownname	1 NAME	2 DIFFERENCES	3 SEQUENCE	4 SPECIES	5 BEGIN	6 END	7 SPECIFICITY	8 REFERENCE
1.	TARGET SEQUENCE	0	a a c t g g					
2.	CLL4	0	a a c t g g	HUMAN	3	5	UNKNOWN	CAI,J.,HUMPHRIES,C-,RICHARDSON,A.&,TUCKER,F.W. (1992)-,J.EXP.MED.,176,10-,73-1081.
3.	257-D	0	a a c t g g	HUMAN	32	33	ANTI-HIV TYPE 1 SPECIFIC FOR THE PRINCIPAL NEUTRALIZING DOMAIN OF gp120 OF IFN AND MAF TO RESIDUES KRIHI	ANDRIS,J.S.,JOHNSON,S.,ZOLLA-PAZNER,S. & CAPRA,J.D. (1991) PROC.NATL.ACAD.SCI.USA,88,7783--7787.
4.	VHVI	0	a a c t g g	HUMAN	35B	36	UNKNOWN	BUJWELA,L. & RABBITTS,T.H. (1988) EUR.J.IMMUNOL.,18,1-843-1845.
5.	CLL-27	0	a a c t g g	HUMAN	44	46	UNKNOWN	BERMAN,J.E.,HUMPHRIES,C.G.,BARTH,J.,ALT,F.W. & TUCKER,P.W. (1991) J.EXP.MED.,175,1529-1535.
6.	Ab21	0	a a c t g g	HUMAN	50	52	POLYREACTIVE AUTOANTIBODY	SANZ,I.,CASALI,P.,THOMAS,J.W,NOTKINS,A.L. & CAPRA,J.D-. (1989) J.IMMUNOL-.,142,4054-4061.
7.	4m6	0	a a c t g g	MOUSE	93	95	UNKNOWN	GU,H.,TARLINTON,D.,MUELLER,W.,RAJEWS-KI,K.& FORSTER,I.-(1991) J.EXP.MED.-,173,1357-1371.

				HUMAN	100E	100F	AUTOANTIBODY	
8.	L22	0	a a c t g g	HUMAN				KIPPS,T.J.,& DUFFY-,S.F. (1991) J.CLI-N.INVST.,87,2087--2096.
9.	4G11	0	a a c t g g	MOUSE	102	103	ANTI-IDIOTYPIC ANT-IBODY AGAINST THE-THYROTROPIN (TSH)-RECEPTOR	TAUB,R.,HSU,J.-C.,GARSKY,V.M.,HILL,B-.L.,ERLANGER,B.F.,& KOHN,L.D. (1992)-J.BIOL.CHEM.,267,-5977-5984.

Fig. 3. Matching of a segment of the human D-minigene, DHQ52 (TARGET SEQUENCE) with different regions of mouse and human H chains.

9

Rowname	NAME	SEQUENCE	SPECIES	SPECIFICITY	REFERENCE
1.	BAT123	--- gaa gtg cag ctt cag gag tcg gga cct ggc ctg gt- g aaa cct tct cag tct ctg tcc ctc acc tgc act gtc - act ggc tac tca atc acc agt gat tat gcc tgg tgg -- - tgg atc cgg cag ttt cca gga aac ctg gag tgg --- t acc tac aac cca tct ctc aaa agt cga atc tct atc - act cga gac aca tcc aag aac ctg ttc ttc ctg cag tt- g agt tct gtg act gct gag gac aca gcc aca tat tac - tgt gca agg ggg agt ttc gga gac --- --- tgg ggc caa - ggg act ctg gtc act gtc tct gct	MOUSE	ANTI-GLYCOPR- OTEIN gp120- OF HTLV-IIIb- STRAIN OF H- IV TYPE 1.	LIOU,R.-S.,ROSEN,E.M.- ,FUNG,M.S.C.,SUN,W.- N.C.,SUN,C.,GORDON,W- .,CHANG,N.T. & CHANG- ,T.W. (1989) J.IMMUN- OL.,143,3967-3975.
2.	CB-mab-p24/ 13-5	--- cag gtc aaa ctg cag gag tct ggg gga ggc tta gt- g agg cct gga ggg tcc ctg aaa ctc tct tgt gca gcc - tct gga ttc act ttc agt agc tat acc atg tct --- -- g tgg ttc cgc cag act cca ggg aag agg ctg gag ttg - gtc gca gct att aat agt --- aat ggt ggt agc acc go- c tac tat cca gac agt gtg aag ggc cga ttc acc atc - tcc aga gac aat gcc aag aac acc ctg tac ctg caa at- g agc agt ctg agg tct gag gac acg gcc ttg tat tac - tgt gca aga cta ccc ctt --- --- gac tac tgg ggt caa - ggg acc acg gtc acc gtc tcc tca	MOUSE	ANTI-P24 COR- E PROTEIN OF- HIV-1	KUTTNER,G.,GIEBMANN, E.,NIEMANN,B.,WINKLE- R,K.,GRUHOW,R.,HINKU- LA,J.,ROSEN,J.,WAHRE- N,B. & VON BAEHR,P. - (1992) MOL.IMMUNOL., 29,561-564.
3.	0.5-BETA	--- cag gtt cag ctg cag cag tct ggg gct gag ctg gt- g agg cct ggg gcc tca gtg aag atg tcc tgc aag gct - tct ggc tac acc ttc act act tac cca atg cat tgg gtg - aag cag aga cat gga aag ggc cta gag tgg att gga - tat att aat cct tac aat gat ggt act aag tac aat ga- g aag ttc aaa ggc aag gcc aca ctg act gca gac aaa - tcc tcc agc aca gcc tac atg caa ctg agc agc ctg aca tct - gag gac tct gcg gtc tat tac tgt gca aga --- --- - --- gac tac --- --- tgg ggc caa - ggc acc acc ctc aca gtc tcc tca	MOUSE	ANTI-PRINCIP- AL NEUTRALIZ- ING DOMAIN (- PND) OF HIV- 1 gp120	MATSUSHITA,S.,MAEDA, H.,KIMACHI,K.,EDA,Y.- ,MAEDA,Y.,MURAKAMI,T- .,TOKIYOSHI,S. & TAK- ATSUKI,K. (1992) AID- S RES.HUMAN RETROVIR- USES,8,1107-1115.
4.	257-D	--- gag gtg cag ctg gtg gag tct ggg gca gga gtg aa- a aag ccg ggg gag tct ctg aag atc tcc tgt aag ggt - tct gga tac acc ttt aac gac aac tgg atc tgg ggc -- - tgg gtg cgc cag atg ccc ggg aaa ggc ctg gag tgg - atg ggg atc ata tat cct --- --- gat gac tct gac ag- c aca gcc agt ccg tca ttc caa ggc cag gtc acc atc - tca gcc gac acg tcc agc acc tac ctg cag tgg agc ag- t ctg cag aca cta tgg acc acc gct gat att cc- c tat acg --- --- tac ttt gac tat tgg ggt cag - gga acc acg gtc acc gtc tcc tca	HUMAN	ANTI-HIV TYP- E 1 SPECIFIC- FOR THE PRI- NCIPAL NEUTR- ALIZING DOMA- IN OF gp120 - OF MN AND HA- P TO RESIDUE- S KRIHI	ANDRIS,J.S.,JOHNSON,- S.,ZOLLA-FAINER,S. &- CAPRA,J.D. (1991) P- ROC.NATL.ACAD.SCI.US- A,88,7783-7787.
5.	71-31	--- cag gtg cag ctg cag gag tct ggg gct gag gtg ag- g aag cct ggg gcc tca gtg aag gtt tcc tgc aag gca - tct ggt tac tcc ttc acc agc tat ggt atc agc tgg gtg - cga cag gcc cct gga cag ggg ctt gag tgg --- - atg gga gga atc atc --- --- cct gtt gtg gtt cac --- - a acc tac gca cag aag ttc cag ggc aga gtc acc atg - acc agg gac acg tcc acg agc aca gtc tat atg gaa ct- g agc agc ctg aga tct gta gac acg gcc gta tat tac - tgt gct gga gtt cag ggg gtg ccc cgg ccc tta ggg ga- c --- --- tac ttt gac tat tgg ggc cag - gga acc ctg gtc acc gtc tcc tca	HUMAN	ANTI-HIV TYP- E 1 SFECIFIC- FOR p24	ANDRIS,J.S.,JOHNSON,- S.,ZOLLA-FAINER,S. &- CAPRA,J.D. (1991) P- ROC.NATL.ACAD.SCI.US- A,88,7783-7787.

| 6. | 3D6 | --- gaa gtg cag ctg gtg gag tct ggg gga ggc ttg gt-
a cag cct ggc agg tcc ctg aga ctc tcc tgt gca gcc ---
tct gga ttc acc ttt aat gat tat gcc atg cac ---
-tgg gtc cgg caa gct cca ggg aag ggc ctg gag tgg -
gtc tca ggt ata agt tgg ---gat agt agt agt at-
a ggc tat gcg gac tct gtg aag ggc cga ttc acc atc --
tcc aga gac aac gcc aag aac tcc ctg tat ctg caa at-
g aac agt ctg aga gct gag gac atg ggc ttt tat tac tg-
t gta aaa gat ---- got ttt gat atc tgg ggc caa --
t ttc acg gtt ----got ttt gat atc tgg ggc caa ---
ggg aca atg gtc acc gtc tct tca | HUMAN | ANTI-HIV gp41 | ANTI-HIV TYP-E 1 SPECIFIC- FOR AMINO A-CIDS 644-663- OF gp41 | FELGENHAUER,M.,KOHL,-J. & RUKER,F. (1990)-NUCL.ACIDS RES., 18-,4927. |
| 7. | 120-16 | --- otc ctg caa cta cag gag tcc ggc tca gga ctg gt-
g aag cct tca cag acc ctg tcc ctc acc tgc act gtc -
tct ggt ggc tcc atc agg agt ggt ggt tat ggc ---
- tgg acc tgg atc cgg cag cca cca ggg aag ggc ctg -
gag tgg att ggt tcc atc tat --- tat tat ggg ggc go-
c tct tac aac ccg tcc ctc aag agt cga gtc acc ttg -
tca gca gac act tcc aag aac caa gcc tcc ctg ---
tgt gcc aga toc ttt ggc gtc tat ttt --------
agc acc ctg gtc tct gtc tcc tca | HUMAN | ANTI-HIV gp41 | ANTI-HIV TYP-E 1 SPECIFIC- FOR AMINO A-CIDS 644-663- OF gp41 | ANDRIS,J.S.,JOHNSON,-S.,ZOLLA-PAZNER,S.,-CAPRA,J.D. (1991) P-ROC.NATL.ACAD.SCI.US-A, 88, 7783-7787. |

Fig. 4. Immunoglobulin H chains with anti-HIV activity. This search looked for the pattern "HIV" in the antibody specificity field, as shown in column 4. Name, sequence, species, and reference for each sequence are listed in columns 1, 2, 3, and 5, respectively.

3.3 Region Analysis (see Notes 4 and 5)

Along with sequence, name, antibody specificity, and reference matching, the fully implemented SEQHUNT can perform region analysis on one or more stretches of sequence from any group of similarly aligned sequences. Figure 5 shows the partial output of a region analysis for CDRL1, positions 24–34 of the L-chain immunoglobulin, performed on all species. This analysis was done allowing no mismatches. Identical matches with the same specificity are represented by a single entry. Sequences with no known specificity were omitted. Figure 6 is the output of a region analysis done on the three CDRs (positions 24–34, 50–56, and 89–97, respectively) of the immunoglobulin L chain. The pipe symbol (|) delineates each CDR in consecutive order (CDR1 | CDR2 | CDR3 |). As in Fig. 5, sequences with identical specificities are represented by a single entry, and those with unknown specificity are omitted. The same CDR associated with antibodies having different specificities had been noted previously *(9)*. Similar instances were found for CDRL2, CDRL3, CDRH1, and CDRH2. In the case of CDRH3, a given sequence is nearly always associated with a unique antibody specificity *(8)*.

4. Notes

1. SEQHUNT is an improved version of SQUERY *(9)*. It has been a valuable tool for the collection and analysis of nucleotide and amino acid sequences of proteins of immunological interest *(1)*. Before entering a recently published sequence into our database, SEQHUNT is used to locate closely related sequences *(see* Fig. 1). Indeed, one of the goldfish H-chain nucleotide sequences, Goldfish 5A *(10)*, was found to be nearly identical to two human sequences, 63P1 and 60P2 *(11)*. It is not certain whether this finding has evolutionary implications or may be an artifact of polymerase chain reactions.

2. SEQHUNT is also useful for designing artificial antibodies with required specificities. Searches for a desired specificity can be made, and all known antibodies with that specificity can be found *(see* Fig. 4). Sequences of these antibodies or their segments may be used as starting materials for detailed designing *(8)*. Thorough analyses of these sequences may provide some insight into the fine structures of interaction between antigen and antibody molecules.

3. The question of why segments of human D-minigenes occur at locations other than CDRH$_3$ in H-chain variable regions is unanswered *(6)*. Even more puzzling is the finding that these segments can appear in H chains of other species *(see* Fig. 3). Without SEQHUNT, such occurrences might never have been found.

```
R    S    S    Q    S    L    V    H    S         N    G    N    T    Y    L    H
aga  tct  agt  cag  agc  ctt  gta  cac  agt  ---  aat  gga  aac  acc  tat  tta  cat
```

9-40
ANTI-FLUORESCEIN (Ka=3.7X10EXP7)
BEDZYK,W.D.,HERRON,J.N.,EDMUNDSON,A.B. & VOSS,E.W.,JR. (1990) J.BIOL. CHEM.,265,133-138.

10VA2
AUTOANTIBODY TO THYROGLOBULIN
GLEASON,S.L.,GEARHART,P.,ROSE,N.R. & KUPPERS,R.C. (1990) J.IMMUNOL., 145,1768-1775.

H146-24B3
ANTI-INFLUENZA VIRUS HEMAGGLUTININ HYBRIDOMA
CATON,A.J.,BROWNLEE,G.G.,STAUDT,L.M. & GERHARD,W. (1986) EMBO J.,5, 1577-1587.

T17
ANTI-(T,G)-A--L
PINCUS,S. & CARMACK,C.E. (1992) MOL.IMMUNOL.,29,811-819.

BV16-19
ANTI-dsDNA (12%), ssDNA (90%), POLY(dT), POLY(dU)
SMITH,R.G. & VOSS,E.W.,JR. (1990) MOL.IMMUNOL.,27,463-470.

GP138-10
ANTI-POLY(GLU50,TYR50)(Ka=3.68X10EXP7),DNA(Ka=2.42X10EXP6),SMITH
ANTIGEN(Ka=2.56X10EXP6),IGG2a(Ka=3.84X10EXP6)
BAILEY,N.C.,FIDANZA,V.,MAYER,R.,MAZZA,G.,FOUGEREAU,M. & BONA,C. (1989)
J.CLIN.INVEST.,84,744-756.

11/32
ANTI-PROGESTERONE HYBRIDOMA
DEVERSON,E.,BEREK,C.,TAUSSIG,M. & FEINSTEIN,A. (1987) EUR.J.IMMUNOL.,17,9-13. (CHECKED
BY AUTHOR 07/02/87)

40-60
ANTI-DIGOXIN HYBRIDOMA(BINDING CONSTANT=6.7X10EXP9)
HUDSON,N.W.,BRUCCOLERI,R.E.,STEINRAUF,L.K.,HAMILTON,J.A.,MUDGETT-HUNTER,M. &
MARGOLIES,M.N. (1990) J,IMMUNOL.,145,2718-2724. (CHECKED WITH GENBANK 02/11/91)

9A6
ANTI-TRINITROPHENYL HYBRIDOMA
REININGER,L.,SPERTINI,F.,SHIBATA,T.,JATON,J.-C. & IZUI,S. (1989) EUR.J.
IMMUNOL.,19,2123-2130.

MRA5K
ANTI-HISTONE
MONESTIER,M. (1991) EUR.J.IMMUNOL.,21,1725-1731.

NL-112-9
ANTI-AMINOPHENYL-BETA-N-ACETYLGLUCOSAMINIDE, BETA(1-6)POLY-D-COUPLED TO BSA
BONILLA,F.A.,ZAGHOUANI,H.,RUBIN,M. & BONA,C. (1990) J.IMMUNOL.,145,616-622.

Fig. 5. Identical matching of a nucleotide sequence of CDRL1 shown at the top with other CDRL1 sequences in the same region. For each match, the name, antibody specificity, and reference are given. In this listing, only sequences with distinct specificities are included. The translated amino acid sequence is shown in single-letter code above the nucleotide sequence.

```
R    S    S    Q    S    I    V    H    S         N    G    N    T    Y    L    E
aga  tct  agt  cag  agc  att  gta  cat  agt  ---  aat  gga  aac  acc  tat  tta  gaa
K    V    S    N    R    F    S         F    Q    G    S    H    V    P
aaa  gtt  tcc  aac  cga  ttt  tct  |    ttt  caa  ggt  tca  cat  gtt  cct  ---  ---  ---
          R    T
---  ---  ---  cgg  acg  |
```

VS1
ANTI-IGG1 MONOCLONAL AUTOANTIBODY (RHEUMATOID FACTOR)
SHLOMCHIK,M.,NEMAZEE,D.,VAN SNICK,J. & WEIGERT,M. (1987) J.EXP.MED., 165,970-987.

D2
ANTI-IDIOTYPIC ANTIBODY AGAINST THE THYROTROPIN (TSH) RECEPTOR
TAUB,R.,HSU,J.-C.,GARSKY,V.M.,HILL,B.L.,ERLANGER,B.F. & KOHN,L.D. (1992)
J.BIOL.CHEM.,267,5977-5984.

NQ19.16.37
ANTI-2-PHENYL OXAZOLONE HYBRIDOMA
BEREK,C.,JARVIS,J.M. & MILSTEIN,C. (1987) EUR.J.IMMUNOL.,17,1121-1129.

Fig. 6. Same as Fig. 5, except that the regions searched are CDRL1, CDRL2, and CDRL3 together.

4. Matching sequences in a given region or combination of regions (Figs. 5 and 6) have provided a unique tool for studying the underlying mechanisms of antibody specificity. Based on the idea of random assortment of the six CDRs generating the antibody repertoire, a given CDR, e.g., CDRL1, should be associated with randomly assorted CDRL2, CDRL3, CDRH1, CDRH2, and CDRH3, which can lead to many different specificities, as illustrated in Fig. 5. However, CDRH3 seems exceptional, since a given CDRH3 sequence is nearly always associated with a unique specificity (9). Specificities associated with identical CDRL1, CDRL2, and CDRL3 together are more limited (see Fig. 6). If amino acid sequences are searched, more specificities will be found for a given CDR or combination of CDRs.

5. Our collection of nucleotide and amino acid sequences of proteins of immunological interest (1) is distinct from other databases because of the alignment of sequences. This alignment is essential for the study of the structure and functions of these proteins. SEQHUNT is the only computer program that can analyze this large aligned database. Additional features will be incorporated into the program when other analyses become important.

References

1. Kabat, E. A., Wu, T. T., Perry, H. M., Gottesman, K. S., and Foeller, C. (1991) *Sequences of Proteins of Immunological Interest,* 5th ed. US Department of Health and Human Services, NIH Publication No. 91-3242.
2. Raub, W. F. (1974) The PROPHET system and resource sharing. *Fed. Proc.* **33,** 2390–2392.

3. Hollister, C. (1988) PROPHET—a national computing resource for life science research. *Nucleic Acids Res.* **16,** 1873–1875.
4. Brinkmann, U., Gallo, M., Brinkmann, E., Kunwar, S., and Pastan, I. (1993) A recombinant immunotoxin that is active on prostate cancer cells that is composed of the F_V region of monoclonal antibody PR1 and a truncated form of Pseudomonas exotoxin. *Proc. Natl. Acad. Sci. USA* **90,** 547–551.
5. Siebenlist, U., Ravetch, J. V., Korsmeyer, S., Waldmann, T., and Leder, P. (1981) Human immunoglobulin D segments encoded in tandem multigenic families. *Nature* **294,** 631–635.
6. Wu, T. T. and Kabat, E. A. (1982) Fourteen nucleotides in the second complementarity-determining region of human heavy-chain variable region gene are identical with a sequence in a human D minigene. *Proc. Natl. Acad. Sci. USA* **79,** 5031–5032.
7. Taylor, L. D., Carmack, C. E., Schramm, S. R., Mashayekh, R., Higgins, K. M., Kuo, C.-C., Woodhouse, C., Kay, R. M., and Lonberg, N. (1992) A transgenic mouse that expresses a diversity of human heavy and light chain immunoglobulins. *Nucleic Acids Res.* **20,** 6287–6295.
8. Wu, T. T., Johnson, G., and Kabat, E. A. (1993) Length distributions of CDRH3 in antibodies. *Proteins: Struct. Funct. Genet.* **16,** 1–7.
9. Wu, T. T. and Kabat, E. A. (1992) Possible use of similar framework region amino acid sequences between human and mouse immunoglobulins for humanizing mouse antibodies. *Mol. Immunol.* **29,** 1141–1146.
10. Wilson, M. R., Middleton, D., and Warr, G. W. (1988) Immunoglobulin heavy-chain-variable region gene evolution: Structure and family relationships of two genes and pseudogenes in teleost fish. *Proc. Natl. Acad. Sci. USA* **85,** 1566–1570.
11. Schroeder, H. W., Jr., Hillson, J. L., and Perlmutter, R. M. (1987) Early restriction of the human antibody repertoire. *Science* **238,** 791–793.

CHAPTER 2

Molecular Modeling
of Antibody-Combining Sites

David M. Webster and Anthony R. Rees

1. Introduction

Antibodies possess a vast repertoire of specificity and affinity. To understand the molecular basis of antibody function, we require high-resolution X-ray crystallographic structures and good solution structures of free and antigen-bound antibodies. The number of reported antibody structures grows each year. Yet the number of structures deposited with the Brookhaven Protein Database (PDB) *(1)* remains relatively small, with 43 deposited entries at the time of writing, when compared to the available sequence data. It is therefore important to develop an effective method of predicting the structure of antibody-combining sites. The validity of predicted structures can then be confirmed by mutagenesis in the combining site. The models can also provide valuable structural information to "humanize" antibodies for therapy effectively, to develop immunosensors, and even for the complete *de novo* design of new antibodies with different functions.

This chapter outlines the structure of antibodies and methods currently available for modeling antibodies. An example of the modeling of an anti-*N*-(P-cyanophenyl)-*N'*-(diphenylemethyl)guanidineacetic acid antibody (1CGS) is also provided *(2)*. The method used to model this antibody is based on the CAMAL algorithm *(3–9)* that combines structural and *ab initio* approaches to determine antibody structure, and is embodied in the commercial version of the program AbM *(10)*.

From: *Methods in Molecular Biology, Vol. 51: Antibody Engineering Protocols*
Edited by: S. Paul Humana Press Inc., Totowa, NJ

1.1. Antibody Structure

1.1.1. The Antibody Fold

Antibodies have a distinctive structure often depicted as a Y or T shape with the two distal arms (Fab) containing the sites for antigen binding (Fig. 1). An antibody consists of two identical light (L) chains and two identical heavy (H) chains that fold into domains. The structure of the now classic immunoglobulin fold was established with the determination of the structure of a Fab fragment by Poljak and coworkers *(11)*, and the presence of this fold in the F_c fragment was shown by Deisenhofer and coworkers *(12)*. This fold and its variants have also been observed in nonantibody molecules, including T-cell receptors. The Fab contains a variable domain (V_L/V_H) and a constant domain (C_L/C_H1), with the two halves of each domain formed from the two H chains.

Since the antibody contains two Fab arms, two antigen molecules may be bound by the same antibody. The constant domains for L and H chains are constant for their particular class. L chains may be one of two classes, κ or λ, and H chains, one of five classes, α, γ, δ, ε, and μ. The two Fabs are attached to the F_c region by a flexible hinge, giving the antibody an intrinsic flexibility.

1.1.2. The Variable Domain

The variable domains (V_L/V_H) associate noncovalently to form a twisted antiparallel β-sheet structure. Although the framework is well conserved between known antibody structures (Table 1A and B), variations in the packing of β-sheets and strands do occur. The sheets may vary in their orientation with respect to one another by as much as 30° ± 18° *(13,14)*, and the strands at the interface are inclined to each other by 50° *(15)*. The β-sheet strands are interspaced with six segments that are the most variable regions of the antibody both in sequence and in structure. These regions are known as the hypervariable or complementarity determining regions (CDRs). Each CDR interconnects a β-strand, with three CDRs (L1, L2, L3) derived from the L chain and three from the H chain (H1, H2, H3). This interconnection of the antiparallel β-strands brings the CDRs close together in space at the distal end of the antibody. Some or all of the CDR loops may be involved in antigen binding. Three classes of antibody-combining-site topology are recognized: a cavity type that typically binds haptens, a groove type that binds peptides, carbohydrates, or nucleic acids, and a planar type that binds proteins *(16)*.

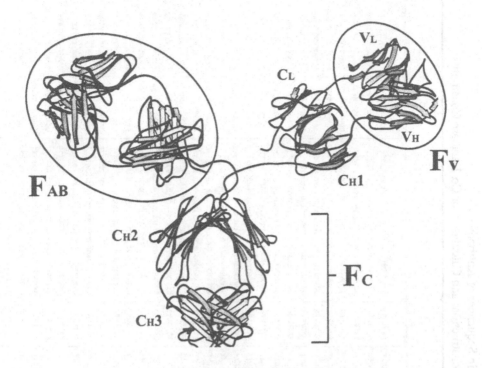

Fig. 1. A cartoon of an IgG antibody displaying two L chains and two H chains. These two chains fold to form a series of antiparallel β-sheet domains that are classed as either variable (V_L and V_H) or constant (C_L and C_H). Association of V_L and V_H domains gives rise to the F_v or variable region. The complementarity determining regions interspace the β-strands of this domain. A larger fragment is the Fab region, which contains the variable domain and a constant domain. The circle depicting the Fab is merely illustrative since it does not include all of the Fab region. The F_c region consists of two constant domains. The hinge and elbow angles for the Fab are different, illustrating potential flexibility in this region.

2. Antibody Modeling

2.1. General Methods

Antibody modeling has attracted increased interest over the past few years *(3,8,9,17–20)*, in part owing to an explosion in the number of published antibody sequences *(21)*, a gradual increase in availability of good crystal structures *(1)*, and availability of fast work stations capable of addressing problems encountered in molecular modeling. The first

Table 1

(A) L-Chain and (B) H-Chain Sequences of Antibodies Used for Framework Construction, Canonical Structure Construction, and Calculation of Cα Database Constraints[a]

Structure	LFR1	L1	LFR2	L2	LFR3	L3	LFR4
A							
glb2	DIQMTQSPSSLSASLGERVSLTC	RASQEISG------YLS	WLQQKP DGTI KRLIT	AASTLDS	GVPKRFSGRRSGSDYSLTISSLESED FADYTC	LQYLS--YPLT	FGAGT KLELKRA
2hfl	DIVLTQSPAIMSASPGEKVTMTC	SASSSVN------YMY	WYQQKS GTSP KRWIY	DTSKLAS	GVPVRFSGSGSGTSYSLTISSMETED AAEYYC	QQWGR--NP-T	FGSGT KLEIKRA
3hfm	DIVLTQSPATLSVTPGNSVSLSC	RASQSIGN------NLH	WYQQKS HESP RLLIK	YASQSIS	GIPSRFSGSGSGTDFTLSINSVETED FGMYFC	QQSNS--WPYT	FGQGT KLEIKRA
2fbj	EIVLTQSPAITAASLGQKVTITC	SASSSVS------SLH	WYQQKS GTSP KPWIY	EISKLAS	GVPARFSGSGSGTSYSLTINTMEAED AAIYYC	QQWTY--PLIT	FGAGT KLELKRA
2fb4	QSVLTQPPSASG-TPGQRVTISC	SGTSSNIG------SSTVN	WYQQLP GMAP KLLIY	RDAMRFS	GVPDRFSGSKSGASLAIGGLLQSED KTDYTC	AAWDVSLNAYV	FGTGT KVTVLGQ
1fh4	ESVLTQPPSASG-TPGQRVTISC	TGTSSNIG------SITVN	WYQQLP GMAP KLLIY	RDAMRFS	GVPTRFSGSKSGTSASLAISGLEARD ESDYTC	ASWNSSDNSYV	FGTGT KVTVLGQ
2mcp	DIVMTQSPSSLSVSAGERVTMSC	KSSQSLLNSGNQKNFLA	WYQQKP GQPP KLLIY	GASTRES	GVPDRFTGSGSGTDFTLTISSVQAED LAVYYC	QNDHS--YPLT	FGAGT KLEIKRA
1rei	DIQMTQSPSSLSASVGDRVTITC	QASQDII------KYLN	WYQQTP GKAP KLLIY	EASNLQA	GVPSRFSGSGSGTDYYFTISSLQPED IATTYC	QQYQS--LPYT	FGQGT KLQIT--
2rhe	ESVLTQPPSASG-TPGQRVTISC	TGSATDIG------SNSVI	WYQVP GKAP KLLIY	YNDLLPS	GVSDRFSASKGTSALAISGLESED ELDYTC	AAWNDSLDBPG	PGGGT KLTVLGQ
4fab	DVVMTQTPLSLPVSLGDQASISC	RSSQSLVHS-QGNTYLR	WYLQKP GQSP NVLIY	KVSNRFS	GVPDRFSGSGSGTDFTLKISRVEARD LGVYFC	SQSTH--VPWT	PGGGT KLEIKRA
2f19	DIQMTQTTSSLSASLGDRVTITC	RASQDISN------YLN	WYQQKP DGTV KLLIY	YTSRLHS	GVSRFSGSGSGTDYSLTISNLEHED IATFC	MSYLS-DASFV	FGSGT KVTVLRQ
1mcw	-SALTQPASVSG-SPGQSITVSC	AGHTSDVA--DSNSIS	WFQQHP DKAP KLLIY	AVTFRFS	GIPLRFSGSKSGNTASLTISGLLPDD RADYTC	SSYEGSD-NFV	FGTGT KVTVLGQ
3mcg	-SALTQPPSASG-SLGQSVTISC	TGTSSDVG--GYNYVS	WYQQHA GKAP KLLIY	EVNKRPS	GVPDRFSGSKSGNTASLTVSGLQAED RADYTC	SSYAGSD-NFV	FGTGT KVTVLGQ
1mam	DIQMTQTSSLSASLGDRVTISC	RASQDIYN------YLN	WYQQKP DGTV KLLIY	YTSRLHS	GVPSRFSGSGSGTSYSLTISRMEARD MATIC	QQGNT--LPPT	FGSGT KLEIKRA
1baf	QIVLTQSPAIMSASPGEKVTMTC	SASSSVY------YMY	WYQQKP GSSP KLLIY	DTSNLAS	GVPVRFSGSGSGTSYSLTISRMEARD AATYYC	QQWSSYP-PIT	FGVGT KLELKRA
1hil	DIVMTQSPSSLTVAGEKVTMSC	TSSQSLFNSGKQKNYLT	WYQQKP GQPP KVLIT	WASTRES	GVPDRFTGSGSGTDFTLTISGVQAED LAVYC	QNDYS--NPLT	FGGGT KLELKRA
8fab	--ELTQPPSVSV-SPGQTARIFC	SANALPNQ------YAY	WYQQKP GRAP VWVII	KDTQRPS	GIPQRFSSSTSGTTVTLTISGVQARD EADYYC	QAWDN--SASI	FGGGT KLTVLGQ
1dfb	DIQMTQSPSTLSASVGDRVTITC	RASQSISR------WLA	WYQQKP GKVP KLLIY	KASSLES	GVPSRFSGSGSGTEFTLTISSLQPDD FATTYC	QQYNS---YS	FGPGT KVDIKRT
1fdl	DIQMTQSPASLSASVGETVTITC	RASGNIHN------YLA	WYQKQ GKSP QLLVY	YTTTLAD	GVPSRFSGSGSGTQYSLKINSLQPED FGNYTC	QHFWS--TPRT	FGGGT KLEIKRA
1igf	DVLMTQTPLSLPVSLGDQASISC	RSNQTILLS-DGDTYLE	WYLQKP GQSP KLLIY	KVSNRFS	GVPDRFSGSGSGTDFTLKISRVEAED LGIYYC	FQGSH--VPPT	FGGGT KLEIKRA
6fab	DIQMTQIPSSLSASLGDRVSISC	RASQDINN------FLN	WYQQKP DGTI KLLIY	FTSRSQS	GVPSRFSGSGSGTDYSLTISNLBQED IAFYYC	QQGNA--LPRT	FGGGT KLEIKRA
7fab	ASVLTQPPSVSG-APGQRVTISC	TGSSSNIG------AGHNVK	WYQQLP GTAP KLLIY	HNNA---	----RFSVKSGTSATLAITGLQAED EADYYC	QSYDR--SLRV	FGGGT KLTVLRQ
1igm	DIQMTQSPSSLSASVGDRVTITC	QASQDISN------YLA	WYQQKP GKAP KLLIY	DASNLET	GVPSRFSGSGSGTDFTFTISSLQPED IATTYC	QQYQN--LPLT	FGPGT KVDIKRT
1bbj	DIQMTQSPASLSVSVGETVTITC	RASENIYS------NLA	WYQKQ GKSP QLLVY	AATNLAD	GVPSRFSGSGSGTQYSLKINSLQSED PGSIYC	QHFWG--TPYT	FGGGP KLEIKRA
1bbd	DIVMTQSPSSLTVTGEKVTMTC	KSSQSLLNSRTQKNYLT	WYQQKP GQSP KLLIY	WASTRES	GVPDRFTGSGSGTDYLTISSVQARD LAVYYC	QNNYN--YPLT	FGAGT KLELKRA
1ncd	DIVMTQSPKFMSTSVGDRVTITC	RASQDVST------AVV	WYQQKP GQSP KLLIY	WASTRHI	GVPDRFAGSGSGTDYTLTISSVQARD LALYYC	QQHYS--PPWT	FGGGT KLEIKRA
1fvc	DIVMTQSPSSLSASVGDRVTITC	RASQDVNT------AVA	WYQQKP GKAP KLLIY	SASFLYS	GVPSRFSGSRSGTDFTLTISSLQPED FATTYC	QQHYT--TPPT	FGQGT KVEIKAT
1igi	DVVMTQTPLSLPVSLGDQASISC	RSSQSLVHS-NGNTYLN	WTLQD. GQSP KLLIY	KVSNRFS	GVPDRFSGSGSGTDFTLKISRVEARD LGIYFC	SQYTH--VPPT	FGGGT KLEIKRA
1ggi	DIVLTQSPGSLAVSLGQRATISC	RASESVDD--DGNSFLH	WTQQKP GQPP KLLIY	RSSNLIS	GIPDRFSGSGSRFDFTLTINFVEADD VAITYC	QQSNE--DPLT	FGAGT KLEIKRA

20

B

Structure	HFR1	H1	HFR2	H2	HFR3	H3	HFR4
glb2	QVQLQQSGTELARPGASVRLSCKASGYTFT	T··FGIT	WVKQ RTQQ GLEWIG	EIFPGNS··KTY	YAERFKGKATLTADKSSTAYMGLSLLTSEDSAV	E···········IRY	WG QGTTLTVS
2hfl	·VQLQQSGAELMKPGASVKISCKASGYTFS	D··YWIE	WVKQ RPGH GLEWIG	EILPGSG··STN	YHERFKGKATFTADTSSSTAYMQLNSLTSEDSGV	···········FDG	WG QGTTLTVS
3hfm	DVQLQESGPSLVKPSQTLSLTCSVTGQ3IT	S··DYWS	WIRK FPGN GLEYMG	YVSVSG···STY	YNPSLKSRISITRDTSKNQYILDLNSVTEDTAT	MD···········GDY	WG QGTLVTVS
2fbj	EVKLLESGGGLVQPGGSLKLSCAASGFDFS	K··YMMS	MVRQ APGK GLEWVA	EIRHPDSG··TIN	YTPSLKDFIISRDNAKNSLYLQMSKVRSEDTAL	LHYGY···········NAY	WG QGTLVTVS
2fb4	EVQLVQSGGGVVQPGRSLRLSCSSSGFIFS	S··YAMY	MVRQ APGK GLEWVA	IIWDDGS··DQH	YADSVKGRFTISRDNSKNTLFLQMDSLRPEDTGV	DGGHGFCSSASCFGPDY	WG QGTPVTVS
2mcp	EVKLVESGGGLVQPGGSLRLSCATSGFTFS	D··FYME	WVRQ PPGK GLEWIA	ASRNKGNKYTE	YSASVKGRFIVSRDTSQSILYLQMNALRAEDTAI	NYYGSTWY·····FDV	WG QCTPVTVS
4fab	EVKLDETGGGLVQPGRPMKLSCVASGFTFS	D··YGMH	WVRQ SPEK GLEWVA	QIRNKPYNEYT	YSDSVKGRFTISRDDSKSSVLQMDNLRVEDMGI	SYG···········MDY	WG QCTSVTVS
2fl9	QVQLQQSGAELVRAGSSVKMSCKASGYTFT	D··YYMH	WVKQ RPGQ GLEWIG	YINPGKG··YLS	YNEKFKGKTTLTVDKSSSTAYMQLSRLTSEDSAV	SFYGGSDLA·VYYFDS	WG QGTTLTVS
1mam	EVKLVESGGGLVQPGGSLRLSCATSCFTFT	D··YYMS	WVRQ PPGK AlGKLIG	FIRNKADGYTE	YNASVKGRFTISRDNSQSILYLQMSTLRAEDSAT	DPYGP·······LAY	WG QGTLVTVS
1baf	DVQLQESGPGLVKPSQSLSLTCTVTGYSIT	S··DYAWN	WIRQ FPGN KLEWMG	YMSYSGG··YTY	YNPSLRSRISITRDTSKNQFFLQLKSVTEDTAT	GMP················	WG QGTLVTVS
1hil	EVQLVESGGDLVKPGGSLRLSCAASGFSFS	S··YGMS	WVRQ TPDK GLEWVA	TISNGGG··YTY	YPDSVKGRFTISRDNAKNTLYLQMSSLKSEDSAM	REYDENG······FAY	WG QGVLVTVS
8fab	AVKLVQAGGGVVQPGRSLRLSCIASGFTFS	N··YGMH	WVRQ APGK GLEWVG	VIWYNGS··RTY	YGDSVKGRFTISRDNSKRTLYMQHNSLRTEDTAV	DPDILTAFS·····FDY	WG QGCMVTVS
1dfb	EVQLVESGGGLVQPGRSLRLSCAASGFTFN	D··YAMH	WVRQ APGK GLEWVS	GISWDSS··SIG	YADSVKGRFTISRDNAKNSLYLQMNSLRAEDMAL	GRDYDYDSGGYFTVAFDI	WG QGCMVTVS
1dfl	QVQLKESGPGLVAPSQSLSITCTVSGFSLT	G··YGVN	WVRQ PPGK GLEWLG	MIWGDGN··TD	YNSALKSRLSISKIDNSKSQVFLKMNSLHTDDTAR	ERDYR·········LDY	WG QGTTLTVS
1igf	EVQLVESGGDLVKPGGSLKLSCAAS3FTFS	R··CAMS	WVRQ TPEK RLEWVA	GISSGGS··YTF	YPDTVKGRFIISRNNARNTLSLQMSSLRSEDTAI	YSSDPFY·····FDY	WG QGTTLTVS
6fab	EVQLVESGGVELVRAGSSVKMSCKASGYTFT	S··NGIN	WVKQ RPGQ GLEWIG	YNNPGNG··YIA	YNEKFKGKTTLTVDKSSSTAYMQLRSLTSEDSAV	SEYYGGSYK·····FDY	WG QGSLVTVS
7fab	AVQLEQSGPGLVRPSQTLSLTCTVSGGTSFD	S··YYWT	WIRQ PPGK GLEWIG	YVFYTG···TTL	LDPSLRGRVTNLVNTSKNQTSLRLSSVTAADTAV	NLIAGG········IDV	WG QGSLVTVS
1igm	EVHLLESGGNLVQPGGSLRLSCAASGFKTN	I··FVMS	WVRQ APGK GLEWVG	GVFGSGG··NTD	YADAVKGRFTITRDNSKNTLYLQMNSLRAEDTAI	HRVSYVLTG·····FDS	WG QGTTLTVS
1bbj	·VQLLSGCNLVQPGGSLRLSCAASGFFTN	D··HAIH	WAKQ KPEQ GLEWIG	YISPGND··DIK	YNEKFKGKATLTADKSSSTAYLQLSSLTSEDTAV	SY··········YGH	WG QGTTLTVS
1bbd	EVQLQQSGAELVRPGASVKLSCTTSGFNIK	D··IYIH	WVKQ RPEQ GLEWIG	RLDPANG··YTK	YDPKFQGKATITVDTSSNTAYLHLSSLTSEDTAV	MDY··········MDY	WG PGTSVTVS
1ncd	QIQLVQSGPELKKPGETVKISCKASGYTFT	N··YGMN	WVKQ APGK GLKWMG	WINTNTG··EPT	YGEEFKGRFAFSLETSASTANLQINNLKNEDTAT	GEDNFGSL·····SDY	WG QGTTVTVS
1fvc	EVQLVESGGGLVQPGGSLRLSCAASGFNIK	D··TYIH	WVRQ APGK GLEWVA	RIYPTNG··YTR	YADSVKGRFTISADFSKNTAVLQMNSLRAEDTAV	WGDGFYA······MDY	WG QGTLVTVS
1igi	·VQLQQSGPELVKPGASVRMSCKSGYIFT	D··FYMM	WVRQ SHGK GLEWIG	YISPYSG··VYG	YNQKFKGKATLTVDKSSSTAYMELRSLTSEDSAV	SSGNKWA······MDY	WG HGASVTVS
1ggi	QVQLKESGPGILQPSQTLSLTCSFSGFSLS	TYGHGVS	WIRQ PSGK GLEWLA	HIFWDG···DKR	YNPSLKSRLKIASKDTSNNQWFLKITSVDYTADTAT	EG···········YIY	WG QOTSVTVS

aSequence tracts in the framework regions used for fitting of structures for R.M.S.D. calculations are highlighted in dark gray.
1baf: *(94)*, 1bbd: *(95)*, 1bbj: *(96)*, 1dfb: *(97)*, 1fdl: *(98)*, 1fvc: *(99)*, 1ggi: *(100)*, 1hil: *(90)*, 1igf: *(101)*, 1igi: *(85)*, 1igm: *(102)*, 1mcw: *(104)*, 1ncd: *(105)*, 1rel: *(106)*, 2fl9: *(107)*, 1fb4 and 2fb4: *(108)*, 2fbj: *(109)*, 2hfl: *(86)*, 2mcp: *(110)*, 2rhe: *(111)*, 3hfm: *(112)*, 3mcg: *(113)*, 4fab: *(114)*, 6fab: *(115)*, 7fab: *(116)*, 8fab: *(117)*, glb2: *(118)*.

attempts at antibody modeling were based on simple homology-based methods *(22,23)*. Soon, rules began to emerge governing the conformations of short antibody loops *(24,25)*. Later, improvements were made in the accuracy of longer loops. These methods can broadly be grouped into knowledge-based approaches *(26–31)* and *ab initio*-based approaches that include methods such as conformational searching *(32–35)*, simulated annealing *(36,37)*, multicopy sampling *(38–40)*, and molecular dynamics *(41,42)*.

2.1.1. Framework Construction

As outlined in Section 2.2., the antiparallel β-sheet structure forming the F_v β-barrel framework is well conserved in structure. Most modeling studies of antibody F_vs have relied on the conserved nature of the β-barrel framework to construct a scaffold on which the CDR loops are built. In this method, an F_v β-barrel framework most identical in sequence to the antibody structure being modeled is chosen as the starting structure. The method relies on the premise that the framework is conserved between different antibodies, but a recent analysis of a set of 12 antibody structures has revealed that the spatial orientation of all strands of the F_v framework may not always be conserved *(4)*. Strands 1–6 are highly conserved, but strands 7 and 8 from the heavy chain are more variable. It is interesting to note that these strands interconnect CDRH3, the most variable CDR loop in both sequence and structure. Incorrect orientation of the framework strands can have important consequences for the construction of CDR loops, particularly where strand orientation affects the take-off trajectories from the F_v framework. The AbM protocol described in Section 2.2.1. attempts to minimize this problem by selecting the most homologous light and heavy chain from the database of known structures. If these are not derived from the same antibody, the respective chains are fitted by their most homologous regions (*see* Table 1) to an averaged hyperboloid function derived from known antibody structures.

2.1.2. CDR Construction

Proteins are not static entities. They exist in a fluid aqueous environment in which backbone loops and side chains may adopt many well-packed conformations that are energetically feasible. The conformations of protein loops are dependent on their length, their packing with other loops or secondary structural elements, the formation of salt bridges, covalent bonds, hydrogen bonds, and their interactions with solvent. Many algorithms have been developed for the construction of protein loops, all of which are applicable to the modeling of CDR loops *(26–42)*. CDRH3 presents unique problems because of the structural diversity of its loop conformations and takeoff angles from the F_v framework. Long H3 loops are particularly difficult to predict accurately. Since most H3 loops fall into this category *(9)*, much effort has been invested in developing suitable construction methods to model this loop.

2.1.2.1. CANONICAL LOOPS

Although the conformations of the CDR loops vary, a relationship between the structure of loop conformations and loop length has been noted *(26,27)*. Chothia and coworkers *(28,29,43–47, see also 48,49)* have established the concept of "canonical families" for five of the six CDR loops (L1–L3, H1, and H2). Canonical loops are defined on the basis of their length, and the position of key residues in the loop and in the framework *(see* Table 2). The distribution of canonical loops among the various classes used in the modeling protocol is shown in Fig. 2. Canonical loops adopt their conserved configuration as a result of their length, their packing with other CDR loops or part of the framework regions, the formation of conserved hydrogen bonding patterns, and even their ability to adopt unusual backbone configurations. Unfortunately, not all loops are canonical and these loops must be constructed by other means.

Useful as the canonical concept is, it has been noted that not all loops classified as canonical obey the "canonical rules" *(4,50)*. CDRL1 of HyHEL10 *(51)* and REI *(52)*, for example, both belong to canonical class 2 loops, but have different conformations owing to a 1→4 peptide flip between the central four residues *(see* ref. *4* for further examples). Furthermore, there is the question of whether all possible pairings of canonical loops are permitted in nature *(6,50)*. It is possible that particular pairings of canonical loops may disrupt the association of V_L–V_H domains, thus limiting the repertoire of canonical pairings.

2.1.2.2. DATABASE/KNOWLEDGE-BASED METHOD

As the database of antibody structures has increased, the use of knowledge-based methods in determining loop conformations has gained in importance *(3,31)*. The advantage of knowledge-based approaches is twofold. First, the starting structures are known to exist in nature. Sec-

Table 2
The Canonical Loops L1, L2, L3, H1, and H2 Defined
on the Basis of Length and the Occurrence of Canonical Residues at the Indicated Positions[a]

CDR	Loop	Class	Loop Length	Key Residues	Pattern	Structures
L1	24-40†	1	10	2,23,25,29,39,41,77	I-x(20)-C(1)-x(1)-A-x(3)-V-x(9)-[LM]-x(9)-W(1)-x(35)-Y	2hfl,2fbj,1baf
	24-34¶	2	11	2,23,25,29,39,41,77	I-x(20)-C(1)-x(1)-A-x(3)-[IV]-x(9)-L-x(1)-W(1)-x(35)-[YF]	glb2,3hfm,1rei,1igm,2f19,1mam,1fdl,6lab,1dfb
		3	17	2,23,25,29,39,41,77	I-x(20)-C(1)-x(1)-S-x(3)-L-x(9)-L-x(1)-W(1)-x(35)-[YF]	2mcp,1hil,1bbd,1bbj
		4	16	2,23,25,29,39,41,77	V-x(20)-C(1)-x(1)-S-x(3)-L-x(9)-L-x(1)-W(1)-x(35)-[YF]	1lgl,4fab
		5	13	2,23,25,30,39,41,77	S-x(20)-C(1)-x(1)-G-x(4)-I-x(8)-V-x(1)-W(1)-x(35)-[A]	2fb4,1fb4,2rhe
		6	11	3,23,25,29,39,41,77	E-x(19)-C(1)-x(1)-[SA]-x(3)-P-x(9)-A-x(1)-W-x(35)-[VSA]	8fab
L2	56-62†	1	7	54,70	[IV]-x(15)-G	2hfl,2fbj,1baf,glb2,3hfm,1rei,1igm,2f19,1mam, 6lab,1ncd,1fvc,2mcp,1hil,1bbd,4fab,1lgl,1lgi, 2fb4,1ggi,1bbj,1dfb,1fb4,1fdl,1mow,3mcg
	50-56¶					
L3	95-105†	1	9	94,96,102,103	C(1)-x(1)-[QNH]-x(6)-P	glb2,3hfm,1rei,1igm,2f19,1mam,6fab,1fvc, 2mcp,1hil,1bbd,4fab,1lgl,1lgi,1ggi,1bbj,1ncd
	89-97¶					1fdl,1rei
		2	9	94,96,102,103	C(1)-x(1)-Q-x(5)-P-[P]	2fbj
		3	8	94,96,103	C(1)-x(1)-Q-x(6)-P	2hfl
H1	26-37†	1	10	26,27,29,36,100,100,102	G-[GFY]-x(1)-[FLV]-x(6)-[MIVLT]-x(63) C(1)-x(1)-[RGHTKE]	2f19,1fdl,1lgf,1mam,2fb4,2fbj,2hfl,2mcp,4fab, 6fab,8fab,glb2,1igm,1bbd,1ncd,1lgl,1fvc,1hil
	31-35B¶					1bbj,1dfb
		2	10	26,27,29,36,100,102	G-[TD]-x(1)-[FI]-x(6)-[WS]-x(63)-C(1)-x(1)-[RN]	3hfm, 7fab
		3	11	26,27,29,36,100,102	G-[FGY]-x(1)-[LI]-x(6)-[WV]-x(63)-C(1)-x(1)-[RH]	1baf
H2	52-63†	1	9	57,76	[DG]-x(18)-[KRI]	1fdl,1baf,1ggi,3hfm
	50-65¶	2	10	55,58,76	[PTA]-x(2)-[GS]-x(17)-[ALT]	2hfl,glb2,1fvc,1ncd
		3	10	57,76	[GSND]-x(18)-R	1lgl,2fb4,1igm,1hil,2fbj,1dfb,8lab
		4	12	59,60,76	[GKN]-Y-x(15)-R	2mcp,4fab,1mam

[a]The first residue of the canonical pattern corresponds to the first canonical in the list of key residues. Residues in square brackets indicate sites where more than one residue type may be present, and x(n) denotes the number of residues linking the preceding and succeeding residues. Residues in braces { } mean "not this residue" in that position. The AbM (10) numbering and Kabat et al. (21) numbering are shown for loops L1–H2. The numbering for H3 is 101–119 (AbM) and 95–102 (Kabat). See Table 1 for references.

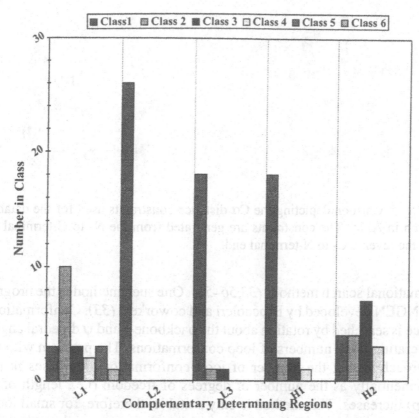

Fig. 2. Distribution of the number of complementarity determining loops falling into canonical L1, L2, L3, H1, and H2 classes. Antibodies used for this analysis are listed in Table 1.

ond, these approaches are computationally more efficient in saturating conformational space when compared with *ab initio* methods. The method of Jones and Thirup *(53)*, for example, identifies useful database loops by searching for loops that satisfy a set of α-carbon distance constraints (Fig. 3). This method is implemented in AbM and is described in more detail in Section 2.2.6. Other methods include those of Sutcliffe and coworkers *(54)*, who use a high-resolution database to identify structurally conserved regions, and of Stanford and Wu *(55)* who generate backbones from an analysis of tripeptides from β-sheet proteins.

2.1.2.3. AB INITIO METHODS

These methods provide an alternative way to saturate conformational space. The generation of all possible loops may be accomplished by con-

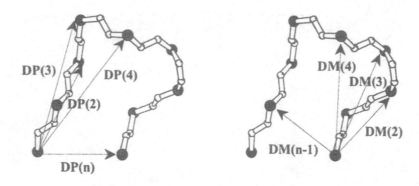

Fig. 3. Cartoon depicting the Cα distance constraints used for the database search in AbM. The constraints are generated from the N- to C-terminal end and the reverse C- to N-terminal end.

formational search methods *(33,56–58)*. One such method is the program CONGEN developed by Bruccoleri and coworkers *(33)*. Conformational space is searched by rotation about the backbone φ and ψ dihedral angles, generating large numbers of loop conformations. The problem with this approach is that the number of loop conformations increases in size exponentially as the number of degrees of freedom (i.e., length of the loop) increases. This method is only suitable, therefore, for small loops. Conformational searching has two advantages over random methods, such as Monte Carlo, simulated annealing *(36,37)*, or molecular dynamics methods *(41,42)*. First, conformational search methods search on a regular grid (in some cases, this may be a disadvantage, since discrete regular search steps may miss some conformations), unlike dynamics or Monte Carlo methods, which sequentially perturb one conformation into another by small increments and, hence, may sample the same space many times. Second, conformational searching does not entail the cost of determining energy derivatives as in molecular dynamics, and permits the examination of noncontinuous energy surfaces *(33)*.

The *ab initio* methods generate multiple conformations that must be evaluated at some stage by an objective function, usually consisting of an energy term. A problem exists in that many low-energy conformations are produced that differ only slightly from each other. The development of force fields and the inclusion of solvation models in free-energy calculations is an area of continuing development *(59–64)*.

2.1.2.4. COMBINED METHOD

A combined approach to the construction of antibody loops was proposed by Martin and coworkers *(3,65)* to overcome some of the deficiencies of the above methods. Loops are constructed using database methods and conformational searching is applied to the central region of the loop. When insufficient loops are found using database methods, the number of loops can be increased by conformational searching of the region of the loop that is most likely to be variable. When the loops are long, conformational searching alone is computationally intractable. By first building the base of the loop by database methods, the computational cost is kept within reasonable bounds. This method is described in Section 2.2.

2.1.3. Side-Chain Construction

The simplest and most cost-effective method of side-chain construction has been the use of rotamer libraries, which depend on a statistical distribution of side-chain χ angles from known protein structures. Analysis of such distributions has shown that side-chain dihedral angles cluster around preferred χ angles. This property has been exploited in a number of side-chain rotamer libraries *(66–70)*. Where the structure of the backbone is known, homologous templates can be used, overlaying as many atoms as possible in the side chains that show correspondence *(71,72)*. It should be noted that the accuracy of side-chain prediction is dependent on availability of good backbone coordinates. With the increasing numbers of high-resolution structures in the PDB, rotamer libraries have been generated that take into account the preferred χ angle distribution of side chains with respect to particular backbone conformations *(73–76)*. Reid and Thornton *(77)* used a rotamer library and performed manual adjustment of side-chain χ angles from the preferred distributions when clashes occurred, followed by energy minimization. The CONGEN method *(33,78)* used in the AbM modeling protocol *(see* Section 2.2.) searches conformational space by rotation about χ angles on a rotational grid concurrent with energy evaluation. Approximate solutions to the placement of side chains have been achieved using optimization techniques, such as simulated annealing *(79,80)*. Genetic algorithms *(70)* have been used to search conformational space. Other approaches that attempt to include the influence of all side-chain positions are the use of the dead-end theorem *(81,82)*, molecular dynamics *(83)*, and self-consistent mean field theory *(84)*.

Surface side chains, unlike core side chains, present particular problems since they are unlikely to adopt a unique conformation due to a lack of packing constraints and their accessibility to solvent. This is particularly true of the longer side-chain amino acids. Consideration must also be given to the packing of bulky hydrophobic residues found on the surfaces of proteins often shielded from solvent by hydrophilic residues. Objective functions to evaluate side-chain positions would ideally contain terms that include the effects of solvent and hydrophobicity *(59–64)*.

2.2. Methods for Modeling Antibody 1CGS
2.2.1. Modeling According to AbM Protocol

The modeling presented here was done with the commercial version of AbM v2.0 *(10)*. Where deviations occur in the research version of the modeling program, these will be noted in the text. The AbM protocol takes a holistic view of available antibody construction methods and utilizes canonical structures, database, and conformational searching, or a combination of the database approach with conformational searching where appropriate. This approach takes advantage of the wealth of crystallographic information and maintains the ability to saturate space using *ab initio* methods.

2.2.2. Methods and Test Example

The anti-*N*-(P-cyanophenyl)-*N*-(diphenylmethyl)guanidine acetic acid antibody (1CGS) *(2)* was chosen for modeling. Its structure has been solved at an average resolution of 2.6 Å, and it contains different types of hypervariable loops that may be modeled using the canonical loop, database, and combined database/CONGEN approaches. This antibody has been chosen here to demonstrate the need for an understanding of antibody structure when interpreting the results of the automated assembly method. The 1CGS antibody was not present in the database of structures used for the construction of the model.

2.2.3. Sequence Alignment

The variable domain sequences of the L and H chains of 1CGS are aligned against a database of antibody sequences that contains 29 L-chain sequences and 24 H-chain sequences (Table 1). Insertions are introduced into the CDR regions at positions of highest sequence variability. The numbering scheme followed in this text is according to AbM, which differs from that of Kabat and coworkers *(21)*. The numbering scheme is outlined in Table 2. Loop L1 is defined as six residues greater than the Kabat et al. definition, having a maximum length of 17 residues. CDRH2, with a maximum of 12 residues, is shorter than the Kabat et al. H2 definition, since residues 61–65 in H2 in the Kabat definition are conserved in structure. The AbM protocol allows redefinition of CDR regions if required.

2.2.4. Framework Construction

The interface of the V_L/V_H framework is known to be well conserved. Small variations in V_L/V_H orientations combined with differences in packing may cause large errors in the positioning of CDR loops on the framework, particularly when the incorrect orientation affects CDR take-off points on the F_v. L and H chains are chosen based on greatest homology from a database of antibody structures. Where these chains are not derived from the same antibody, a fitting procedure is used to reconstruct a new F_v framework. The L and H chains of the 1CGS antibody show greatest homology with the corresponding subunits derived from two different antibodies. Therefore, the model framework for 1CGS was constructed as a chimera of the L chain from 1igi (*[85]*; 2.7-Å resolution) and the H chain from 2hfl (*[86]*; 2.54-Å resolution). As outlined in Section 2.1., the positioning of strands 1–6 is well conserved. The two chosen domains are least-square fitted to an averaged hyperboloid based on 12 antibody structures *(4)* using the most conserved regions of strands 1–6 (Table 1). Strands 7 and 8 are not used in the fitting procedure. These take their position in the model from the fitted database structure. The sequence of the framework is adjusted to the model, and side chains are added using a template-based approach, where side-chain torsions of the model are adjusted to match the equivalent parent torsions of the crystal structure. Nonequivalent atoms are positioned using the iterative conformational search program CONGEN.

2.2.5. CDR Construction

Because of the conserved structure of canonical loops, they are given highest priority in the construction process and are generated first. For short loops less than six residues in length, the conformational search method CONGEN is employed to saturate conformational space. For loops of greater length, conformational searching becomes restrictive in computer time, and either the database or the combined method is used. If sufficient numbers of database loops are found for loops of six or seven residues in length, the database method is preferred because of its computational efficiency. For loops greater than seven residues in length, a combined approach may be used to construct the base of the loop using a database of structures, followed by reconstruction of the central portion of the loop using the *ab initio* search method CONGEN. Each of the methods (CONGEN, database, or combined method) overlaps in its useful range with other methods. Thus, the choice of a particular method depends to some degree on the best judgment of the researcher. Side chains are constructed using a template-based approach in which nonequivalent atoms are positioned using the conformational search algorithms of CONGEN. The objective function of this procedure uses a solvent-modified energy term in which the electrostatic and attractive nonbond terms have been removed. The force field used in the energy evaluation is the Eureka force field of Osguthorpe and coworkers, which is derived from the CVFF force-field *(87,88)*.

As described in Section 2.1.3., side chains in protein cores are well packed and can be evaluated adequately using a simple energy function. However, surface side chains, owing to their lack of packing constraints and accessibility to solvent, may occupy many low-energy sites. The use of a simple energy term may not be appropriate in this case. The packing of bulky hydrophobic side chains is particularly important when they are found at the surface, since they are normally shielded from solvent by hydrophilic side chains. In the research version of AbM (and future releases of the software) *(see ref. 4)*, the use of Monte Carlo simulated annealing with an energetic function that contains a full nonbond term and a simple torsional term:

$$E = \xi_0 \sum_{i=1}^{n} [(r_0/r)^6 - 2(r_0/r)^{12}] + \kappa_0\cos(3\varpi) \tag{1}$$

with postsimulation screening using a hydrophobic function:

$$f_a = - \sum A_{rel} \cdot H_{rel} f_a \varepsilon \ (-1{:}1) \tag{2}$$

has been found to be effective in accurately placing such side chains.

2.2.6. CDR Modeling Protocol

Analysis of the 1CGS sequence shows that CDR loops L2, L3, H1, and H2 are canonical loops (Table 2). The CDR loop L1 is long (16 residues) and was constructed using the combined database/CONGEN approach. The CDRH3 loop (seven residues) was constructed using only the database approach. CDR loops are assembled in a particular order, starting with the canonical loops. The remaining loops are generated from the outside of the combining site inward to the center, with CDRH3 always constructed last. For antibody 1CGS, CDR loop L1 was built onto the framework in the presence of the four canonical loop backbones. The AbM protocol offers the option to include side chains from the other CDRs, though this was not done in the present model. CDR loop H3 was built in the presence of the other five CDR loop backbones, after construction of the L1 loop (Table 3).

2.2.6.1 MODELING CANONICAL LOOPS L2-H2 (*SEE* NOTE 1)

Since the structure of the canonical loops L2–H2 is well conserved, these loops are constructed first. A canonical loop from the database of antibodies (Table 2) is chosen on the basis of sequence homology and placed onto the framework (*see also* ref. *4*) taking into account the take-off angle of the base of the CDR with the framework. Each loop is built on a bare framework in isolation of the other canonical loops. Side chains are constructed as described in Section 2.2.5.

2.2.6.2. MODELING THE L1 LOOP (*SEE* NOTE 2)

CDR loop L1 is constructed using the combined database/CONGEN method. The base of the loop is constructed using the database method that utilizes information from known structures to saturate conformational space. Database searching has the advantage over purely *ab initio*-based approaches such as those employed in CONGEN, of being computationally efficient as well as generating structures that are already known to exist in nature. This method uses a predetermined set of α-carbon distance constraints. These are derived from all of the CDR loops from known antibody structures. The α-carbon constraints specify the geometry of CDR loops of a particular length within a tolerance of $\bar{\chi} = 3.5\sigma$. An α-carbon database containing all structures from the Brookhaven PDB is searched for loops of the same length and geometric fit. Selected loops are clustered to eliminate redundant structures, and the central portion of the remaining loops is removed for construction by the CONGEN method.

A 16-residue loop has very tight α-carbon distance constraints. Only three database loops were selected that conformed to the required geometry for the L1 loop of antibody 1CGS. The central five residues corresponding to [V(HSN)G] in the model were removed from each of the selected loops and reconstructed using CONGEN. Conformational space was searched by rotation of the backbone ϕ and ψ angles restricted by

Table 3
Outline of the Protocol for the Initial Modeling and Subsequent Remodeling of the L1 and H3 Loops[a]

CDR	Sequence	Length	Build method	Priority	Database hits	CONGEN[e]
Initial Model						
L1	RPSQSL[V(HS–N)G]NTYLH	16	Combined database CONGEN	2	3	3567
L2	RVSNRFS	7	Canonical (class 1)	1	b	b
L3	SQGTH–VPYT	9	Canonical (class 1)	1	b	b
H1	GYTFSE–YWIE	10	Canonical (class 1)	1	b	b
H2	EILPGSG–RTN	10	Canonical (class 2)	1	b	b
H3	GYSS——MDY	7	Database	3	29978[c]/5712[d]	b
Remodel						
H3	GYSS——M	5	Database search only	2	67998[c]/4110[d]	b

[a]The H3 loop was shortened at the base of the loop, and the five-residue loop reconstructed using the database method in the presence of the original L1 backbone and canonical loops. The shoulder region of the L1 loop was reconstructed in the presence of the remodeled H3 and canonical backbones using the combined database/CONGEN method. The square brackets [] indicate the region to be constructed, and the round brackets indicate the region of chain closure using the Gö and Scheraga (89) algorithm.

[b]Does not apply.

[c]Total number of database hits.

[d]Number remaining after initial clustering.

[e]Number of loops after reconstruction of central portion using CONGEN.

Ramachandran energies of a specified cutoff values. Conformational searching was also used in side-chain construction (*see* Section 2.2.6.1.). Chain closure of the central three residues (HSN) was performed using the chain-closure algorithm of Gö and Scheraga *(89)*. Each of the resulting 3567 putative loops was screened using the solvent-modified energy function. The loops were clustered, and the five lowest energy unique conformations were selected. Loops derived from database searches were filtered by the structural determining region algorithm of Sutcliffe and coworkers *(54)* (*see* ref. *41*). If only a CONGEN search is made, then the lowest energy structure would be selected.

2.2.6.3. MODELING THE H3 LOOP

CDR loop H3 is generally the most difficult loop to model accurately because of variability in its structure and takeoff angle from the framework. It was noted in Section 2.1.1. that strands 7 and 8 interconnecting CDRH3 vary in their positioning in different antibodies. It is important to model the takeoff trajectory accurately, since small differences can produce large variations in the placement and, hence, the overall structure of the CDRH3 loop. The AbM protocol attempts to take this variability into account by defining four H3 families *(8,9)* that differ in length, the position of key residues, and loop takeoff angles. Currently, seven H3 structural classes are incorporated in our research version of the AbM program and will be included in the next planned release of the commercial version.

The CDRH3 loop of antibody 1CGS is seven residues in length (GYSSMDY). This loop was constructed using the database method without reconstruction of the central region. Because of the structural variability of H3 loops, the constraints on their modeling are weak. For CDRH3 of 1CGS, a large number of database loops were identified (29978). This number was reduced by the structurally determining region algorithm of Sutcliffe and coworkers *(54)*, the loops were clustered, and evaluation of putative structures was as described in Section 2.2.6.2. A comparison of the initial model with the crystal structure is shown in Fig. 4.

2.2.7. Remodeling of H3 (see Note 3)

Examination of the sequence of the H3 loop revealed an aspartic acid at position 105 (AbM numbering) and a conserved arginine at position 100 in the framework. In known structures containing this configuration, a salt bridge is formed between the two charged residues, tying down the

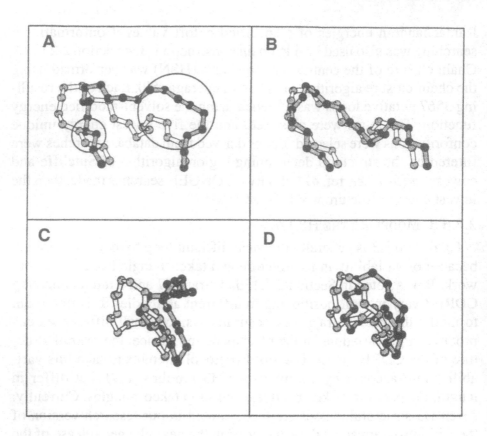

Fig. 4. Panels A and C show orthogonal views of the backbone of the initial model of H3 with the crystal structure in white and the model in dark gray. The smaller circle indicates the region near the N-terminal Section of the loop where the chain deviates from the crystal structure. The larger circle indicates a bulge characteristic of H3 loops that do not make a salt bridge between Arg-212 and Asp-218 (AbM numbering). Panels B and D show orthogonal views of the remodeled H3 loop.

base of the H3 loop. The 1CGS modeled loop did not possess this salt bridge. In addition, the H3 loop displayed a bulge (Fig. 4) often seen when a salt bridge is absent at the base of the loop. These observations do not inspire confidence in the initial model of the H3 loop. The H3 loop was therefore remodeled in the presence of the other five loops by moving the region defined as framework by two residues (framework underlined):

TR [GYSSMDY] **WG** → TR [GYSSM] **DYWG**

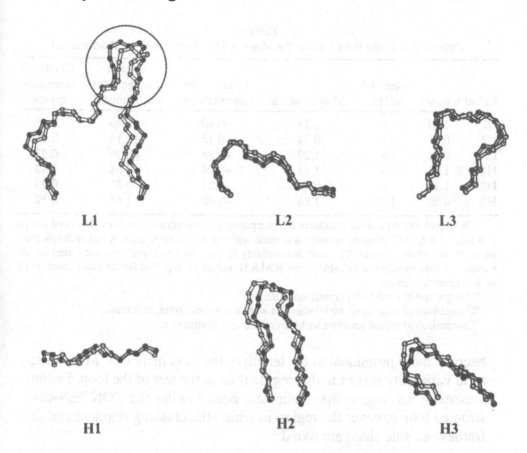

Fig. 5. Comparison of the backbone of the final six modeled CDR loops. The crystal structure is depicted in white, and the model in dark gray. The region that showed a clash in L1 is circled *(see text)*. All figures were aligned along the axis joining the N- and C-terminus and the axis entering the page and the plane of the loop orthogonal to the base of the page. The loops were then rotated, so that they are orthogonal to the first view. This representation does not bias the viewing in favor of any particular orientation.

so that the conformation of the base of the loop is now derived from a known antibody structure. Construction of the shortened five-residue loop proceeded as before (Section 2.2.6.3.).

2.2.8. Remodeling Considerations (see Note 4)

The region near the C-terminus of the L1 loop (Fig. 5) showed a small clash with part of a side chain from the light chain of the F_v framework. This region lends characteristic structural features to L1 loops that

Table 4
Comparison of the R.M.S.D. of the Model CDRs from the Crystal Structure [a]

Initial model[a]	Remodel of H3[b]	Minimization[a]	Change after minimization[c]	Overall change from initial model	Crystal to minimized crystal[d]
L1	1.63	>	1.23	−0.40	−0.40	0.51
L2	0.61	>	0.74	+0.13	+0.13	0.58
L3	0.94	>	1.20	+0.26	+0.26	0.53
H1	1.29	>	1.33	+0.04	+0.04	0.42
H2	1.18	>	0.97	−0.21	−0.21	0.43
H3	4.29	1.72	1.66	−0.06	−2.63	0.52

[a]The initial and remodeled structures are compared with the crystal structure. The final model was minimized, and further comparison was made with the crystal structure that had undergone the same minimization protocol. The modeled antibody is fitted to the crystal structure based on the framework regions outlined in Table 1, and R.M.S.D. values are reported for the loops constructed on this fitted framework.
[b]Comparison of model with crystal structure.
[c]Comparison of minimized model structure with minimized crystal structure.
[d]Comparison of crystal structure with minimized crystal structure.

become more prominent as the length of the loop increases. More structural variability is seen in this region than in the rest of the loop. Serious clashes in this region may indicate a need to alter the CONGEN-constructed loop to cover the region in which the clashing segment and the framework side chain are found:

RPSQSL[V(HS-N)G]NTYLH → RPSQSLVH[S-(NGN)T]YLH

It is sometimes as important to decide when not to remodel a region as when to remodel. The L1 loop was **not** remodeled for the following reasons.

1. The clash was small, and would probably be eliminated by energy minimization or molecular dynamics.
2. Remodeling of L1 would probably not be affected by the newly constructed H3 loop, since they are quite distant from each other in the combining site.
3. The question of where to place the reconstruction region is still very much a subjective one. Good guidelines on this point have yet to emerge from the literature despite many attempts to define such rules. Under these circumstances, reconstruction of the CONGEN-built region would merely reflect a subjective judgment without any strong underlying rationale.

2.2.9. Minimization

Construction of the framework, CDR loops, and side chains may result in some steric clashes as noted above in Section 2.2.8. These clashes may

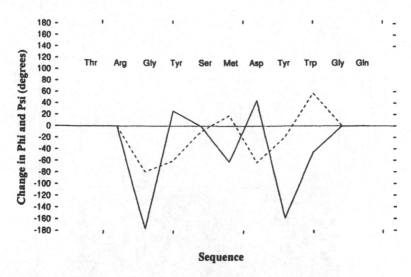

Fig. 6. Plot of the difference in φ and ψ angles of the initial and final models of CDR H3 loop. Differences in φ and ψ angles are calculated as positive if the change from crystal to model is clockwise when viewed along the N to Cα axis and negative if the rotation is counterclockwise.

be eliminated by energy minimization or molecular dynamics using a program like Discover *(90)*. The protocol followed here to this end fixed all heavy atoms and allowed hydrogen atoms to relax using steepest descent minimization for 50 cycles. The tethering force was then reduced on all side-chain atoms (both loop and framework) for 50 further cycles of steepest descent minimization. The tethering force on CDR loop backbone atoms was reduced in steps over 100 further cycles. Finally, 100 cycles of conjugate gradient minimization without any tethering force on the CDR backbones or framework and CDR side-chains were performed. Typically, the backbone framework atoms remain fixed during the minimization. This protocol is followed to allow regions that are most likely to contain clashes (such as hydrogens) to relax their conformation without affecting other regions of the model unduly during the initial stages of minimization. In order to compare the crystal and model structures, both of these structures were subjected to the same minimization protocol.

3. Notes

1. As expected, the canonical loops (L2–H2) are modeled well using the yardstick of similarity to the crystal structure, with root mean square deviations (R.M.S.D.) of 0.61–1.29 Å for the initial model (Table 4, *see* previous page).

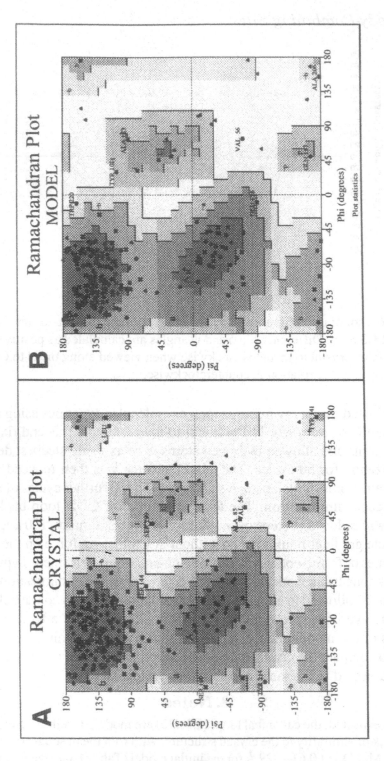

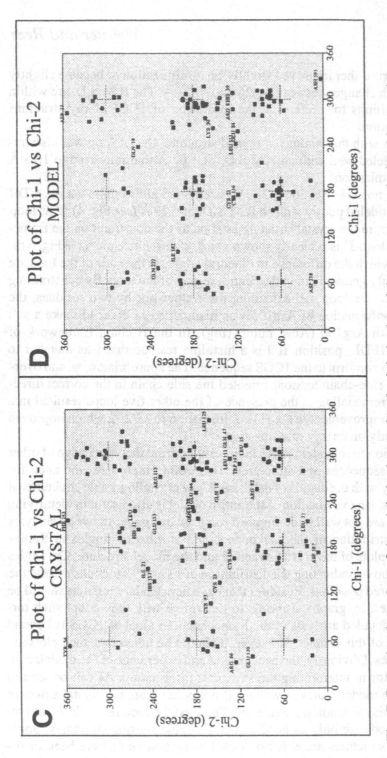

Fig. 7. Ramachandran plots of the minimized crystal and minimized model structures are depicted in A and B, respectively. The dark gray areas show the most favored regions. Plots C and D show the χ^1/χ^2 side-chain distributions of the crystal and model structures, respectively. Tighter clustering of the points around the crosses indicates that the distribution of side-chain χ angles more closely approximates ideal χ angle distribution determined from statistical distributions of side-chains from known structures.

These loops either improved slightly on minimization or became slightly worse with changes between +0.26 and -0.21 Å. The R.M.S.D. are within the error limits for proteins at the resolution of 1CGS X-ray structure determination.

2. Compared with the minimized crystal structure, the L1 loop was also initially modeled well with an R.M.S.D. of 1.63 Å that improved to 1.23 Å after minimization.

3. The clash noted in Section 2.2.7. was removed after minimization. CDR H3 was modeled poorly with an R.M.S.D. of 4.29 Å (*see* Fig. 4). This loop deviated from the crystal structure as soon as the constraint on the framework was lost. This is clearly shown in a ϕ, ψ difference plot (*see* Fig. 6 on p. 37) in which the difference in dihedral angles at the ends of the loop are significantly greater than in the central region of the loop. By constraining the base of the loop and extending the framework by two residues, the correct conformation of Asp105 was maintained in order to make a salt bridge with Arg100 (AbM numbering). In the H-chain framework of antibody 1FDL, position 100 is a histidine residue that was mutated to arginine to conform to the 1CGS sequence. The appropriate ϕ, ψ, and overlapping χ side-chain torsions oriented the side chain in the correct direction. The remodeling in the presence of the other five loops resulted in a dramatic improvement in the H3 conformation to 1.72 Å, which improved only slightly on energy minimization.

4. The decision to remodel the H3 loop resulted from the knowledge of other antibody sequences and structures. This point emphasizes the need for familiarity with the details of database X-ray crystallographic structures of antibodies. An examination of the entire model is also useful in identifying areas that are not well built. Figure 7 *(on previous page)* shows an analysis of the distribution of the backbone ϕ and ψ dihedral angles in Ramachandran plots of the crystal structure and the model structure. Chi angles are also shown indicating the distribution of $\chi 1$ and $\chi 2$ torsions around the most favored positions. Residues that have nonstandard torsions should be investigated by graphical means to determine why they adopt such torsions. A detailed analysis of the Ramachandran plots of 1CGS is beyond the scope of this chapter. However, it should be noted that such plots are only guides. Obviously, the background and experience of the modeler are a key factor in interpreting the structural information. As can be seen in Fig. 7, the model scores as well as, if not better than, the crystal structure on the basis of standard parameters. The model structures built by homology methods are only as good as the available starting structures. Some antibody structures are either of such low resolution or have been incorrectly built that their use in modeling must be suspect. It should also be

noted that crystallographic structures may be influenced by crystal-packing interactions, giving rise to conformations that would not exist if it were not for these contacts or if the antibody were in solution.

5. This chapter can be used as a brief introduction to the extensive literature available on antibody modeling. With increasing need for good-quality antibody structures, molecular modeling can be expected to play an increasing role in several types of investigations of antibody function. Regardless of the method of modeling, an intimate knowledge of antibody structure is required when using any automated method. Continued improvement of objective energy functions that include the effect of solvent is currently an important challenge in developing modeling protocols. In addition, recent reports *(91–93)* of induced fit in some antibodies pose new challenges in modeling changes occurring on antigen–antibody complexation and in predicting which antibodies undergo induced structural transformations and which do not. Figures 3–5 were generated using MOLSCRIPT *(119)* and Fig. 7 was generated using PROCHECK *(120)*.

References

1. Bernstein, F. C., Koetzle, T. F., Williams, G. J. B., Meyer, E. F., Brice, M. D., Rodgers, J. R., Kennard, O., Shimanouchi, T., and Tasumi, M. (1977) The protein data bank. A computer based archival file for macromolecular structures.*J. Mol. Biol.* **112,** 535–542.
2. Guddat, L. W., Shan, L., Anchin, J. M., Linthicum, D. S., and Edmundson, A. B. (1994) Local and transmitted conformational changes on complexation of an anti-sweetener Fab. *J. Mol. Biol.* **236,** 247–274.
3. Martin, C. R., Cheetham, J. C., and Rees, A. R. (1991) Molecular modeling of antibody combining sites. *Methods Enzymol.* **203,** 121–153.
4. Pedersen, J., Searle, S., Henry, A., and Rees, A. R. (1992) Antibody modeling: Beyond homology. *ImmunoMethods* **1,** 126–136.
5. Rees, A. R., Pedersen, J. T., Searle, S. J., Henry, A. H., and Webster, D. M. (1993) Towards rational antibody engineering, in *Protein Engineering II* (Goodenough, P., ed.), CPL, Newbury, pp. 95–111.
6. Rees, A. R., Staunton, D., Webster, D. M., Searle, S. J., Henry, A. H., and Pedersen, J. T. (1994) Antibody design: beyond the limits.*Trends Biotechnol.* **12,** 199–206.
7. Webster, D. M., Pedersen, J., Staunton, D., Jones, A., and Rees, A. R. (1994) Antibody combining sites: extending the natural limits. *Appl. Biochem. Biotechnol.* **47,** 119–134.
8. Searle, S. J., Pedersen, J. T., Henry, A. H., Webster, D. M., and Rees, A. R. (1995) Antibody structure and function, in *Antibody Engineering Manual* (Borrebaeck, K., ed.), Oxford University Press, Oxford, UK, pp. 3–51.
9. Rees, A. R., Pedersen, J. T., Searle, S. J., Henry, A. H., and Webster, D. M. (1994) Antibody structure from X-ray crystallography and molecular modeling, in *Immunochemistry* (van Oss, C. J. and van Regenmortel, H. V., eds.), Marcel Dekker, New York, pp. 616–650.

10. AbM. A computer program for modeling variable regions of antibodies. Oxford Molecular Ltd., Oxford, UK.
11. Poljak, R. J., Amzel, L. M., Avery, H. P., Chen B. L., Phizackerley, R. P., and Daul, F. (1973) Three-dimensional structure of the Fab fragment of a human immunoglobulin at 2.8 Å. *Proc. Natl. Acad. Sci. USA* **70,** 3305–3310.
12. Deisenhofer, J., Colman, P. M., and Huber, R. (1976) Crystallographic structural studies of a human F_c fragment. I. An electron density map at 4 Å resolution and a partial model. *Hoppe-Seyler's Z Physiol. Chem.* **357,** 435–445.
13. Lesk, A. M. and Chothia, C. (1982) Evolution of proteins formed by β-sheets. 2. The core of the immunoglobulin domains. *J. Mol. Biol.* **160,** 325–342.
14. Chothia, C. and Janin, J. (1981) Relative orientation of close-packed β-pleated sheets in proteins. *Proc. Natl. Acad. Sci. USA* **78,** 4146–4150.
15. Novotny, J., Bruccoleri, R., Newell, J., Murphy, D., Haber, E., and Karplus, M. (1983) Molecular anatomy of the antibody-binding site. *J. Biol. Chem.* **258,** 14,433–14,437.
16. Webster, D. M., Henry, A. H., and Rees, A. R. (1994) Antibody–antigen interactions. *Curr. Opin. Struct. Biol.* **4,** 123–129.
17. Bolger, M. B. and Sherman, M. A. (1991) Computer modeling of combining site structure of anti-hapten monoclonal antibodies. *Methods Enzymol.* **203,** 21–45.
18. Padlan, E. A. and Kabat, E. A. (1991) Modeling antibody combining sites. *Methods Enzymol.* **203,** 3–21.
19. Anchin, J. M. and Linthicum, D. S. (1992) Molecular and computational techniques for modelling antibody combining sites. *J. Clin. Immunoassay* **15,** 42–50.
20. Mandal, C. and Linthicum, D. S. (1992) Computer-aided modeling of complete antibody Fab structures using alpha carbon atomic coordinates. *J. Clin. Immunoassay* **15,** 42–50.
21. Kabat, E. A., Wu, T. T., Reid-Miller, M., Perry, H. M., and Gottesman, K. S. (1992) *Sequences of Proteins of Immunological Interest,* 5th ed. US Department of Health and Human Services, National Institutes of Health, NIH publication no. 91-3242.
22. Padlan, E. A., Davies, D. R., Pecht, I., Givol, D., and Wright, C. (1976) Model building studies of antigen binding sites: the hapten binding site of MOPc315. *Cold. Spring Harbor Symp. Quant. Biol.* **41,** 627–637.
23. Mainhart, C. R, Potter, M., and Feldmann, R. J. (1984) A refined model for the variable domains (F_v) of the J539 β(1,6)-D-galactan-binding immunoglobulin. *Mol. Immunol.* **21,** 469–478.
24. Wilmot, C. M. and Thornton, J. M. (1988) Analysis and prediction of the different types of β-turns in proteins. *J. Mol. Biol.* **203,** 221–232.
25. Rose, G. D., Gierasch, L. M., and Smith, J. A. (1985) Turns in peptides and proteins. *Adv. Prot. Chem.* **37,** 1–109.
26. Darsley, M. J., Phillips, B. C., Rees, A. R., Sutton, B. J., and de la Paz, P. (1985) An approach to the study of anti-protein antibody combining sites, in *Investigation and Exploitation of Antibody Combining Sites.* Plenum, New York, pp. 63–68.
27. de la Paz, P., Sutton, B. J., Darsley, M. J., and Rees, A. R. (1986) Modeling of the combining sites of three anti-lysozyme monoclonal-antibodies and of the complex between one of the antibodies and its epitope. *EMBO J* **5,** 415–425.

28. Chothia, C. and Lesk, A. M. (1987) Canonical structures for the hypervariable regions of immunoglobulins. *J. Mol. Biol.* **196,** 901–917.
29. Chothia, C., Lesk, A. M., Tramontano, A., Levitt, M., Smith-Gill, S. J., Air, G., Sheriff, S., Padlan, E. A., Davies, D., Tulip, W. R., Colman, P. M., Spinelli, S., Alzari, P. M., and Poljak, R. J. (1989) Conformations of immunoglobulin hypervariable regions. *Nature* **342,** 877–883.
30. Snow, M. E. and Amzel, L. M. (1986) Calculation of the three dimensional changes in protein structure due to amino acid substitutions: the variable region of immunoglobulins. *Proteins: Struct. Funct. Genet.* **1,** 267–279.
31. Bajorath, J., Stenkemp, R., and Aruffo, A. (1993) Knowledge-based model building of proteins: concepts and examples. *Protein Sci.* **2,** 1798–1810.
32. Shenkin, P. S., Yarmush, D. L., Fine, R. M., Wang, H., and Levinthal, C. (1987) Predicting the antibody hypervariable loop conformation. I. Ensembles of random conformations for ringlike structures. *Biopolymers* **26,** 2053–2085.
33. Bruccoleri, R. E., Haber, E., and Novotny, J. (1988) Structure of antibody hypervariable loops reproduced by a conformational search algorithm. *Nature* **335,** 564–568.
34. Bruccoleri, R. E. (1993) Application of systematic conformational search to protein modeling. *Mol. Simulation* **10,** 151–174.
35. Bassolino-Klimas, D., Bruccoleri, R. E., and Subramaniam, S. (1992) Modeling the antigen combining site of an anti-dinitrophenyl antibody, AN02. *Protein Sci.* **10,** 1465–1476.
36. Higo, J., Collura, V., and Garnier, J. (1992) Development of an extended simulated annealing method: application to the modeling of complementary determining regions of immunoglobulins. *Biopolymers* **32,** 33–43.
37. Collura, V., Higo, J., and Garnier, J. (1993) Modeling of protein loops by simulated annealing. *Protein Sci.* **2,** 1502–1510.
38. Zheng, Q., Rosenfeld, R., Vajda, S., and deLisi, C. (1993) Determining protein loop conformation using scaling-relaxation techniques. *Protein Sci.* **2,** 1242–1248.
39. Zheng, Q., Rosenfeld, R., deLisi, C., and Kyle, D. J. (1994) Multiple copy sampling in protein loop modeling: computational efficiency and sensitivity to dihedral angle perturbations. *Protein Sci.* **3,** 493–506.
40. Miranker, A. and Karplus, M. (1991) Functionality maps of binding sites: a multicopy simultaneous search method. *Proteins: Struct. Funct. Genet.* **11,** 29–34.
41. Fine, R. M., Wang, H., Shenkin, P. S., Yarmush, D. L., and Levinthal, C. (1986) Predicting antibody hypervariable loop conformations II: minimization and molecular dynamics studies of McPC603 from many randomly generated loop conformations. *Proteins: Struct. Funct. Genet.* **1,** 342–362.
42. van Gelder, C. W. G., Leusen, F. J. J., Leunissen, J. A. M., and Noordik, J. H. (1994) A molecular dynamics approach for the generation of complete protein structures from limited coordinate data. *Proteins: Struct. Funct. Genet.* **18,** 174–185.
43. Chothia, C. and Lesk, A. M. (1987) Canonical structures for the hypervariable regions of immunoglobulins. *J. Mol. Biol.* **196,** 901–917.

44. Chothia, C., Lesk, A. M., Tramontano, A., Levitt, M., Smith-Gill, S. J., Air, G., Sheriff, S., Padlan, E. A., Davies, D., Tulip, W. R., Colman, P. M., Spinelli, S., Alzari, P. M., and Poljak, R. J. (1989) Conformations of immunoglobulin hypervariable regions. *Nature* **342,** 877–883.
45. Tramontano, A., Chothia, C., and Lesk, A. M. (1989) Structural determinants of the conformations of medium-sized loops in proteins. *Proteins: Struct. Funct. Genet.* **6,** 382–394.
46. Tramontano, A., Chothia, C., and Lesk, A. M. (1990) Framework residue 71 is a major determinant of the position and conformation of the second hypervariable region in the V_H, domains of immunoglobulins. *J. Mol. Biol.* **215,** 175–182.
47. Chothia, C., Lesk, A. M., Gherardi, E., Tomlinson, I. M., Walter, G., Marks, J. D., Llewelyn, M. B., and Winter, G. (1992) Structural repertoire of the human V_H segments. *J. Mol. Biol.* **227,** 799–817.
48. Tramontano, A. and Lesk, A. M. (1992) Common features of the conformations of antigen-binding loops in immunoglobulins and application to modeling loop conformations. *Proteins: Struct. Funct. Genet.* **13,** 231–245.
49. Wu, S. and Cygler, M. (1993) Conformation of complementarity determining region L1 loop in murine IgG λ light chain extends the repertoire of canonical forms. *J. Mol. Biol.* **229,** 597–601.
50. Steipe, B., Plückthun, A., and Huber, R. (1992) Refined crystal structure of a recombinant immunoglobulin domain and a complementary-determining region 1-grafted mutant. *J. Mol. Biol.* **225,** 739–753.
51. Padlan, E. A., Sliverton, E. W., Sheriff, S., Cohen, G. H., Smith-Gill, S. J., and Davies, D. R. (1989) Structure of an antibody–antigen complex: crystal structure of the HyHEL-10 Fab-lysozyme complex. *Proc. Natl. Acad. Sci. USA* **86,** 5938–5942.
52. Epp, O., Lattman, E. E., Schiffer, M., Huber, R., and Palm, W. (1975) The molecular structure of a dimer composed of the variable portions of the Bence-Jones protein/REI refined at 2.O Å resolution. *Biochemistry* **14,** 4943–4952.
53. Jones, T. A. and Thirup, S. (1986) Using known substructures in protein model building and crystallography. *EMBO J.* **5,** 819–822.
54. Sutcliffe, M. J., Hancef, I., Camey, D., and Blundell, T. L. (1987) Knowledge-based modelling of homologous proteins, Part 1: three-dimensional frameworks derived from the simultaneous superposition of multiple structures. *Protein Eng.* **1,** 377–384.
55. Stanford, J. M. and Wu, T. T. (1981) A predictive method for determining possible three-dimensional foldings of immunoglobulin backbones around antibody combining sites. *J. Theor. Biol.* **88,** 421–439.
56. Moult, J. and James, M. N. G. (1986) An algorithm for determining the conformation of polypeptide segments in proteins by systematic search. *Proteins: Struct. Funct. Genet.* **1,** 146–163.
57. Dammkoehler, R. A, Karasek, S. F., Berkley Shands, E. F., and Marshall, G. R. (1989) Constrained search of conformational hyperspace. *J. Comput. Aided Mol. Des.* **3,** 3–21.

58. Havel, T. F., Kuntz, I. D., and Crippen, G. M. (1983) The combinatorial distance geometry method for the calculation of molecular conformations. I. A new approach to an old problem. *J. Theor. Biol.* **104,** 359–381.

59. Novotny, J., Rashin, A. A., and Bruccoleri, R. E. (1988) Criteria that discriminate between native proteins and incorrectly folded models. *Proteins: Struct. Funct. Genet.* **4,** 19–30.

60. Novotny, J., Bruccoleri, R. E., and Saul, F. (1989) On the attribution of binding energy in antigen-antibody complexes McPC603, D1.3 and HyHEL-5. *Biochemistry* **28,** 4735–4749.

61. Vila, J., Williams, R. L., Vásquez, M., and Scheraga, H. A. (1991) Empirical solvation models can be used to differentiate native from near-native conformations of bovine pancreatic trypsin inhibitor. *Proteins: Struct. Funct. Genet.* **10,** 199–218.

62. Schiffer, C. A., Caldwell, J. W., Kollman, P. A., and Stroud, R. M. (1993) Protein structure prediction with a combined solvation free energy-molecular mechanics force field. *Mol. Simulation* **102,** 121–149.

63. Smith, K. C. and Honig, B. (1994) Evaluation of the conformational free energies of loops in proteins. *Proteins: Struct. Funct. Genet.* **18,** 119–132.

64. Jackson, R.M. and Sternberg, M. J. E. (1994) Application of scaled particle theory to model the hydrophobic effect: implications for molecular association and protein stability. *Protein Eng.* **7,** 371–383.

65. Martin, A. C. R., Cheetham, J. C., and Rees, A. R. (1989) Modeling antibody hypervariable loops: a combined algorithm. *Proc. Natl. Acad. Sci. USA* **86,** 9268–9272.

66. Janin, J., Wodak, S., Levitt, M., and Maigret, B. (1978) Conformation of amino acid side-chains in proteins. *J. Mol. Biol.* **125,** 357–386.

67. Ponder, J. W. and Richards, F. M. (1987) Tertiary templates for proteins. Use of packing criteria in the enumeration of allowed sequences for different structural classes. *J. Mol. Biol.* **193,** 775–791.

68. Bhat, T. N., Sasisekheran, V., and Vijayan, M. (1979) An analysis of side-chain conformations in proteins. *Int. J. Pept. Protein Res.* **13,** 170–184.

69. Benedetti, E., Morelli, G., Nemethy, G.. and Scheraga, H. A. (1983) Statistical and energetic analysis of side-chain conformations in oligopeptides. *Int. J. Pept. Protein Res.* **22,** 1–15.

70. Tuffery, P., Etchebest, C., Hazout, S., and Lavery, R. (1991) A new approach to the rapid determination of protein sidechain conformations. *J. Biomol. Struct. Dynam.* **8,** 1267–1289.

71. Blundell, T. L., Sibanda, B. L., Sternberg, M. J. E., and Thornton, J. M. (1987) Knowledge-based prediction of protein structures and the design of novel molecules. *Nature* **326,** 347–352.

72. Summers, N. L. and Karplus, M. (1989) Construction of side-chains in homology modelling. Application to the C-terminal lobe of rhizopuspepsin. *J. Mol. Biol.* **216,** 991–1016.

73. McGregor, M. J., Islam, S. A., and Sternberg, M. J. E. (1987) Analysis of the relationship between sidechain conformation and secondary structure in globular proteins. *J. Mol. Biol.* **198,** 295–310.

74. Dunbrack, R. L. Jr. and Karplus, M. (1993) Backbone-dependent rotamer library for proteins. Application to side-chain prediction. *J. Mol. Biol.* **230,** 543–574.

75. Dunbrack, R. L. Jr. and Karplus, M. (1994) Conformational analysis of the backbone-dependent rotamer preferences of protein sidechains. *Nature: Struct. Biol.* **5,** 334–339.

76. Schrauber, H., Eisenhaber, F., and Argos, P. (1993) Rotamers: to be or not to be? An analysis of amino acid side-chain conformations in globular proteins. *J. Mol. Biol.* **230,** 592–612.

77. Reid, L. S. and Thornton, J. M. (1989) Rebuilding flavodoxin from Ca coordinates: a test study. *Proteins: Struct. Funct. Genet.* **5,** 170–182.

78. Bruccoleri, R. E. and Karplus, M. (1987) Prediction of the folding of short polypeptide segments by uniform conformational sampling. *Biopolymers* **26,** 137–168.

79. Lee, C. and Subbiah, S. (1991) Prediction of protein side-chain conformation by packing optimization. *J. Mol. Biol.* **217,** 373–388.

80. Holm, L. and Sander, C. (1992) Fast and simple Monte Carlo algorithm for side chain optimization in Proteins: Applications to model building by homology. *Proteins: Struct. Funct. Genet.* **14,** 213–223.

81. Desmet, J, DeMaeyer, M., Hazes, B., and Lasters, I. (1992) The dead-end elimination theorem and its use in protein side-chain positioning. *Nature* **356,** 539–542.

82. Lasters, I. and Desmet, J. (1993) The fuzzy-end elimination theorem: correctly implementing the side chain placement algorithm based on the dead-end elimination theorem. *Protein Eng.* **6,** 717–722.

83. Koehl, P. and Delarue, M. (1994) Application of a self-consistent mean field theory to predict protein side-chains conformation and estimate their conformational entropy. *J. Mol. Biol.* **239,** 249–275.

84. van Gelder, C. W. G., Leusen, F. J. J., Leunissen, J. A. M., and Noordik, J. H. (1994) A molecular dynamics approach for the generation of complete protein structures from limited coordinate data. *Proteins: Struct. Funct. Genet.* **18,** 174–185.

85. Jeffrey, P. D., Strong, R. K., Sieker, L. C., Chang, C. Y. Y., Campbell, R. L., Petsko, G. A., Haber, E., Margolies, M. N., and Sheriff, S. (1993) 26-10 Fab-digoxin complex: Affinity and specificity due to surface complementarity. *Proc. Natl. Acad. Sci. USA* **90,** 10,310–10,314.

86. Sheriff, S., Silverton, E. W., Padlan, E. A., Cohen, G. H., Smith-Gill, S. G., Finzel, B. C., and Davies, D. R. (1987) Three dimensional structure of an antibody–antigen complex. *Proc. Natl. Acad. Sci. USA* **84,** 8075–9079.

87. Viner, R. C. (1989) The derivation of a valence forcefield for carbohydrates. Ph.D. thesis, University of Bath, UK.

88. Dauber-Osguthorpe, P, Roberts, V. A., Osguthorpe, D. J., Wolff, J., Genest, M., and Hagler, A. T. (1988) Structure and energetics of ligand binding to proteins: *Escherichia coli* dihydrofolate reductase-trimethoprim, a drug-receptor system. *Proteins: Struct. Funct. Genet.* **4,** 31–47.

89. Gö, N. and Scheraga, H. A. (1970) Ring closure and local conformational deformations of chain molecules. *Macromolecules* **3,** 178–187.

90. Discover. A molecular dynamics program. Biosym Technologies. San Diego.
91. Rini, J. M., Schulze-Gahmen, U., Wilson, I. A. (1992) Structural evidence for induced fit as a mechanism for antibody–antigen recognition. *Science* 255, 959–965.
92. Herron, J. N., He, X. M., Ballard, D. W., Blier, P. R., Pace, P. E., Bothwell, A. L. M., Voss, E. W., and Edmundson, A. B. (1989) An auto-antibody to single stranded DNA: comparison of the three-dimensional structures of the unliganded Fab and a deoxynucleotide-Fab complex. *Proteins: Struct. Funct. Genet.* 5, 271–280.
93. Stanfield, R. L., Takimoto-Kamimura, M., Rini, J. M., Profy, A. T., and Wilson, I. A. (1993) Major antigen-induced domain rearrangements in an antibody.*Structure* 1, 83–93.
94. Brunger, A. T., Leahy, D. J, Hynes, T. R., and Fox, R. O. (1991) 2.9 Å resolution structure of an anti-dinitrophenyl-spin-label monoclonal antibody.*J. Mol. Biol.* 221, 231–256.
95. Tormo, J., Stadler, E., Skern, T., Auer, H., Kanzler, O., Betzel, C., Blaas, D., and Fita, I. (1992) 3-dimensional structure of the Fab fragment of a neutralizing antibody to human rhinovirus serotype-2.*Protein Sci.* 1, 1154–1161.
96. Brady, R. L., Edwards, D. J., Hubbard, R. E., Jiang, J.-S., Lange, G., Roberts, S. M., Todd, R. J., Adair, J. R, Emtage, J. S., King, D. J., and Low, D. C. (1992) Crystal structure of a chimeric Fab fragment of an antibody binding tumor cells. *J. Mol. Biol.* 227, 253–264.
97. He, X. M., Rueker, F., Casale, E., and Carter, D. C. (1992) Structure of a human monoclonal antibody Fab fragment against gp41 of human immunodeficiency virus type-1. *Proc. Natl. Acad. Sci. USA* 89, 7154–7158.
98. Amit, A. G, Mariuzza, R. A., Phillips, S. E. V., and Poljak, R. J. (1986) The three-dimensional structure of an antibody-antigen complex at 2.8 Å resolution.*Science* 233, 747–753.
99. Eigenbrot, C., Randal, M., Kossiakoff, A. A., and Presta, L. (1993) X-ray structures of the antigen binding domains from three variants of humanized anti-P185HER2 antibody 4DS and comparison with molecular modeling.*J. Mol. Biol.* 229, 969–995.
100. Rini, J. M., Stanfield, R. L., Stura, E. A., Salinas, P. A., Profy, A. T., and Wilson, I. A. (1993) Crystal structure of a human immunodeficiency virus type-1 neutralizing antibody, 50.1, in complex with its V3 loop peptide antigen.*Proc. Natl. Acad. Sci. USA* 90, 6325–6329.
101. Stanfield, R. L., Fieser, T. M., Lerner, R. A., and Wilson, I. A. (1990) Crystal structures of an antibody to a peptide and its complex with peptide antigen at 2.8 Å. *J. Mol. Biol.* 248, 712–719.
102. Fan, Z. C., Shan, L., Guddat, L. W., He, X. M., Gray, W. R., Raison, R. L., and Edmundson, A. (1992) 3-Dimensional structure of an F$_v$ from a human-IgM immunoglobulin. *J. Mol. Biol.* 228, 188–207.
103. Rose, D. R., Przybyska, M., To, R. J., Kayden, C. S., Oomen, R. P., Vorberg, E., Young, M. N., and Bundle, D. R. (1993) Crystal structure at 2.45 Å resolution of a monoclonal Fab specific for the Brucella-A cell wall polysaccharide moiety. *Protein Sci.* 2, 1106–1113.

104. Ely, K. R., Wood, M. K., Rajan, S. S., Hodsdon, J. M., Abola, E. E., Deutsch, H. F., and Edmundson, A. B. (1985) Unexpected similarities in the crystal-structures of the MCG light-chain dimer and its hybrid with the WEIR protein. *Mol. Immunol.* **22,** 93–100.

105. Tulip, W. R., Varghese, J. N., Laver, W. G., Webster, R. G., and Coleman, P. M. (1992) Refined crystal structure of the Influenza virus N9 neuraminidase-NC41 Fab complex. *J. Mol. Biol.* **227,** 122–148.

106. Epp, O., Lattman, E. E., Schiffer, M., Huber, R., and Palm, W. (1975) The molecular structure of a dimer composed of the variable portions of the Bence-Jones protein /REI refined at 2.0 Å resolution. *Biochemistry* **14,** 4943–4952.

107. Lascombe, M. B., Alzari, P. M., Boulot, G., Saludjian, P., Tougard, P., Berek, C., Haba, S., Rosen, E. M., Nisonoff, A., and Poljak, R. J. (1989) Three-dimensional structure of Fab R19.9, a monoclonal murine antibody specific for the p-azobenzenearsonate group. *Proc. Natl. Acad. Sci. USA* **86,** 607–611.

108. Marquart, M., Diesenhofer, J., and Huber, R. (1980) Crystallographic refinement and atomic models of the intact immunoglobulin KOL and its antigen-binding fragment at 3.0 Å and 1.9 Å resolution. *J. Mol. Biol.* **141,** 369–391.

109. Mainhart, C. R., Potter, M., and Feldmann, R. J. (1984) A refined model for the variable domains (F$_v$) of the J539 β(1,6)-D-galactan-binding immunoglobulin. *Mol. Immunol.* **21,** 469–479.

110. Segal, D., Padlan, E. A., Cohen, G., Rudikoff, S., Potter, M., and Davies, D. R. (1974) The three-dimensional structure of a phosphocholine binding mouse immunoglobulin Fab and the nature of the binding site. *Proc. Natl. Acad. Sci. USA* **71,** 4298–4302.

111. Furey, W., Jr., Wang, B. C., Yoo, C. S., and Sax, M. (1983) Structure of a novel Bence-Jones protein (rhe) fragment at 1.6 Å resolution. *J. Mol. Biol.* **167,** 661–692.

112. Padlan, E. A., Silverton, E. W., Sheriff, S., Cohen, G. H., Smith-Gill, S. J., and Davies, D. R. (1989) Structure of an antibody–antigen complex: crystal structure of the HyHEL-10 Fab-lysozyme complex. *Proc. Natl. Acad. Sci. USA* **86,** 5938–5942.

113. Ely, K. R., Herron, J. N., Harker, M., and Edmundson, A. B. (1989) Three-dimensional structure of a light chain dimer crystallized in water. Conformational flexibility of a molecule in two crystal forms. *J. Mol. Biol.* **210,** 601–615.

114. Herron, J. N., He, X. M., Mason, M. L., Voss, E. W., and Edmundson, A. B. (1989) Three-dimensional structure of a fluorescein Fab complex crystallized in 2-methyl-2,4pentanediol. *Proteins: Struct. Funct. Genet.* **5,** 271–280.

115. Rose, D. R., Strong, R. K., Margolies, M. N., Gefter, M. L., and Petsko, G. A. (1990) Crystal structure of the antigen-binding fragment of the murine antiarsonate monoclonal antibody 36-71 at 2.9 Å resolution. *Proc. Natl. Acad. Sci. USA* **87,** 338–342.

116. Saul, F. A. and Poljak, R. J. (1992) Crystal structure of human immunoglobulin fragment Fab New at 2.0 Å Resolution. *Proteins: Struct Funct Genet* **14,** 363–371.

117. Saul, F. A. and Poljak, R. J. (1992) Crystal structure of the Fab fragment from the myeloma immunoglobulin IgG HIL at 1.8 Å resolution. Preliminary structure entry deposited in the Brookhaven protein data bank. In preparation.

118. Jeffrey, P. D. (1989) The structure and specificity of immunoglobulins. Ph.D. thesis. University of Oxford, UK.
119. Kraulis, J. (1991) MOLSCRIPT: a program to produce both detailed and schematic plots of protein structures. *J. Appl. Crystall.* **24,** 946–950.
120. Laskowski, R. A., MacArthur, M. W., Moss, D. S., and Thornton, J. M. (1993) PROCHECK—A program to check the stereochemical quality of protein structures. *J. Appl. Crystall.* **26,** 283–291.

CHAPTER 3

Structure and Properties
of Human Immunoglobulin
Light-Chain Dimers

Fred J. Stevens and Marianne Schiffer

1. Introduction

Antibodies are multisubunit proteins, but unlike many other multi-subunit proteins, it is possible to study structural and functional properties of an antibody subunit free of the others. Thus, antibodies are singular proteins in that they are highly amenable to analysis by a fundamental scientific research strategy, i.e., investigation of complex systems by study of its parts. The metabolism of even a superficially simple bacterial cell cannot be understood without a rigorous understanding of the kinetic properties of each of the enzymes involved. In much the same way, the quaternary interactions of protein subunits cannot be understood except in those relatively rare cases in which the subunit and individual domain components of a complex protein can be examined individually, yielding structural and biophysical information.

The production of free antibody light (L) chains and intact immunoglobulins in multiple myeloma, a cancer of the immune system, provided chemically homogeneous proteins that were used for analysis of primary and tertiary/quaternary structure of antibodies (*see* ref. *1* for review). Prior to production of monoclonal antibodies (MAb), human proteins obtained from myeloma patients, and analogous proteins produced in mice in which plasmacytomas had been induced, provided the bulk of the data characterizing structural, functional, and genetic aspects of antibodies.

From: *Methods in Molecular Biology, Vol. 51: Antibody Engineering Protocols*
Edited by: S. Paul Humana Press Inc., Totowa, NJ

At the time of this writing, approx 30 structures of antibody antigen-binding fragments (Fabs), many of them complexed with antigen or hapten, have been described. Nevertheless, several issues remain that justify study of the L-chain component. The most fundamental perhaps is the concept that it is constructive to think of an antibody not as a protein, but rather as a collaboration of two separate proteins, heavy (H) chain and L chain, that have evolved to work together. The separate identity of these two proteins is consistent with the observation that the L chain and the H chain are genetically encoded on separate chromosomes, and that the L chain and the H chain are in fact consortia of related proteins that are shuffled as essentially interchangeable modules in the generation of a diverse immune system. The structures of the interfaces involved in L-chain and H-chain interactions are highly conserved in order to achieve this intercompatibility, but this conservation is not absolute. Variations between germ-line genes occur, and further variations may be acquired by somatic mutation during the maturation of an immune response. Interspecies differences are also found. Since amino acid side chains in the complementarity determining regions (CDRs) can also influence domain interactions, transferring murine CDRs to a human L- and H-chain framework is not always sufficient to transfer specificity, an important issue for the "humanization" of mouse MAb.

The intact L chain consists of two domains, termed variable (V) and constant (C), which are both β-sandwich structures that exhibit some differences in the arrangement of their β-strands. As such, the structure of the L chain encompasses both structural strategies found throughout the immunoglobulin superfamily, which includes antibodies, T-cell receptors, MHC proteins, HLA, numerous cell-surface receptors, cell-adhesion molecules, and others. Many of the amino acids involved in domain–domain interactions in the formation of Fabs contribute to the formation of the L-chain dimer, which closely resembles an Fab. As a consequence, detailed understanding of the structural and functional similarities and differences found in Fabs and L-chain dimers will provide important information by which to understand and anticipate the interaction properties of the broad array of superfamily members.

Although the study of L chains contributes to understanding the structural basis of the functional properties of antibodies and their cousins, it is becoming increasingly valuable to study L chains irrespective of their immunological relevance. Free L chains are produced in large quantities during various plasma cell dyscrasias, and it is important to study the structure and functional properties of these proteins in order to understand the basis of the pathological aggregation and tissue deposition that occurs in approximately half of these patients *(2–7)*. In some cases, L-chain proteins form casts in tubules of the nephron; in other cases, punctate deposits are found on basement membranes in a condition termed L-chain deposition disease. One of the most striking aggregation processes is the formation of amyloid fibrils. By a mechanism that is not understood, some L chains spontaneously form noncovalently combined assemblies that are highly regular in structure and extremely stable. Formation and deposition of these fibrils are regarded as irreversible and are not treatable. In some patients, fibrils accumulate in specific organs, such as the kidney, heart, or liver. In others, amyloid deposition is systemic, and fibrils are found in tissues throughout the body.

2. Crystallographic Studies of Bence Jones Proteins

The three-dimensional structures of more than 40 immunoglobulin L chains have been determined to date; for a detailed review, *see (8)*. The majority of the L-chain proteins have been characterized in conjunction with H chain as Fabs produced from murine MAb. A dozen human L chains have been described in varying degrees of detail. L-chains **New, Kol**, and **Dob** were determined in conjunction with H chains in crystallographic studies of Fabs or intact IgGs. The structure of protein **Pot** was determined in an Fv obtained from a myeloma IgM *(9)*. Table 1 summarizes results of published crystallographic analyses of free human L chains. As will be discussed below, the protein products of most of the genes that code for human L chains have not been crystallographically analyzed.

2.1. λ L Chains

Protein **Mcg** was an amyloid-forming λII protein and was the first Bence Jones protein for which a crystallographic structure was determined *(19)*. Together with the contemporaneous conformations of Fabs **New** *(20)* and **McPC603** *(21)*, these early conformations provided insight into the structural basis of antibody function. The important features revealed by these structures confirmed the hypothesis of Wu and Kabat *(22)* that the hypervariable segments of the L- and H-chain-variable domains were spatially contiguous in the folded protein, although dispersed in the primary structure. These structures also validated the proposal, based on sequence analysis, that the L chain and H chain were

Table 1
Crystallographic Studies of Human L Chains

Subgroup	Protein	Medium	Space group	Res.	R-factor, %	Ref.
λ1	Loc VC	H_2O	$P2_12_12_1$	2.4	16	(10)
		$(NH_4)_2SO_4$	$P2_12_12_1$	2.3	17	(11)
		$NaKSO_4$	$P2_12_12_1$	2.2	16	Schiffer et al.[b]
	Rhe V	$(NH_4)_2SO_4$	$P2_12_12_1$	1.6	15	(12)
λ2	Mcg VC	$(NH_4)_2SO_4$	$P3_121$	2.3	14	(13)
	Mcg VC	H_2O	$P2_12_12_1$	2.3	21	(14)
	Weir VC[a]	$(NH_4)_2SO_4$	$P3_121$	3.5	22	(15)
λ3						
λ4						
λ6						
λ8						
κ1	Au V	$(NH_4)_2SO_4$	$P6_122$	2.5	31	(16)
	Rei V	$(NH_4)_2SO_4$	$P6_1$	2.0	24	(17)
	Roy V	$(NH_4)_2SO_4$	$P6_122$	3.0	33	(18)
	Wat V	$(NH_4)_2SO_4$	$P6_4$	1.9	15	(25a)
κ2						
κ3						
κ4	Len V	$(NH_4)_2SO_4$	$C222_1$	1.8	24	Chang et al.[b]

[a]As a heterodimer with Mcg.
[b]Unpublished results.

each organized as two independently folded domains. In addition to confirming hypotheses derived from the amino acid sequences of human myeloma and mouse plasmacytoma proteins, the crystallographic structures also revealed what has become known as the "immunoglobulin fold," the β-barrel or β-sandwich, which typified both the variable and constant domains of both L and H chain. Both types of domains were generally similar, but differed in their detailed arrangement of β-strands. Additionally, the interfaces used in V–V domain interactions were opposite those found in C–C interactions, a relationship described as "rotational allomerism" (23). The principal observations obtained from these original crystallographic investigations have not been contradicted.

Subsequently, the structure of the **Mcg** L chain was determined in the myeloma IgG and in a heterodimer formed with another λII protein, **Weir**, allowing an evaluation of the influence of quaternary interactions on tertiary structure. In addition, crystals of **Mcg** were obtained from both water and ammonium sulfate solvents (14). Interestingly, modest rearrangements of the variable domain relationships were observed in the two-solvent systems. However, the significance of this observation was not immediately apparent. The issue of whether the crystallization conditions or the crystal lattice itself substantially alters the structure of the molecule relative to that found in dilute solution was addressed by neutron-scattering studies *(24)*. The radius of gyration measured by neutron scattering was consistent with that calculated from the **Mcg** atomic coordinates determined by X-ray crystallography, suggesting that no major rearrangement or alteration of relative positions of variable domains had taken place as a result of crystallizing this flexible protein.

The second λ L chain to be crystallographically analyzed was the λI protein **Rhe,** for which crystals of the variable domain were obtained *(12)*. In contrast to the similarity of the V_L–V_L interaction in **Mcg** compared to the reference Fab, **New,** the quaternary interactions of **Rhe** V_Ls were completely different. Although **Rhe** is a dimer, it differs significantly from the "normal" **Rei** or **Mcg** structure. When one of the domains is superimposed on another, to juxtapose the remaining domains requires a 61° rotation and a 19-Åtranslation. The interactions between the domains are dominated by interactions between aromatic and Pro residues. Residues Phe98, Pro96, and Trp91 from one monomer interact with Tyr49, Tyr50, and Pro55 of the other monomer. The unusual substitutions at positions 50 and 96 in combination with the Trp at 91 might promote this novel dimer pair.

The domain–domain interaction in **Rhe** is further strengthened by a local conformation change in a 15-residue loop of FR2 (37–51) in such a manner that they now can form hydrogen bonds with each other at the dimer interface. It is very clear that the binding site formed by **Rhe** complementarity determing segments could not be formed by simply replacing residues in the CDRs.

It is perhaps fair to assert that the unique **Rhe** structure was thought of as a laboratory novelty, but not likely to be of immunochemical significance, because similar quaternary relationships were not to be expected in Fabs. Yet, in another sense, protein **Rhe** may represent one of the more immunochemically significant L chains. The fact that the structural basis of the **Rhe** conformation has not been explained to date reveals our lack of complete understanding of antibody domain interactions. Although we can easily tabulate the frequently observed amino acids involved in interdomain contacts of V_L–V_L and V_L–V_H assemblies, we

Table 2
Comparative Crystallographic Data for Protein **Loc** in Three Crystal Forms

Form	Unit cell dimensions, Å			Space group	% Protein	Res, Å	R-factor, %
Loc W	118.9	73.6	49.8	$P2_12_12_1$	0.52	2.4	16.3
Loc NaKS	83.9	72.6	63.6	$P2_12_12_1$	0.58	2.2	17.2
Loc AS	149.3	72.4	46.5	$P2_12_12_1$	0.45	2.3	16.2

are still unable to predict with confidence the consequences of alterations of the amino acids involved in the interactions. Some of these amino acids are found in the CDR segments that vary significantly from protein to protein. A definitive explanation of the quaternary interactions in protein **Rhe** would represent a significant development in our understanding of the structural basis of immunoglobulin domain interactions and would have importance for biotechnological and pharmaceutical applications.

The third λ protein to be crystallographically analyzed was the cast-forming λI protein **Loc**. The structure of this protein was initially determined from crystals obtained from ammonium sulfate solution (**Loc AS**) *(10)*. The nature of the conformation obtained was not anticipated and led to analyses of two additional crystal forms obtained under different solvent compositions (Table 2). In contrast to the classical antigen-binding "pocket" formed by the variable domains in the **Mcg** protein and other immunogobulins, the variable domain association in **Loc AS** resulted in a central protusion in the binding site, with grooves on two sides of the protrusion. Subsequently, the structure was determined in a second crystal form grown from distilled water (**Loc W**). This form has an antigen-binding pocket similar to that found in the **Mcg** protein and free antigen-binding fragment structures *(11)*. Structures have been refined in two crystal forms: the R-factor is 16.3% for 2.4-Å data for **Loc W** and 16.2% for 2.3-Å data for **Loc AS**.

A third crystal form has been determined with a current R-factor of 17.2% with 2.2-Å data (unpublished results). The third crystalline form of protein **Loc** was obtained from a sodium potassium sulfate medium (**Loc NaKS**) at pH 8. The structure of **Loc NaKS** also differed from the structures of **Loc AS** and **Loc W** by an altered arrangement of the variable domains. The relative domain positions in **Loc NaKS** were intermediate between the almost canonical orientation present in **Loc W** and the large-scale shift in domain positions in **Loc AS**. **Loc** protein has a His residue at position 38, which is usually occupied by a Gln. Because the pK_a of the His side chain is approx 6.5, the interdomain hydrogen-bonding pattern between **Loc** domains is more susceptible to variations in pH than other L chains. A Trp residue at position 91 probably contributes to a domain arrangement that depends on ionic strength. The Trp residues from the two domains interact in the high-salt crystal forms. These substitutions, although uncommon, are not unique to the **Loc** protein, suggesting that: (1) the functional properties of some naturally occurring antibodies might be determined (or be determinable) by pH and ionic-strength modulation of L-chain- and H-chain-variable domain interactions, and (2) introduction of appropriate amino acids to the interfaces of L-chain- and H-chain-variable domains may provide a means to influence antibody diversity and self-association affinities for biotechnological applications.

2.2. κ L Chains

To date, structural analyses of human κ L chains have been restricted to crystals of V_L domains. Although preliminary crystallographic data from one intact κII protein were reported *(25)*, the quality of these crystals has not been satisfactory for collecting the data required to solve the structure.

Protein **Rei** was crystallized as a V_L dimer and its structure determined to high resolution *(17)*. No clinical information concerning the pathological properties of protein **Rei** is available. Because of the high quality of the crystallographic data obtained for this Bence Jones protein, a detailed description of the network of hydrogen bonds between backbone atoms, between backbone and side chain, and between side chains of different amino acids was possible. The tertiary and quaternary structures of protein **Rei** were very similar to those observed in **Mcg** and Fabs **New** and **Kol**. Similar structures were observed in two other κI proteins, **Au** and **Roy**. The **Au** and **Roy** models were not refined, and information concerning detailed arrangements of the side chains in these proteins is not available. The conformation of **Rei** has served as a prototype V_L domain, and has been used as the starting point of several modeling studies to predict structures of antibodies and other molecules in the immunoglobulin superfamily.

The structure of cast-forming κI protein **Wat** was recently completed. Protein **Wat** is the second human κI protein conformationally character-

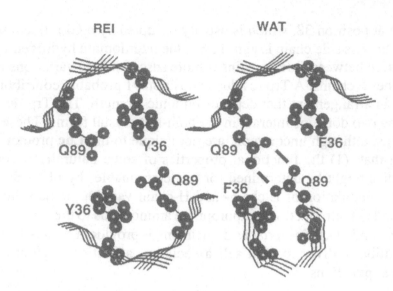

Fig. 1. Comparison of κI proteins **Rei** and **Wat** interface structures, illustrating the amino acids thought to account for different domain interactions. In **Wat,** the highly conserved Tyr36 is replaced by Phe, resulting in altered hydrogen-bonding capabilities; a rotation and translation of one domain brings two Gln89 side chains into position to form a double hydrogen bond. In the figure, domains in the upper portion of the diagram are positioned in the same orientation. Comparison of the ribbon backbone segments in the lower portion clearly indicates differences in the monomer orientations in the two proteins.

ized at high resolution, and the determination of its three-dimensional structure enabled a detailed comparison *(25)* with that of protein **Rei** *(17)*. The peptide backbones of proteins **Wat** and **Rei** were virtually identical to each other and are consistent with the V_L domain structure seen in other antibodies. However, the arrangement of the domains in **Wat** differs from that seen in **Rei**. When reference domains of **Wat** and **Rei** are superimposed, both an 11.8° rotation and a 1.3-Å translation of the second domain of **Wat** are required to align it with the corresponding domain of **Rei**.

The principal reason for this variation is believed to be a substitution at position 36, located in the center of the domain–domain interface (Fig. 1). At this position, **Wat** has a Phe residue in contrast to the Tyr found in **Rei** and most L-chain monomers. In effect, this removes a single oxygen atom from the interfacial surface of each monomer and removes the hydrogen-bonding capability contributed by Tyr. This loss of hydrogen bonding is compensated for by the observed shift in relative domain positions, which brings two Glu residues located at position 89 into orientations that permit the formation of a double hydrogen bond across the domain interface. Although it is highly likely that the Tyr ⇒ Phe substitution is the "trigger" that generates the altered domain arrangement, a second substitution, Tyr ⇒ Leu at position 96, appears to be a prerequisite for the domain shift. Modeling analysis indicates that insufficient space is available for the bulkier Tyr side chain in the arrangement found in the **Wat** dimer. Fortuitously, Leu96 was present in protein **Roy**, for which crystallographic analysis demonstrated a "standard" domain relationship *(18)*. Therefore, Leu96 may be necessary, but is not sufficient, to engender the domain arrangement observed in protein **Wat**. This illustrates that domain–domain interactions, like other protein–protein interactions, involve the cooperative contributions of several amino acids located on the surfaces involved. To understand these interactions, especially in considering the differences in properties of naturally occurring human L chains (which all differ at numerous sites), requires consideration of the consequences of multiple differences.

The two cast-forming proteins that have been crystallographically characterized, **Wat** and **Loc**, both show unusual domain interactions. However, it is not yet clear if this observation is of direct importance for understanding cast formation. Although only a limited number of cast-forming L chains have been sequenced, a cast-forming λIII protein, **Cle**, has a standard set of amino acids at the domain interface; crystallographic analysis of protein **Cle** is under way in this laboratory. Of more significance is that protein **Wat**, like proteins **Loc** and the amyloid-associated λII protein **Mcg**, has a domain structure that is superimposible on the V_L domain of **Rei**. Thus, if the structures observed in crystals are pertinent to the form of the protein undergoing pathology-related aggregation and deposition, then these phenomena are not dependent on amino acid substitutions that generate large-scale conformational perturbations.

The κIV protein **Len** is the first crystallographically analyzed Bence Jones protein whose "benign" nature is well established. This protein was produced by the patient at levels of 50 g/d without apparent clinical consequences. Protein **Len** is also the first representative of the κIV subgroup to have been crystallographically characterized. This protein is notable among Bence Jones proteins in that it differs from the sequence encoded by the germ-line gene by only one amino acid substitution, Asn ⇒ Ser at position 29. Although the refinement of the **Len** conformation is still under way, the domain structure of the κIV protein is effectively identical to that found for κI structures, with the exception of the existence of the extended CDR1 loop that characterizes κIV and κII L chains.

2.3. Unanswered Structural Questions

Thirteen germ-line genes have been identified that encode the four human κ L-chain subgroups. Of these genes, one accounts for the κIV subgroup, and two and three more for subgroups κIII and κII, respectively. The remaining seven genes generate the proteins categorized as κI. A similar pattern is present for the λ proteins. Although the λ germ-line genes are less completely characterized, between 20 and 30 functional germ-line genes seem to encompass the inherited human λ L-chain repertoire. The existence of this genome data enables an evaluation of the completeness of our understanding of L-chain conformational properties and should provide guidance by which future structural work can address possible signficance of specific germ-line substitutions. The κ germline-encoded amino acid sequences of 13 genes for which corresponding functional L chains have been identified are summarized in Table 3. Note that the gk** identifiers are not the original terminology of Klein et al. *(26)*, but have been assigned for the purposes of this chapter to indicate correspondence to the standard κ subgroups. Also, note that although the alignment of these sequences essentially follows that of Wu and Kabat *(22)*, the insert in CDR1 has been placed to start at position 27c rather than 27a. This two-residue shift is suggested by the structure of the κIV protein **Len**, the first human L chain with an extended CDR1 to be crystallographically analyzed.

The κV exon encompasses 101 positions, including the six amino acid insert in CDR1. Of these, 38 sites are invariant throughout the κ gene repertoire. As summarized in Table 4, it is possible, based on the structures of **Rei** and **Wat**, to propose reasonable rationales for the contribution of the particular conserved side chain to the conformation and stability of the variable domain. An interesting exception is position 27, at which a Gln is present in all κ germ-line genes. In both **Rei** and **Wat**, the Gln side chain is apparently extended into the solvent, and it is difficult to perceive any interaction with other atoms in the domain. The Gln

Table 3
Aligned Human κ Germ-line Gene-Encoded Amino Acid Sequences

```
       01_         11_         21_         27d         35_
gkla:  DIQMTQSPST  LSASVGDRVT  ITCRASQSI.  .....SSWLA  WYQQKPGKAP
gklb:      S                   Q   D            NY N
gklc:      S                                    Y  N
gkld:      S                       G            RND G
gkle:      S                       G            NY      F
gklf:  A L S                       G            A
gklg:      S V                     G
gk2a:    V   T LS  PVTP EPAS   S S SLL    DSDDGNTY D  L    QS
gk2b:    V     LS  PVTP EPAS   S S SLL    HS NGYNY D  L    QS
gk2c:    V   T LS  VTP QPAS    S KS SLL   HS DGKTY Y  L    QP
gk3a:  E V     A     V P E A   LS   SV       DNV          Q
gk3b:  E VL    G     L P E A   LS   SV       S  Y         Q
gk4 :    V    DS   AV L E A    N KS SVL   YSSNNKNY        QP

       45_         55_         65_         75_         85_         95_
gkla:  KLLIYKASSL  ESGVPSRFSG  SGSGTEFTLT  ISSLQPDDFA  TYYCQQYNSY  S
gklb:         D N     T             D F         E I           DNL  P
gklc:         A       Q             D           E           SY T   P
gkld:  R       A      Q             D           E         L H      P
gkle:  S       A      Q             D           E                  P
gklf:          D                    D           E           F N    P
gklg:          A      Q             D           E           A F P
gk2a:  Q     TL YR A     D          D K     RVEAE VG V  M RIEF P
gk2b:  Q     LG NR A     D          D K     RVEAE VG V  M ALQT P
gk2c:  Q     EV NR F     D          D K     RVEAE VG V  M SIQL P
gk3a:  R      G TR AT I A                   SE    V      NW P
gk3b:  R      G R  AT I D           D       R E E V      G S P
gk4 :        W TR       D           D       AE V  V      Y T P
```

Sequence data from Klein et al. *(26)*. From top to bottom, sequences are L12a, 018-08, 012-02, A30, L1, L18, L5, 011-01, A19-A3, A2,L12-L16, A27, and B3.

side chain is not positioned to interact with a V_H in an Fab. Of 74 V_L sequences obtained from Bence Jones proteins or myeloma Igs, 69 contain Gln at position 27. In three of the five variants, Leu is present. Three L chains, κI protein **Ise** *(27)* and κIV protein **Blu**, were all associated with L-chain deposition disease *(28)*; κI protein **And** formed amyloid *(29)*. The fifth variant, protein **Ree**, had a Glu for Gln substitution. No clinical information about this protein is available. The relationship, if any, between particular amino acid substitutions and L-chain pathologies has not yet been established.

Table 4
Conserved Residues in Human K
Germ-line Genes and Possible Origins of Selection

Pos.	Res.	Apparent role	Contacts	Rei	Wat	Len
2	Ile	Packing				
5	Thr	Hydrogen bond	(Gln 3)			
6	Gln	Hydrogen bond	(Thr 102); 88-N,O;101-N			
8	Pro	Turn				
16	Gly	Turn				
23	Cys	Disulfide	Cys-88			
26	Ser	Hydrogen bond	3-N,O			
27	Gln	None obvious				
35	Trp	Internal H$_2$O				
		Packing	Ile 48; (Leu 73); (Ile 21)			
38	Gln	Hydrogen bond	42-O			
		Interface	Gln-38			
39	Lys	Hydrogen bond	81-O;83-O	Thr	Arg	
40	Pro	Turn				
41	Gly	Turn				
44	Pro	Turn				
47	Leu	Packing	Ile 48; Tyr 86			
48	Ile	Packing	Leu 47;Tyr 86;Trp 35;(Leu 54)			
49	Tyr	Interface	(Leu 94)			
52	Ser	Hydro. bond, turn	50-O			
57	Gly	Packing				
59	Pro	Turn				
61	Arg	Salt bridge	Asp 82			
62	Phe	Packing	(Val 58); (Leu 73); Ile 75			
63	Ser	Hydrogen bond	74-O			
64	Gly	Packing				
65	Ser	Hydrogen bond	72-O			
66	Gly	Packing				
67	Ser	Hydrogen bond	30-O			
68	Gly	Turn				
69	Thr	Hydrogen bond	25-O			
71	Phe	Packing		Tyr		
72	Thr	None obvious				
75	Ile	Packing	Phe 62; (Leu 73); Tyr 86			
76	Ser	Hydrogen bond	61-O			
82	Asp	Salt bridge	Arg 61			
86	Tyr	Hydrogen bond	(Gln 37); 82-O			
87	Tyr	Packing	Ile 75; (Leu 73); (Ile 21)			
88	Cys	Disulfide	Cys-23			
90	Gln	Hydrogen bond	(Asp 1);92-N;93-N;95-O			

N: backbone nitrogen; O: backbone oxygen; contacts identified in parentheses are residues found at positions of restricted variability; amino acid variations found in **Rei, Wat,** and **Len** are listed.

Table 5 lists sites where variation is observed. A number of these variations are conserved within subgroups; the residue found most frequently in the κI germ-line genes is identified. In several of these instances, subgroup-associated compensatory substitutions can be identified. For instance, the κI germ-line genes all encode Ala at position 13 and Val at position 19. In all of the non-κI genes, the side chains are reversed. These two side chains are involved in internal packing of the domain and are in contact with each other. Therefore, in all of the κ chains, the internal packing at this position is effectively equivalent, although the atoms occupying equivalent sites are connected to different α carbons. Another example involves positions 75 and 77, which span a β-turn. In the κI, κIIIa, and κIV genes, these two positions are stabilized by hydrogen bonding between a Ser and a Gln. In κII and κIIIb, a salt bridge involving an Arg and a Glu at these sites accomplishes the same task.

The rationalization of other subgroup-associated substitutions is less clear. In the κI subgroup, a Gln at position 3 forms an external hydrogen bond with Thr at position 5. In the other κ chains, position 3 is replaced by a Val, nominally leaving the hydrogen-bonding capacity of position 5 unsatisfied. Position 42 is the positively charged residue Lys in all κI, but is the neutral Gln in all other κ genes, whereas a Leu residue at position 54 in the κI set is replaced by an Arg. The appearance of Arg at position 54 is most often accompanied by a negatively charged Asp at nearby position 60, providing the possibility of an external salt bridge and maintaining charge balance. In contrast, the side chain at position 42 extends into the solvent and does not appear to interact with any other side chain in the V_L.

It is possible that rationalization of the conservation of either Lys or Gln at position 42 may be found in unapparent interaction with the C domain. In other cases, the lack of obvious structurally correlated substitutions might reflect a need to examine some combination of three or more replacements to rationalize the substitutions. To the extent that the amino acid interchanges listed in Table 4 reflect different evolutionary solutions that relate alternative primary structures to the same tertiary structure, it should be possible to find the "rules" that explain the particular substitutions. In some cases, no specific structural role may be obvious from the crystal structure, possibly reflecting an important contribution to the folding pathway or stability *(30)*.

Table 5
Positions of Restricted Variability in Human K Germ-line Genes

Pos.	Res.	Apparent role	Contacts	Rei	Wat	Len
1	Asp	None obvious				
3	**Gln**	Hydrogen bond	Thr 5			Val
4	Met	Packing				
7	Ser	Hydrogen bond	(Arg 24)			
9	**Ser**	None obvious				Asp
10	Ser	Hydrogen bond	(Gln 105)			
11	Leu	Packing	(Val 19); (Ala 13)			
12	**Ser**	Hydrogen bond	(Lys 107)			Ala
13	**Ala**	Packing	(Val 19); (Leu 11)			Val
14	Ser	Hydrogen bond	(Lys 107)			
15	**Val**	None obvious				Leu
17	Asp	Hydrogen bond	14-N			Glu
18	**Arg**	Hydrogen bond	76-O			
19	**Val**	Packing	(Leu 11); (Ala 13)			Ala
20	Thr	Hydrogen bond	(Thr 74)			
21	Ile	Packing	Trp 35			
22	Thr	Hydrogen bond	7-O			Asn
24	Arg	Hydrogen bond	5-O; (Ser 77)	Gln		Lys
		Salt bridge	(Asp 70)			
25	**Ala**	Packing	((Ile29))			Ser
27b	Ile	Packing	Phe 71			Val
33	Leu	Packing	((Ile29)); Phe 71		Val	
36	Tyr	Interface			Phe	

(continued)

Table 6 summarizes the sites that can be considered truly variable. Although positions 27c and 27d are actually invariant among the germ-line genes where these positions are occupied, they are included in this list to indicate the variations in length that occur between positions 27b and 30. Most of the variable positions are in loops and constitute CDRs of the L chain. The segments identified as hypervariable or complementarity-determining are 24–34, 50–56, and 89–97. Of the positions identified in Table 6, only position 46 is not conventionally considered to be complementarity determining. However, position 46 is located at the base of the binding site, and its side chain is accessible to solvent. The three residues encoded in the germ-line provide one hydrophobic, one ionic, and one hydrogen-bonding partner at this site.

Table 5 *(continued)*

Pos.	Res.	Apparent role	Contacts	Rei	Wat	Len
37	**Gln**	Hydrogen bond	Tyr 86; (Lys 45)			
42	**Lys**	None obvious			Gln	
43	**Ala**	None obvious				Pro
45	**Lys**	Hydrogen bond	(Gln 37)			
51	**Ala**	Turn				
54	**Leu**	None obvious				Arg
56	Ser	None obvious		Ala	Thr	
58	Val	Packing	Phe 62			
60	**Ser**	None obvious				Asp
70	Asp	Salt bridge	(Arg 24)			
73	Leu	Packing	Phe 62; Tyr 86	Phe	Phe	
74	**Thr**	None obvious				
77	Ser	Hydrogen bond	(Gln 79)			
78	Leu	Packing	Ile 75; (Leu 104); (Ala 13); (Ile 106)			
79	**Gln**	Hydrogen bond	Arg 61; Glu 81			
80	**Pro**	Turn				Ala
81	Glu	Salt bridge	Arg 61			
83	Phe	Packing	(Ile 106)	Ile	Ile	Val
84	Ala	None obvious				
85	**Thr**	None obvious				Val
89	**Gln**	Hydrogen bond	(Tyr 36')			
95	Pro	Turn				

Residues identified in bold indicate positions where chemically distinctive side chains are found in different germ-line-encoded proteins; double parentheses indicate high variability contacts.

As indicated in Tables 4 and 5, several positions within the hypervariable segments are invariant at the germ-line level or are conserved within subgroups. For instance, positions 26, 27, 52, and 90 are invariant. As noted above, position 54 is Leu in all κI and Arg in the other germ-line genes. If one considers position 46 to be a noncontiguous element of CDR2, then of the 39 CDR segments encoded by the germ-line genes, only one example of duplication of CDR segments is found. CDR2 of gk1c is identical to that in the rarely observed gk1g. It is therefore likely that the primary selective pressure directing the evolution of the variable domain genes is, as might be expected, is the generation of CDR diversity. Variations in the framework segments may reflect genetic drift, generating structurally equivalent β-domain structures rather than sub-

Table 6
Positions of Most Variability
Among K Germ-line Genes

Pos.	Res.
27a	Asp, Gly, Ser
27c	Leu[a]
27d	Asp, His, Tyr
27e	Ser[a]
27f	Asp, Ser
28	Asn, Asp, Gly, Ser
29	Asn, Gly, Ile, Ser
30	Arg, Asn, Lys, Ser,Tyr
31	Asn, Asp, Ser, Thr
32	Ala, Asn, Asp, Trp, Tyr
34	Ala, Asn, Asp, Gly, Tyr
46	Arg, Leu, Ser
50	Asp, Glu, Gly, Leu, Lys, Thr, Trp
53	Asn, Ser, Tyr, Thr
55	Ala, Gln, Glu, Phe
91	Ala, Arg, His, Phe, Ser, Tyr
92	Asn, Asp, Gly, Ile, Leu, Tyr
93	Asn, Gln, Glu, Ser
94	Leu, Phe, Ser, Thr, Trp ,Tyr

[a]Positions 27c and 27e are included in this listing to reflect their presence in the CDR1 insert present in some but not all κ chains.

group-specific immunological roles. More detailed scrutiny of these structures and implications of observed variations will be needed. A thorough understanding of the structural implications of conserved and varied portions of κ, λ, and H-chain-variable domains will provide a solid foundation for homology modeling of other members of the immunoglobulin superfamily, as well as protein engineering to optimize technological application of antibodies.

According to the analysis of Klein et al. *(26)*, both proteins **Wat** and **Rei** appear to be descendants of the same germ-line gene (gk2b). Thus, only 2 of the 13 κ genes have been directly studied crystallographically. However, examination of the germ-line sequences in Table 3 suggests that the κIV protein **Len** might be considered a structural prototype of the κII subset. Similarly, most of the framework of the two κIII genes is also similar to κIV. The most striking difference between κIII and κIV is found in CDR1, in which the length of the κIII segment more closely corresponds to that of κI. Therefore, the three existing well-refined κ structures may provide a reasonably complete sampling of human κ V_L structures, although little information is available regarding κ C_L conformation.

In contrast, two λ subgroups are distinguished by structural features that may be important immunologically or clinically. The λVI subgroup is rarely observed and is thought to be encoded by a single (or possibly two) germ-line genes *(31)*. In all cases for which clinical data are available for λVI proteins, the L chain is associated with the formation of amyloid fibrils. No other L-chain subgroup is so invariantly associated with a single clinical consequence of its overproduction. Although λVI proteins have several unusual amino acid substitutions when compared to other λ proteins, the most striking feature is a two amino acid insert following position 66. This insert would be expected to extend a loop that abuts the CDR segments of the domain. Because the composition of positions 66–66b varies among λVI proteins, it is tempting to consider this loop to be a fourth CDR segment that is unique to this rare subgroup. The probable immunological significance of this insert is supported by the recent description of a homologous L chain in the repertoire of the mouse *(32)*. The recently described human λVIII subgroup *(33)* is notable for a six-residue extension of CDR2. This insert is particularly intriguing because of the general low degree of variability in L-chain CDR2, which had suggested that this loop contributed relatively little to the generation of antibody diversity. The identification of the λVIII subgroup suggests that there may be a particular antigenic niche for which an extended CDR2 contributes to the mechanism of complementarity. No crystallographic structure of either λVI or λVIII proteins is currently available, and therefore the conformational alterations imposed by the subgroup-associated inserts remain unknown. However, the strategy used to address this issue is likely to be different than that previously used to obtain structural data characterizing human L chains. The most effective route to characterizing specific subgroup features may be to synthesize the complete genes coding for these proteins and to use bacterial expression methods to provide the L chains for crystallographic analysis. In other cases, it may be useful simply to modify genes to incorporate the subgroup feature into another L chain for which crystallization methods have already been developed.

3. Self-Association Properties of Bence Jones Proteins

3.1. L-Chain Dimerization

The natural function of an antibody L chain is to interact with an antibody H chain; together they generate the functional antigen-binding site. Because of the conformational homology of V_H and V_L, many of the interactions involved in V_H-V_L association to form an Fab can be emulated in a self-association interaction. For instance, the V_H-V_L contact between Gln 39(H) and Gln38 (L) is replicated by Gln 38–Gln 38 juxtaposition in V_L dimers. Thus, dimerization of V_L is a functional echo of the formation of an Fab. As a consequence, differences in self-association properties of different antibody L chains are likely to correlate with differences in interaction with V_H.

The dimerization of antibody L chains was initally described by Edelman and Gally *(34)*, Green *(35)*, and Azuma et al. *(36)*. Maeda and coworkers *(37)* took advantage of the Trp residue at position 32 in Bence Jones protein **Au** to use quenching of fluorescence on dimer formation to determine affinity constants for V_L self-association. For V_L dimerization, they reported a dimerization constant of $10^5 M^{-1}$. Independent kinetic measurements indicated an on-rate of $9 \times 10^6 M^{-1}/s$ and an off-rate of $1.5 \times 10^2/s$. In a subsequent study of the interaction properties of the complete L chain, a slightly smaller estimate of equilibrium constant was obtained, indicating that the C_L domain does not contribute to the free energy of interaction between L chains.

Stevens et al. *(38)* used size-exclusion chromatography to compare interaction properties of several κI Bence Jones proteins. Dimerization affinities ranged from $<10^4 M^{-1}$ to $>10^6 M^{-1}$, as reflected by elution positions of the monomer component between that expected for dimer and for monomer based on molecular weight. In a limited number of cases, higher-order aggregation of L chains to form complexes larger than dimer was observed. The variability of dimerization properties was attributed to position 96 in CDR3, and it was suggested that a hydrophobic residue at this position increases dimerization, whereas the presence of a charged group had the opposite effect. The suggestion that position 96 was able to influence dimerization of L chains and, presumably, interactions between L chain and H chain was of particular interest in that: (1) it was the first suggestion that a complementarity determining amino acid substitution might influence domain interactions, and (2) position 96 is the junction between the V domain exon and the J segment. Because the joining of these gene segments can occur at any base within the codon, position 96 is the most variable position in the L chain.

The observation that amino acids in the CDRs influence dimerization suggested that pairs of L chains may exist for which the affinity of heterologous association might exceed that of homologous association. One example of an apparent preferential heterologous association was found with the κI proteins **Kin** and **Und** *(39)*. Although the primary structures of both proteins have been determined (Solomon, personal communication), the origin of the preferential heterologous association is still not readily apparent. Other CDR positions also influence dimerization and, by implication, V_L-V_H interactions. Kolmar et al. *(40)* constructed a gene to produce a recombinant form of the L-chain **Rei** and demonstrated an increased affinity of dimerization of approximately one order of magnitude by replacing Leu at position 94 with an His. The increase in affinity is thought to result from formation of a hydrogen bond between His and the Gln side chain at position 54, another CDR position.

Although V_L-V_L interactions are comparable to those found in V_H-V_L, the C_L domains behave differently. As indicated above, there is little or no affinity of interaction between C_Ls. In contrast, C_L-C_H interactions contribute approximately half of the free energy of interaction between L and H chain in an intact Fab, the affinity of which has been estimated at $10^{12}M^{-1}$ *(41)*. In contrast to V_H-V_L interactions, which are mediated by hydrogen bonds and van der Waals contacts, C_L-C_H docking also incorporates two salt bridges that provide significant free energy *(42)*. In noncovalent dimers of L chains, it is unlikely that the two C_L domains have a well-defined quaternary arrangement.

3.2. High-Order L-Chain Aggregation

The original description of what was to become known as a Bence Jones protein was based on the observation of a precipitate formed in urine that was heated to about 55°C; the precipitate dissolved as the temperature of the solution approached the boiling point *(43)*. The demonstration by Edelman and Gally *(34)* of the equivalence of Bence Jones proteins and antibody L chains was a seminal event in the study of immunology. Neet and Putnam *(44)* used sedimentation techniques to demonstrate that elevated temperatures induced L chains to form large aggregates. In at least one case, sedimentation values corresponded to aggregates of molecular weight in excess of 10^6. Analogously to the precipitation phenomenon, aggregates dispersed as temperatures were further increased. Interestingly, proteins obtained from different patients differed in their aggregation properties.

Of the three forms of L-chain deposition pathologies, amyloid fibril formation is an established product of aggregation. By a mechanism that remains to be determined, L chains spontaneously self-assemble to form a highly ordered fibril approx 10 nm in diameter and of indefinite length. It is not known whether the fibril contains native forms or denatured L chains. However, if the latter, then the fibril subunit must represent an alternative well-defined L-chain conformation. X-ray fiber diffraction study indicates characteristic spacings of β-domains with the β-sheets aligned parallel to the fibril axis (for review, *see* Stone *[45]*). Of additional significance is that the dye Congo Red, when bound to an amyloid fibril, imparts a green birefringence, indicating that the fibril imparts on the dye the structural organization of a crystal in one dimension. The amyloid fibrils are highly stable, but can be dispersed in strong denaturing conditions; therefore, this assembly is likely to involve large surfaces of noncovalent interaction. L-chain amyloid fibrils are also characterized by the general absence of most or all the C domain, for reasons that are not clear. Not all patients who overproduce antibody L chains form amyloid; others suffer from other forms of L-chain deposition. In still other cases, there are no pathological consequences. It is reasonable to suggest that, like the process that leads to amyloid formation, other forms of L-chain deposition disease also represent different forms of L-chain aggreation.

We have completed a study of 40 clinically characterized Bence Jones proteins *(46)*. For most of the proteins, size-exclusion chromatographic analyses in three different buffer systems were performed to examine aggregation at concentrations ranging over two orders of magnitude. Four of the five proteins clinically categorized as nonpathological were scored as nonaggregating, whereas 33 of 35 pathological chains showed varying degrees of aggregation under one or more of the solution conditions used for chromatography. In two of the three apparent discrepancies, the clinical diagnoses were themselves somewhat ambiguous. The κI protein **Borf** showed limited, but observable aggregation in both neutral phosphate and urea-containing buffers, but no apparent pathological consequences were observed during the course of treatment of the patient. However, when tested in an in vivo mouse model *(47)* that had previously been demonstrated to replicate pathological properties of proteins from individual patients, protein **Borf** showed cast formation tendencies and some basement membrane precipitation, and could have been designated as pathological on that basis *(46)*.

Only one "false negative" had been unambiguously diagnosed as a pathological protein by both autopsy and mouse model results. This is λ protein **Loc**, which showed no aggregation *(46)* under the conditions used in these tests. The reasons for this are not known; however, as has been shown by crystallographic analysis of this protein in three solution conditions, ammonium sulfate *(10)*, deionized water *(11)*, and sodium potassium sulfate (Huang and Schiffer, unpublished results), the quaternary interactions of this protein are very sensitive to pH, ionic strength, and solution composition. The sensitivity of this molecule to dissolution is apparently attributable, at least in part, to the presence of a His at position 38, instead of the most frequently found Gln (84% of λ Bence Jones proteins or myeloma protein variable domains). His38 is found in 7% of the λ sequences, occurring in a subset of the λI L chains. In most L-chain dimers, Gln38 side chains from each monomer interact with each other to form dual hydrogen bonds, contributing significantly to the free energy of dimerization and emulating the interaction found between H chain and L chain in an Fab. Although this possibility is not present in λ proteins bearing His at this position, a hydrogen bond with Tyr87 of the other monomer is possible at pH above approx 6.5. Protein **Loc**, like most λ L chains, also has a Trp residue at position 91, which may contribute to the apparent sensitivity to ionic strength.

A limited survey of aggregation dependence on temperature was carried out. Figure 2 summarizes chromatographic data of one of the proteins examined. Protein **Dool** showed extensive aggregation when analyzed at 50°C. When the chromatograms obtained at 24 and 37°C are compared, an apparent small increase in high-mol-wt component is accompanied by an apparent decrease in dimerization. Of the eight proteins tested in this survey, protein **Dool** demonstrated the most dramatic temperature response. The importance of temperature effects was recently demonstrated in a study of the temperature dependence of aggregation by the amyloid-forming variant of cystatin C *(48)*. Although normal cystatin C has no tendency to dimerize or aggregate, the inherited

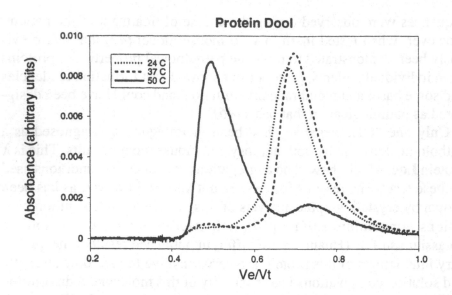

Fig. 2. Size-exclusion chromatograms of κI protein **Dool**. Protein concentration was 2 mg/mL in each run. Ve/Vt indicates eluted volume divided by total column volume (1.77 mL); sample size was 0.005 mL, and flow rate was 0.06 mL/min. Protein elution at the excluded volume of the column is observed at each of the three temperatures (20, 37, and 50°C), indicating the presence of high-mol-wt aggregates on the order of 200,000 Daltons or more, corresponding to complexes involving as many as ten or more L chains. At 50°C, the majority of the sample was clearly involved in formation of aggregates. Protein eluting at Ve/Vt ≈ 0.7 is apparently free L chain showing very little tendency to dimerize.

substitution of a Gln for an Leu at position 68 imparts self-association properties that lead to the formation of amyloid. The authors demonstrated that a small temperature increase, from 37 to 40°C, significantly accelerated aggregation of the protein.

In summary, chromatographic analyses of more than 40 Bence Jones proteins have verified the potential utility of similar methods to provide diagnostically relevant information for the evaluation of an individual's risk for pathological complications arising from in vivo deposition of the protein. The substantial patient-to-patient variation in the conditions that preferentially enhance aggregation suggests that analysis of in vitro aggregation dependencies may provide insights that could be useful in designing optimized patient-specific therapeutic regimens. Results suggest that the aggregation phenomena observed via chromatography may reflect an early step in the process that leads to pathological deposition. If so, then the chromatography technique should prove to be a valuable tool for the rapid screening of compounds that, by inhibition of aggregation, could be useful therapeutic agents for treatment of L-chain-related pathologies.

3.3. Unanswered Interaction Questions

An understanding of the interactions of variable domains is of interest from the perspectives of immunology, pharmacology, biotechnology, and fundamental protein chemistry. The issues involved include interlinkage of Fab assembly and specificity, design of reagents to modify interactions of proteins assembled from immunoglobulin superfamily domains, optimization of production of recombinant antibodies or antibody fragments, and use of these proteins to address basic issues of protein interactions.

It has been clearly demonstrated that at least some residues in contact with antigen also influence quaternary domain interactions. One of the consequences of this is that an amino acid substitution that might appear by modeling to increase affinity between antibody and antigen (by, for instance, contributing an additional hydrogen bond) may in practice actually decrease affinity. If, as has been suggested *(49a)*, V_H and V_L interact in a dynamic manner that generates subpopulations of different antigenic specificity, then the rate of isomerization between the subpopulations is effectively a component of the association rate constant between antibody and antigen. Thus, if an amino acid substitution designed to increase affinity for antigen by decreasing the dissociation rate also has the unintended consequence of stabilizing a V_H–V_L complex that does not bind antigen, then the net consequence could be to generate an antibody with an effectively lowered affinity as determined by the ratio of association and dissociation rate constants. The linkage between structural features responsible for antibody specificity and those involved in controlling domain relationships may be of particular significance in the process of humanization of MAb for immunotherapy. One promising strategy has been to replace human CDRs with the corresponding segments from a mouse MAb that has a high affinity for a relevant antigen into a human framework *(50,51)*. However, if intramolecular interactions between murine CDRs and human framework differ from those in the original mouse antibody, functionally significant differences between the chimeric antibody and the original reagent can be introduced *(52)*.

We have shown that substitutions of certain amino acids on the interfaces can alter the relative positions of CDR segments on the two domains. These amino acids cannot contact the antigen, but can propagate changes in domain interactions that could dramatically affect interactions. The positions involved were highly conserved: Gln38 in V_L, which interacts with Gln39 of the H-chain, and Tyr36, which forms a hydrogen bond with the backbone of the H-chain component of the Fab. Conservation of these positions presumably reflects evolutionary selection based on the need to maintain complementarity of the collaborating proteins. However, what has been observed may not exhaust structural capabilities.

The pathological properties arising from spontaneous self-assembly of L chains provide several opportunities for the development of pharmaceutical reagents to block dimerization or higher-order aggregation. L-chain dimers possess a structural symmetry that sets them apart from other proteins; in principle, antidimer aggregation drug molecules designed to recognize this symmetry might be expected to show relatively little crossreactivity with other proteins of the patient. However, attenuation of dimerization itself might present a more difficult challenge. As noted previously, the amino acids involved in dimer formation are highly conserved. Thus, a drug that worked through a mechanism involving hydrogen bond formation with Gln38, Tyr36, Tyr87, and Gln89 could be a very potent inhibitor of L-chain dimerization. However, it could also disrupt circulating antibodies and lymphocyte surface receptors. If V_H and V_L are capable of transient dissociation (although remaining in close proximity owing to C_L-C_H covalent and noncovalent interactions), then an opportunity for a drug to bind could exist and such binding might have a general immunosuppressive effect. Conceivably, a similar side effect might extend to other receptors and adhesion molecules of the immunoglobulin superfamily.

A drug that distinguishes free L chain from antibody-assembled L chain might be designed to enhance L-chain dimerization by forming a ternary complex with both monomers. If the compound is intercalated between the monomers, the resulting quaternary configuration would be distinct from the normal dimer, thereby rendering it unable to take part in higher-order interactions. Because the same symmetric set of interactions would not be present in an antibody, crossreactions would be minimized. Similarly, little interaction with other superfamily proteins would be expected. Although T-cell receptors and other superfamily proteins are similar to L and H chains, they are not identical. Given sufficient sophistication in understanding the interaction properties of V_H and V_L, it may become possible to develop reagents that disrupt the functional complexes. Such reagents would be new research tools for immunological research and could provide the basis for the development of new drugs for diseases involving inflammation and autoimmunity.

Two biotechnological applications can be mentioned, one in which the L chain is a product, and the other in which the L chain might be considered a device to control a process. Antibodies form the basis of a multibillion-dollar immunodiagnostics industry. This industry was founded on polyclonal antisera obtained from animals. Increasingly, immunodiagnostic assays are based on the use of monoclonal and recombinant antibodies. It is likely that immunotherapeutic antibodies will be predominantly recombinant. Recombinant Fabs and Fvs formed in bacteria are the product of three competing reactions, including self-dimerizations of L and H chains as well as the productive interaction of a L chain with a H chain. In the case of forming an Fab, C_L–C_H interactions successfully drive the reaction to a productive outcome, but at the cost of synthesizing twice as much protein as is needed to generate an antibody-binding site. The formation of a functional Fv from separate V_H and V_L is more problematic. Reactions to form V_H dimers and V_L dimers are comparable in affinity to those forming Fv. These self-associations may lead to formation of higher-order aggregates and precipitates. Therefore, it can be expected that efforts to modify V_H and V_L coordinately by introducing evolutionarily unacceptable substitutions might lead to improved control for formation of recombinant Fv.

A second and entirely novel application of variable domains has been suggested by the work of Kolmar et al. *(40)*, who synthesized a gene for the production of a recombinant form of protein **Rei**. Recombinant **Rei** was fused to the amino-terminal part of the *Vibrio cholerae* ToxR regulator protein. When expressed in an *E. coli* strain in which a cholera toxin::lacZ gene had been constructed, the **Rei** portion of the fusion protein was located on the periplasmic side of the cell membrane, whereas the ToxR protein was present in the cytoplasmic side. Dimerization of **Rei** fusion protein activated the ctx::lacZ gene resulting in β-galactosidase synthesis. A variant V_L was formed in which the affinity of dimerization was increased approx 10-fold by replacement of Leu at position 94 with His resulting in increased production of β-galactosidase.

We have shown that dimerization of L chains is sensitive to pH and salt concentration. It should be possible to synthesize L chains whose dimerization is affected by metal ions or other small molecules. This suggests that it is now possible to design rationally feedback mechanisms into bacteria used in fermentation processes. These bacteria could be modified, as illustrated by Kolmar, such that L-chain fusion proteins are coupled to the expression of an enzyme involved in the fermentation process. Depending on interaction properties of the recombinant V_L, rates of enzyme production would be linked to alterations in the medium composition as they occur. It is also easy to imagine in this scenario replacing V_L dimers with Fv units of defined ligand specificity. If V_H and V_L interfaces were modified to minimize self-dimerization and allow stable Fv formation only on formation of a ternary complex with ligand, then the means would exist to couple internal enzyme production to external molecular signals.

Finally, L chains are proteins. This self-evident fact is sometimes overlooked in that studies of antibodies have traditionally focused on issues of immunochemistry, not protein chemistry. Nevertheless, L chains and V_L domains in particular have several features that could prove useful for basic studies of structural determination of protein physicochemical properties. For instance, they are prime representatives of a major conformational motif, the β-sandwich. The domains are quite stable. One functional attribute, dimerization, is shared by all L chains, and these interactions are measurable by a number of techniques. Thus, dimerization provides a model system for investigating protein recognition properties. Quantitative analysis of higher-order aggregation by some L chains is more problematic, but the development of a working system to analyze the mechanism of amyloid formation could eventually serve as a model for other examples of protein self-assembly, ranging from the interactions of β-domains in viral capsids to the development of various filaments involved in cellular infrastructure.

Well-developed methods exist for production and modification of recombinant antibody components. A large database exists that archives hundreds of immunoglobulin amino acid sequences *(53)*. This archive can be considered a catalog of functionally acceptable amino acid substitutions. Changes in dimerization properties and stability would be expected for many of the substitutions. Changes in the free energy of dimerization are not always a simple function of a single substitution, but also involve the context, i.e., the presence or absence of particular amino acids at other sites as illustrated by the observations of the structural basis for the altered domain relationships in proteins **Loc** and **Wat**. Therefore, the relatively simple mode of recognition involved in dimer formation could provide a valuable system for studying cooperativity of amino acid residues and be particularly appropriate for computer modeling owing to the large conformational database developed from the numerous crystallographic analyses of L-chain structures, both as dimers and in Fabs. L-chain dimerization is altered by changes in pH, ionic strength, and temperature, and therefore, could provide detailed data for future improvements in computer models to address these important issues of solvent composition.

4. Conclusion

Naturally occurring human and murine L chains and immunoglobulins provided much of the early information about the structural and genetic fundamentals of immunity. The principal current reason for work with Bence Jones proteins is to address the structural basis of L-chain pathologies. Amino acid sequence differences between pathological and nonpathological proteins provide the data for constructing hypotheses that may elucidate the disease processes and eventually suggest new therapies. However, natural human L chains probably cannot be used to test these hypotheses rigorously. Because of the large number of amino acid variations among these proteins, many potential rationales can account for the differences observed in dimerization, aggregation, or stability. In addition, although some Bence Jones proteins have been obtained in large quantities, the protein produced by an individual patient is unique and is available in limited quantities that cannot be replenished.

Work to address the clinical properties of L chains requires a broad-based interdisciplinary effort involving clinical researchers to identify and characterize pathological and nonpathological proteins that serve as critical controls, protein chemists to characterize the physicochemical properties of the native proteins, molecular biologists to "immortalize" the protein by cloning the gene and constructing site-specific variants, crystallographers to determine structural changes that result from genetic manipulation, and computational biologists using simulations to rationalize functional changes resulting from structural modification. Such studies build on the foundation of many years of study by a large number of immunochemically motivated researchers. Although a good understanding of the structural basis of antigen recognition by antibodies now exists and the means to exploit these properties for immunodiagnostic and immunotherapeutic purposes are well developed, study of the structural basis of immunoglobulin pathologies has barely begun.

Acknowledgments

This work was supported by the US Department of Energy, Office of Health and Environmental Research, under Contract No. W-31-109-ENG-38; and by US Public Health Service Grant DK43757. The authors would like to thank D. K. Hanson, M. Peak, and P. Wilkins-Stevens for critical reading of the manuscript and helpful suggestions.

References

1. Stevens, F. J., Solomon, A., and Schiffer, M. (1991) Bence Jones proteins: a powerful tool for the fundamental study of protein chemistry and pathophysiology. *Biochemistry* **30,** 6803–6805.
2. Solomon, A. (1982) Bence Jones proteins: malignant or benign? *New Engl. J. Med.* **306,** 605–607.
3. Castano, E. and Frangione, B. (1988) Biology of disease: human amyloidosis, Alzheimer's disease and related disorders. *Lab. Invest.* **58,** 122–132.
4. Feiner, H. (1988) Pathology of dysproteinemia: light chain amyloidosis, non-amyloid immunoglobulin deposition disease, cryoglobulinemia syndromes, and macroglobulinemia of Waldenstrom. *Human Pathol.* **19,** 1255–1272.
5. Solomon, A. and Weiss, D. T. (1988) A perspective of plasma cell dyscrasias: clinical implications of monoclonal light chains in renal disease, in *The Kidney in Plasma Cell Dyscrasias* (Minetti, L., D'Amico, G., and Ponticelli, C., eds.), Kluwer Academic Publishers, Dordrecht, pp. 3–18.
6. Orfila, C., Lepert, J.-C., Modesto, A., Bernadet, P., and Suc, J.-M. (1991) Fanconi's syndrom, kappa light-chain myeloma, non-amyloid fibrils and cytoplasmic crystals in renal tubular epithelium. *Am. J. Nephrol.* **11,** 345–349.
7. Solomon, A. and Weiss, D. T. (1993) Ominous consequences of immunoglobulin deposition. *New Engl. J. Med.* **329,** 1422–1423.
8. Padlan, E. A. (1994) Anatomy of the antibody molecule. *Mol. Immunol.* **31,** 169–217.
9. Fan, Z.-C., Shan, L., Guddat, L. W., He, Z.-M., Gray, W. R., Raison, R. L., and Edmundson, A. B. (1992) Three-dimensional structure of an Fv from a human IgM immunoglobulin. *J. Mol. Biol.* **228,** 188–207.
10. Chang, C.-H, Short, M. T., Westholm, F. A., Stevens, F. J., Wang, B.-C., Furey, W., Solomon, A., and Schiffer, M. (1985) Novel arrangement of immunoglobulin

variable domains: X-ray crystallographic analysis of the lambda-chain dimer Bence Jones protein Loc. *Biochemistry* **24,** 4890–4897.

11. Schiffer, M., Ainsworth, C., Xu, Z.-B., Carperos, W., Olsen, K., Solomon, A., Stevens, F. J., and Chang, C.-H. (1989) Structure of a second crystal form of Bence Jones protein Loc: strikingly different domain associations in two crystal forms of a single protein. *Biochemistry* **28,** 4066–4072.

12. Furey, W., Wang, B. C., Yoo, C. S., and Sax, M. (1983) Structure of a novel Bence Jones protein (Rhe) fragment at 1.6 Å resolution. *J. Mol. Biol.* **167,** 661–692.

13. Xu, Z.-B. and Schiffer, M. (1988) The refinement and structure of Mcg Bence Jones dimer at 2.3 Å resolution. *Ann. Mtg. Amer. Crystal. Assoc. PD28.*

14. Ely, K. R., Herron, J. N., Harker, M., and Edmundson, A. B. (1989) Three-dimensional structure of a light chain dimer crystallized in water: conformational flexibility of a molecule in two crystal forms. *J. Mol. Biol.* **210,** 601–615.

15. Ely, K. R., Herron, J. N., and Edmundson, A. B. (1990) Three-dimensional structure of a hybrid light chain dimer: protein engineering of a binding cavity. *Mol. Immunol.* **27,** 101–114.

16. Fehlhammer H., Schiffer, M., Epp, O., Colman, P. M., Lattman, E. E., Schwager, P., Steigemann, W. S., and Schramm, H. J. (1975) The structure determination of the variable portion of the Bence Jones protein Au. *Biophys. Struct. Mechanism* **1,** 139–146.

17. Epp, O., Lattman, E., Schiffer, M., Huber, R., and Palm, W. (1975) The molecular structure of a dimer composed of the variable portions of the Bence Jones protein Rei refined at 2.0 Å resolution. *Biochemistry* **14,** 4943–4952.

18. Colman, P., Schramm, H., and Guss, J. (1977) Crystal and molecular structure of the dimer of variable domains of the Bence Jones protein Roy. *J. Mol. Biol.* **116,** 73–79.

19. Schiffer, M., Girling, R., Ely, K. R., and Edmundson, A. B. (1973) Structure of a lambda-type Bence Jones protein at 3.5 Å resolution. *Biochemistry* **12,** 4620–4631.

20. Poljak, R. J., Amzel, L. M., Avey, H. P., Chen, B. L., Phizackerley, R. P., and Saul, F. (1973) Three-dimensional structure of the Fab' fragment of a human immunoglobulin at 2.8 Å resolution. *Proc. Natl. Acad. Sci. USA* **70,** 3305–3310.

21. Segal, D. M., Padlan, E. A., Cohen, G. H., Rudikoff, S., Potter, M., and Davies, D. R. (1974) The three-dimensional structure of a phosphorylcholine-binding mouse immunoglobulin Fab and the nature of the antigen binding site. *Proc. Natl. Acad. Sci. USA* **71,** 4298–4302.

22. Wu, T. T. and Kabat, E. A. (1972) An analysis of the sequences of the variable regions of Bence Jones proteins and myeloma light chains and their implications for antibody complementarity. *J. Exp. Med.* **132,** 211–250.

23. Edmundson, A. B., Ely, K. R., Abola, E. E., Schiffer, M., and Panagiotopoulos, N. (1975) Rotational allomerism and divergent evolution of domains in immunoglobulin light chains. *Biochemistry* **14,** 3953–3961.

24. Schiffer, M., Stevens, F. J., Westholm, F. A., Carlson, D., and Schoenborn, B. (1982) Small angle neutron scattering study of Bence Jones protein Mcg: comparison of structures in solution and in crystal. *Biochemistry* **21,** 2874–2878.

25. Schiffer, M., Westholm, F. A., Panagiotopoulos, N., and Solomon, A. (1978) Crystallographic data on a complete κ-type human Bence Jones protein. *J. Mol. Biol.* **124,** 287–290.
25a. Huang, D.-B., Chang, C.-H., Ainsworth, C., Brünger, A. T., Eulite, M., Solomon, A., Stevens, F. J., Schiffer, M. (1994) Comparison of crystal structures of two homologous proteins: structural origin of altered domain interactions in immunoglobulin light-chain dimers. *Biochemistry* **33,** 14,848–14,857.
26. Klein, R., Jaenichen, R., and Zachau, H. G. (1993) Expressed human immunoglobulin κ genes and their hypermutation. *Eur. J. Immunol.* **23,** 3248–3271.
27. Rocca, A., Khamlichi, A. A., Aucouturier, P., Noel, L.-H., Denoryoy, L., and Preud'homme, J. L. (1993) Primary structure of a variable region of the VkI subgroup (ISE) in light chain deposition disease. *Clin. Exp. Immunol.* **91,** 506–509.
28. Cogne, M., Preud'homme, J.-L, Bauwens, M., Touchard, G., and Aucouturier, P. (1991) Structure of a monoclonal kappa chain of the V-kappa-IV subgroup in the kidney and plasma cells in light chain deposition disease. *J. Clin. Invest.* **87,** 2188–2190.
29. Liepnieks, J. J., Dwulet, F. E., and Benson, M. D. (1990) Amino acid sequence of a kappa I primary (AL) amyloid protein (AND). *Mol. Immunol.* **27,** 481–485.
30. Hurle, M. R., Helms, L., Li, L., Chan, W., and Wetzel, R. (1994) A role for destabilizing amino acid replacements in light chain amyloidosis. *Proc. Natl. Acad. Sci. USA* **91,** 5446–5450.
31. Ch'ang, L.-Y., Yen, C.-P., Besl, L., Schell, M., and Solomon, A. (1994) Identification and characterization of a functional human Igλ$_{VI}$ germline gene. *Mol. Immunol.* **31,** 531–536.
32. Reidl, L. S., Kinoshita, C. M., and Steiner, L. A. (1992) Wild mice express an Ig V-lambda gene that differs from any V-lambda in BALB/c but resembles a human V-lambda subgroup. *J. Immunol.* **149,** 471–480.
33. Chuchana, P., Blancher, A., Brockly, F., Alexandre, D., Leranc, G., and Lefranc, M.-P. (1989) Definition of the human immunoglobulin variable lambda (IGLV) gene subgroups. *Eur. J. Immunol.* **20,** 1317–1325.
34. Edelman, G. M. and Gally, J. A. (1962) The nature of Bence Jones proteins: chemical similarities to polypeptide chains of myeloma globulins and normal gamma-globulins. *J. Exp. Med.* **116,** 207–227.
35. Green, R. W. (1973) Conformation and association of the light chain from a homogeneous human immunoglobulin. *Biochemistry* **12,** 3225–3231.
36. Azuma, T., Hamaguchi, K., and Migita, S. (1974) Interactions between immunoglobulin polypeptide chains. *J. Biochem.* **76,** 685–693.
37. Maeda, H., Engel, J., and Schramm, H. J. (1976) Kinetics of dimerization of the variable fragment of the Bence Jones protein Au. *Eur. J. Biochem.*. **69,** 133–139.
38. Stevens, F. Westholm, J., F., Solomon, A., and Schiffer, M. (1980) Self-association of human immunoglobulin κI light chains: role of the third hypervariable region. *Proc. Natl. Acad. Sci. USA* **77,** 1144–1148.
39. Stevens, F. J. and Schiffer, M. (1981) Computer simulation of protein self-association during small-zone gel filtration: estimation of equilibrium constants. *Biochem. J.* **195,** 213–219.

40. Kolmar, H., Frisch, C., Kleemann, G., Gotze, K., Stevens, F. J., and Fritz, H.-J. (1994) Dimerization of Bence Jones proteins: linking the rate of transcription from an *Escherichia coli* promoter to the association constant of REIv. *Biol. Chem. Hoppe-Seyler* **375,** 61–70.
41. Dorrington, K. J. (1978) The structural basis for the functional versatility of immunoglobulin G. *Can. J. Biochem..* **56,** 1087–1101.
42. Schiffer, M., Chang, C.-H., Naik, V. M., and Stevens, F. J. (1988) Analysis of immunoglobulin domain interactions: evidence for a dominant role of salt bridges. *J. Mol. Biol.* **203,** 799–802.
43. Jones, H. B. (1848) On a new substance occurring in the urine of a patient with mollities ossium. *Phil. Trans. R. Soc. Lond.* 55–62.
44. Neet, K. and Putnam, F. W. (1966) Characterization of the thermal denaturation of Bence Jones proteins by ultracentrifugation at elevated temperatures. *J. Biol. Chem.* **241,** 2320–2325.
45. Stone, M. J. (1990) Amyloidosis: a final common pathway for protein deposition in tissues. *Blood* **75,** 531–545.
46. Myatt E., Westholm, F. A., Weiss, D. T., Solomon, A., Schiffer, M., and Stevens, F. J. (1994) Pathogenic potential of human monoclonal immunoglobulin light chains: relationship of *in vitro* aggregation to *in vivo* organ deposition. *Proc. Natl. Acad. Sci. USA* **91,** 3034–3038.
47. Solomon, A., Weiss, D. T., and Kattine, A. (1991) Nephropathological potential of human Bence Jones proteins: experimental and clinical correlates. *N. Engl. J. Med.* **324,** 1845–1851.
48. Abrahamson, M. and Grubb, A. (1994) Increased body temperature accelerates aggregation of the Leu-68 Gln mutant cystatin C, the amyloid-forming protein in hereditary cystatin C amyloid angiopathy. *Proc. Natl. Acad. Sci. USA* **91,** 1416–1420.
49. Stevens, F. J., Chang, C.-H., and Schiffer, M. (1988) Dual conformations of an immunogloublin light-chain dimer: heterogeneity of antigen specificity and idiotope profile may result from multiple variable-domain interaction mechanisms. *Proc. Natl. Acad. Sci. USA* **85,** 6895–6899.
49a. Foote, J. and Molstein, C. (1994) Conformational isomerism and the diversity of antibodies. *Proc. Natl. Acad. Sci. USA* **91,** 10,370–10,374.
50. Jones, P. T., Dear, P. H., Foote, J., Neuberger, M. S., and Winter, G. (1986) Replacing the complementarity-determining regions in a human antibody with those from a mouse. *Nature* **321,** 522–525.
51. Riechmann, L., Clark, M., Waldmann, H., and Winter, G. (1988) Reshaping human antibodies for therapy. *Nature* **332,** 323–327.
52. Foote, J. and Winter, G. (1992) Antibody framework residues affecting the conformation of the hypervariable loops. *J. Mol. Biol.* **224,** 487–499.
53. Kabat, E. A., Wu, T. T., Perry, H. M., Gottesman, K. S., and Foeller, C. (1991) *Sequences of Proteins of Immunological Interest*, 5th ed., Public Health Service National Institutes of Health, Washington, DC.

CHAPTER 4

Crystallographic and Chromatographic Methods for Study of Antibody Light Chains and Other Proteins

Marianne Schiffer and Fred J. Stevens

1. Introduction

A three-dimensional structure of reasonably high resolution is the starting point of any protein engineering project, whether intended to improve the affinity of an antibody, change the specificity of an enzyme, or to test a hypothesis regarding the role of a particular residue in determining structure or stability. The atomic coordinates determined by X-ray crystallography or, increasingly, NMR, provides the means to visualize the shape of a protein as well as the distances between atoms within a protein, or between a protein and ligand or another macromolecule. The free energy changes that determine protein structure, stability, and interaction properties ultimately arise from the distances that separate the various types of atoms involved, including proteins, ligands, and solvent molecules.

One of the most general functional properties of proteins is that of recognition; i.e., the operational role of most proteins involves interactions with one or more components, including metals, ions, ligands, other proteins, and nucleic acids. The potential value of size-exclusion chromatography (gel filtration) to study protein interactions was appreciated very soon after the introduction of porous materials suitable for the separation of proteins on the basis of size. The Hummel-Dreyer and various large-zone methods were rapidly developed *(1–3)*. However, the rela-

From: *Methods in Molecular Biology, Vol. 51: Antibody Engineering Protocols*
Edited by: S. Paul Humana Press Inc., Totowa, NJ

tively low resolution and structural frailty of original separation media made each chromatography run time-consuming because of the requirement for slow solvent flow rates. Substantial quantities of sample were required to establish saturated zones on the large-scale columns. These considerations discouraged widespread application of chromatography as a means to characterize protein interactions rigorously.

The introduction of gel-filtration matrices for operation in high-performance liquid chromatography (HPLC) systems provided much improved efficiency of data collection in terms of rate, reproducibility, and resolution. Commonplace use of computerized data collection systems makes digitized forms of the experimental chromatograms available for detailed analysis. The general availability of computationally powerful work stations makes practical the use of computer simulation to model and analyze affinity dependence of elution profiles, and overcomes previous dependence on large-zone methods for which rigorous mathematical treatments were possible. These reasons for the ubiquity of HPLC systems in biochemistry research laboratories suggest that chromatography methods may become a practical approach for analyzing changes in interaction properties introduced by the structural alterations resulting from site-specific mutagenesis.

1.1. Protein Crystallography

The collection and analysis of X-ray crystallography data is a technically specialized and computationally intensive effort. However, the most important and rate-limiting step in the process that leads to the ultimate elucidation of a protein's three-dimensional structure can be undertaken in any protein chemistry/molecular biology laboratory. Because, almost by definition, any project involving protein engineering is motivated to alter some functional feature of an interesting protein, it is clear that such projects will generate numerous protein variants, each of which, if conformationally analyzed, can make a significant contribution to understanding structural/functional relationships in proteins. Therefore, efforts to crystallize site-specific mutants routinely can be expected to become an increasingly significant aspect of the efforts of molecular biology laboratories (*see* Note 1).

Protein crystallization has been informally referred to as witchcraft and black magic. The descriptive terminology reflects the experience of many workers that it was possible to invest heroic effort and time in the purification of a protein and to screen a myriad of conditions for crystallization without ultimate success. In other cases, frustration resulted not from the lack of crystallization, but from the formation of a multitude of tiny crystals too small for generation of suitable diffraction data.

Persistence and patience are two significant factors in obtaining protein crystals. Purity of the sample is universally considered to be important, and ongoing improvements in protein purification and analytical technologies can be expected to contribute to enhanced success in crystallization (*see* Note 2). Precision in technique is essential for the systematic and reproducible testing of crystallization conditions. Useful methods to crystallize proteins have been detailed *(4)*, and we will not attempt a general review, but will summarize methods specifically used in studies of antibody L chains. One of these proteins, Bence Jones protein **Loc**, ultimately yielded crystals in three different solvent conditions used to generate crystal formation. In each of the crystals, the domain–domain interactions in the L-chain dimer were different (*5,6*, and unpublished results), serving as a reminder that choice of crystallization method is relevant to the outcome of crystallographic analysis, particularly when dealing with multisubunit proteins or protein complexes. When a protein can be crystallized in more than one solvent condition, comparisons of structures may provide useful insight into protein/solvent relationships.

1.2. Chromatography for Interaction Analysis

Size-exclusion chromatography is based on the passage of molecules through a medium that can be considered to be a mesh encompassing pores of various sizes. The interior of a pore is occupied effectively by solvent that is immobile and represents a stationary phase. The mobile phase is represented by the solvent that is being pumped through the column. Molecules in the solvent diffuse between mobile and stationary phases; the relative volumes of each that are accessible determine the elution rate of a particular molecule.

A small molecule, such as water or acetone, is presumed to have access to the entire volume of the pores, whereas a macromolecule, such as a protein, may be able to penetrate some pores, but not others (or may be viewed as penetrating pores partially). Proteins of different sizes have access to different solvent volumes in the chromatography matrix; larger molecules have diminished volumes of stationary phase accessible to them and pass through the column faster than smaller molecules. When two proteins interact and form a complex, then during the lifetime of the complex, the migration rates of the components are faster than those that occur for the same components when uncomplexed.

Therefore, when a size-exclusion chromatogram of a mixture of two proteins, such as a monoclonal antibody (MAb) and its antigen, is compared to an artificial chromatogram generated by the summation of the two chromatograms obtained when the components were analyzed separately, interaction is revealed by differences between the experimental and the synthetic elution profile *(7,8)*. In effect, the synthetic chromatogram represents the elution profile expected if no interaction between the two components takes place *(see* Note 3). The magnitude of change is determined by the relative composition of the interactive sample as complex and free components. These relative concentrations are determined by the affinity of interaction and the concentrations of the interacting molecules. Therefore, the shape of the elution profile is determined by the affinity of interaction and the concentrations of interactants. In addition, the kinetics of interaction also contribute to the ultimate shape of the elution profile by controlling the rate of intermixing between the complexed and free pools during protein migration through the column *(9)*.

Significant information can be obtained from simple examination of the raw data and by qualitative comparisons. In one interesting case *(10)*, no changes in elution behavior were found on mixing a protein and an MAb that had been obtained following immunization by a peptide derived from the protein. Using standard enzyme-linked immunosorbent assay (ELISA) methods for selection of the MAb and characterization of its binding, it was originally inferred that the MAb recognized the native configuration of the protein. Radiolabeled protein assay had indicated that the affinity of the antibody for antigen was in excess of $10^6 M^{-1}$, an interaction that would have been readily detected by chromatography. Chromatography data, which effectively examines bulk intermolecular interactions, indicated that the MAb in fact recognized a nonnative conformation, perhaps generated by solid-phase adsorption during ELISA or resulting from the iodination procedure generating a radiolabeled tracer. Indeed, crystallographic characterization of a complex formed by the peptide and the MAb demonstrated that the configuration of the bound peptide was not that found in the cognate intact protein *(11)*.

Thus, qualitative use of the chromatography method provides a rapid indication of binding properties that avoids some of the possible concerns that are relevant to more indirect methods. Qualitative application can be used to confirm the specificity of an MAb or to compare epitope specificities of two MAbs *(12)*. Epitope "mapping" is based on the premise that if Fabs X and Y bind to identical or overlapping epitopes, a mixture of antigen A with the Fabs generates complexes $A-X$ and $A-Y$; i.e., no increase in mol-wt species is found relative to that obtained when the antigen is reacted with either antibody alone (*see* Note 4). If X and Y bind at different sites, then complexes of the form $X-A-Y$ can be formed leading to a higher mol-wt species. The formation of doubly bound A also leads to an increase in protein eluted at the position of free A.

A variation on this strategy can be used semiquantitatively to estimate dissociation rate constants for antibodies having very high affinity for antigen. This approach exploits "autocompetition" between an antibody and an Fab prepared from itself. Following addition of Fab to an equilibrated mixture of antibody and antigen, serial aliquots of the mixture are chromatographed. To a first approximation, changes in the elution profile reflect replacement of antibody by Fab, which is itself dependent on dissociation of the initial antibody–antigen complex. Therefore, at least in the early stages of re-equilibration, it is possible to use the rate of change of the elution profile to estimate the dissociation rate constants, which tend to be a principal determinant of high affinity.

Quantitative interpretation of small-zone chromatograms requires the use of computer simulation to model the interaction processes that occur on the column. In large-zone chromatography, bulk transport of the sample is primarily determined by a region of constant concentration that remains unchanged throughout the run (*see* Note 5). As a consequence, the elution position of the plateau region can be interpreted as if it reflected the elution of a "virtual" complex of molecular weight between that of free and complexed species. The intermediate molecular weight is determined by the fraction of complex present in the zone, leading to calculation of the affinity constant by the standard relationship, $K = c/ab$, where c, a, and b represent the equilibrium molar concentrations of complex and the two interacting species.

No simple relationship exists between the final elution position of a small zone of interacting proteins and the affinity constant governing interaction. This is a consequence of the fact that the protein concentration throughout the zone is constantly changing during its migration. Change in concentration is driven not only by the standard processes of diffusion and dispersion, but also by the macromolecular interactions that occur within the protein zone. Because protein concentration is not uniform across the zone, the ratio of complexed and free species is also variable with the highest proportion of complex found in the region of highest concentration. Therefore, the average elution rate of the molecules in the central region of an elution band is higher than at either the leading or trailing edge and, as a result, the elution process is continuously "disequilibrating" the elution zone.

We introduced a simple iterative computer simulation of small-zone chromatography to assist in understanding the elution properties of human L chains for which we had observed apparently anomalous elution behavior of the free monomer, i.e., elution positions intermediate between that of the covalent dimer and the position expected for a free monomer. In addition, the peak containing monomer generally was asymmetric, with a consistently sharp leading edge and an extended trailing edge. The simulation was able to emulate the behavior observed experimentally *(13)* and to link both the variability in elution position and asymmetry of elution peak to a rapid self-association process in which L chains obtained from individual patients had different dimerization affinities, presumably arising most often from differences in amino acids in the CDRs that contribute to the interface involved in dimerization or formation of an Fab.

The iterative simulation represents the chromatography process as a repeating series of events, each occurring in a finite time step. In much the same way that calculus integrates a complex function by subdividing the function into an array of small elements each of which are more easily approximated, we assume that given sufficient computing power to enable sufficiently small simulated time steps, and if the mathematical representation of the physical processes occurring during chromatography is sufficiently complete, then simulation is a useful tool by which to interpret quantitatively the physicochemical basis of the chromatograms observed for interacting protein systems (*see* Note 6).

2. Materials

2.1. Crystallization (see *Note 7*)

2.1.1. Buffers

1. Appropriate buffers are determined by pH ranges useful for manipulating protein solubility. Buffers that have been used in various crystallization

efforts include acetate, bicine, citrate, cacodylate, imidazole, HEPES, MES, and Tris.
2. Inappropriate buffers include those that support bacterial and fungal growth. Phosphate buffers should be avoided when possible.

2.1.2. Precipitants

Precipitant reagents are added to solutions of proteins to decrease solubility and induce crystal growth. Precipitating agents (salts, organic compounds, and polymers) include ammonium phosphate, ethanol, ethylene glycol, glycerol, lithium sulfate, magnesium formate, 2-methyl-2,4-pentanediol, polyethylene glycol(s), polyethyleneimine, potassium phosphate, potassium tartrate, iso-propanol, 2-propanol, sodium acetate, sodium citrate, sodium formate, sodium potassium sulfate, sodium tartrate, and numerous others.

2.1.3. Apparatus

1. Various vials, wells, capillary tubes, and dialysis devices have been successfully used for crystallization. In general, the apparatus must be clean, permit observation, and in cases of long-term storage, capable of being tightly sealed.
2. An environment for storage (incubation) of crystallization setups that offers minimal vibration or thermal fluctuations.

2.2. Chromatography

2.2.1. Data Collection System

1. Chromatography matrix: Any HPLC-compatible gel-filtration matrix is acceptable in principle. Considerations include nonspecific interactions with proteins that may interfere with studies of certain proteins. Some matrices tend to bind basic proteins at low ionic strength; other matrices will have characteristic secondary interactions determined by their particular surface chemistries. It is probable that no universal matrix exists that exhibits purely size-mediated separation for all proteins under all solvent conditions.
2. Column dimensions: Based on the objectives of each study, a choice must be made between using commercially available prepacked columns or using smaller user-prepared columns. If commercial columns are chosen, the benefits include: (a) higher resolution resulting from larger volume and, perhaps, higher quality control of packing technique, and (b) convenience. The benefits obtained from small user-prepared columns include the use of smaller samples and increased sensitivity/dynamic range. In

some cases, the conversion of a single column costing several hundred dollars into ten or more small columns may be a consideration.

3. Detector: Continuous UV detection of protein is far superior for analytical chromatography than collection of fractions. The ability to monitor at multiple wavelengths provides for a wider dynamic range of protein concentrations that may be used as well as possibly allowing for correction of some artifacts that might be associated with baseline variations. Protein absorbance at 214 nm is approx 10-fold higher than at 280 nm; however, buffer selection may be restricted at this wavelength, and sensitivity to absorbance by contaminants may also become a problem. Minimization of dead volume between column and detector and use of small flow cells provide for most authentic representation of peak shape, which is a particular consideration for the use of small columns.

4. Data: Elution profiles should be collected by computer and should be supported by software that allows for addition, subtraction, and comparison of experimental and synthetic profiles. These features are readily available in commercial software that operates various HPLC systems. Additional work with these data is facilitated if the values of absorbance as a function of time or elution volume are storable as a text file that can be later transferred over a network connection, or via a floppy disk to another work station for further analysis or comparison to simulated profiles.

3. Methods

3.1. Crystallization

3.1.1. Concentration

Purified protein samples should be concentrated to levels approaching solubility limits. Crystallization of human L chains typically involved starting concentrations ranging from 10–30 mg/mL.

3.1.2. Crystallization by Dialysis

Some proteins (usually euglobulins) will form crystals when slowly dialyzed against a low-ionic-strength solution or deionized water. Dialysis is usually performed using dialysis "buttons" or tubes containing protein solution, and closed off at one end by the dialysis membrane.

3.1.3. Crystallization by Batch Precipitation

1. Varying quantities of selected precipitant(s) are combined with solutions containing protein at various concentrations—creating a matrix of different protein:precipitant ratios.
2. Containers are sealed tightly to avoid evaporation of liquid.

Table 1
Examples of Crystallization Conditions Used in L-Chain Studies

Protein	Class	Method[a]	Starting Solvent	Precipitant	Ref.
Cle	Human λ_{III} VC[b]	B	0.15M NaCl[c]	$(NH_4)_2SO_4$	*(14)*
Loc	Human λ_I VC	B	0.15M NaCl	$(NH_4)_2SO_4$	*(5)*
		B	0.15M NaCl	$NaKSO_4$, pH 8	N.P.[d]
		D	0.15M NaCl	H_2O	*(6)*
Mcg	Human λ_{II} VC	B	0.10M Tris-HCl	$(NH_4)_2SO_4$	*(15)*
		D	0.15M NaCl	H_2O	*(15)*
Pav[e]	Human λ_{III} VC				*(16)*
Rhe[e]	Human λ_I V				*(17)*
Au	Human κ_I V	D	0.05M Tris-HCl, pH 8	$(NH4)_2SO_4$	*(18)*
Fin	Human κ_{II}VC	B	0.15M NaCl	$(NH_4)_2SO_4$, pH 6.5	*(19)*
Len	Human κ_{IV} V	V	0.15M NaCl	$(NH_4)_2SO_4$, pH 6.5	N.P.
Rei	Human κ_IV	D	0.05M Tris-HCl, pH 8	$(NH_4)_2SO_4$	*(20)*
Roy	Human κ_IV	D	0.05M Tris-HCl, pH 8	$(NH_4)_2SO_4$	*(21)*
Wat	Human κ_IV	V	0.15M NaCl	$(NH_4)_2SO_4$, pH6.5	N.P.
McP603	Mouse κV	V	0.10M Acetate, pH 4	$(NH_4)_2SO_4$	*(22)*
M29b	Mouse κV	V	0.10M Acetate, pH 5.8	Iso-propanol + PEG	*(23)*

[a]B: Batch; D: Dialysis; V: Vapor diffusion.
[b]VC: intact L chain; V: variable domain only.
[c]Phosphate buffer to pH 7.5.
[d]N.P. Not published: M. Schiffer, unpublished observations.
[e]Multiple successful crystallization conditions; consult reference.

3. Containers are periodically inspected (usually by microscope) for presence of crystals or other evidence of precipitation/gelation (*see* Note 8).
4. If no crystal development or other evidence of phase transition is observed after a suitable time period, samples are discarded (or repurified), and steps 1–3 are repeated with alternative precipitants and/or buffer composition.
5. If small crystals, gel, or precipitant is observed in one or more containers, steps 1–3 are repeated with the same precipitant, but with a bracketing concentration matrix encompassing smaller step variations in concentrations.

3.1.4. Crystallization by Vapor Diffusion

1. Two independent liquid components are maintained within a single sealed container. A hanging or sitting drop contains a mixture of protein and a subcritical concentration of precipitant. A well/reservoir contains a larger volume of liquid containing a higher concentration of precipitant. A matrix of different protein:precipitant ratios is established. Steps 2–5 listed in Section 3.1.3. are then performed.
2. Refer to Table 1 for a brief synopsis of some of the diverse conditions that have been used to crystallize L chains.

3.2. Chromatography

3.2.1. Homologous Interaction (Dimerization)

1. Check elution position of protein standards (*see* Note 9).
2. Concentrate protein. Ideally, the solubility of the protein will permit concentration to a level high enough to assure that most of the protein is found in a dimerized form.
3. Prepare dilution series. The minimum concentration is determined by the detection limits of the chromatography system that will be used. Ideally, the minimum concentration will be sufficiently low to assure that most of the protein in the sample is present as monomer. Although it may be good practice to have a uniform distribution of dilutions throughout the range of concentrations, the most valuable data points are those occurring in the region in which elution position is most sensitive to concentration. Twelve to 15 dilutions provide an excellent data set for quantitative simulation.
4. Collect data for all samples. Interspersing sample concentrations is generally a better strategy that systematically analyzing from highest concentration to lowest in that it minimizes the impact of slow variations on flow rate on the usefulness of data. It is also useful to repeat analyses of at least some of the samples during the course of a series of runs.
5. Quality control: At low concentrations, protein may be lost owing to adsorption to containers or chromatography apparatus. If sensitivity of the detector is adjusted between runs such that the product of the full-scale deflection and the concentration of the sample remain constant, then inspection of the resulting chromatograms can provide an indication of this (as well as possible dilution error). The area under the elution profile is expected to be constant. If decreases are observed, and if the loss is the result of adsorption to the container in which the diluted protein is stored, then losses may be minimized if dilution is made shortly before injection into the column.
6. Repeat step 1 to verify consistency of chromatography runs.
7. Analyze data as appropriate. Relative affinity constants can be quickly estimated from the fact, that in a dimerization experiment, the peak position is determined by the product of initial concentration and affinity constant. Thus, for two proteins of the same molecular weight, and assuming that the intrinsic elution velocities of dimer and monomer for the two proteins are equal, then the relative association constants are inversely related to the ratio of concentrations that generate equivalent elution positions. Absolute affinity constant determination requires application of the simulation.

3.2.2. Heterologous Interaction

1. Check elution position of protein standards.
2. Determine elution position of component 1.
3. Determine elution position of component 2.
4. Combine components 1 and 2, and incubate for a sufficient period of time to assure equilibration.
5. Determine elution profile of mixture.
6. (Optional) Repeat step 5 to confirm equilibrium had been reached prior to injection of mixture into column. If equilibrium was not obtained, then the two chromatograms generated in steps 5 and 6 will be different.
7. Repeat step 1.
8. Analyze data as appropriate. If the purpose of the experiment was to verify the presence of interaction, and if the interaction is strong, then inspection of the chromatogram generated in step 4, when compared to the chromatograms obtained in steps 2 and 3, will clearly indicate this. Interaction should be characterized by the presence of a higher-mol-wt elution peak than seen in either step 2 or 3. Weak or absent interaction should be distinguished by combining the digital chromatograms obtained in steps 2 and 3, and directly comparing this synthetic chromatogram to the digitized chromatogram of the mixture. Assuming that the concentrations of components were the same when chromatographed freely or in the mixture, and also assuming a perfect experiment, then if no interaction takes place, the synthetic and experimental chromatograms will be superimposable. Deviations from superposition arising from shifts to earlier elution positions are indicative of interaction of moderate to low affinity.

If the purpose of the experiment was to obtain data suitable for estimation of the affinity and kinetics of interaction, then steps 4–6 should be repeated at several concentrations and ratios of the interacting components. The concentration range should be as wide as experimentally convenient, with most data obtained in concentration ranges for which the shape of the elution profile appears to be most sensitive. Some of these chromatograms will be used as "targets" in simulation runs that fit algorithm parameters estimating the rate constants of association/dissociation, the elution velocity of the complex, and, in some cases, the stoichiometry of interaction. Other chromatograms will be used to test the predictive value of the fitted parameters with the presumption that if a single set of parameters can be used to generate simulated chromatograms that emulate the experimental data at all concentrations and ratios, then these predicted rate constants accurately reflect the affinity constant given by the ratio of association and dissociation rates.

3.2.3. Epitope Mapping

1. Check elution position of protein standards.
2. Determine elution positions for antigen *A*.
3. Determine elution positions for antibodies/Fabs *X* and *Y* (*see* Note 10).
4. Combine *A* and *X* at concentrations used in steps 2 and 3.
5. Combine *A* and *Y* at concentrations used in steps 2 and 3.
6. Combine *A* with a mixture of *X* and *Y* at concentrations used in steps 2 and 3.
7. Incubate mixtures for a period sufficient to achieve equilibrium.
8. Determine elution profiles for combinations generated in steps 4–6.
9. Analyze data. If the affinities of *X* and *Y* for *A* are sufficiently high and if the respective epitopes are independent and allow simultaneous binding of *X* and *Y*, the combination generated in step 6 should clearly indicate the existence of higher-mol-wt components than were observed in the mixtures obtained from steps 4 and 5. The quantity of protein eluting at positions corresponding to free *X* and *Y* will be relatively unchanged. If the epitopes of *X* and *Y* overlap or are identical, then there should be no increase in apparent molecular weight, and there should be a significant increase in the quantity of protein eluted at the free *X* and *Y* position(s). If *X* and *Y* affinities are too low to allow saturation of binding sites, then simulation analysis may be necessary to determine the independence of epitopes (*see* Note 11).

3.2.4. Affinity Estimation (*see Note 12*)

1. Develop a model of the chromatography system, i.e., assign values for cell volume, number of cells in column, number of cells in sample, and flow rate.
2. Assign protein molecular weights and best estimates of elution velocities, dispersion factors, and diffusion factors.
3. Simulate free components with adjustments of the parameters set in step 2 to optimize correspondence of simulated and experimental chromatograms.
4. Assign estimated values for elution velocity, dispersion factor, and diffusion factor of complex.
5. Varying only association and dissociation rate constants, attempt to fit elution profile generated for one concentration set of interacting components.
6. Use best rate constants to predict elution profiles that were obtained experimentally at other concentrations/ratios of reactants.
7. Guided by the magnitude and nature of discrepancies between predicted and observed chromatograms, systematically and iteratively adjust kinetic parameters and/or estimated velocity of complex to improve overall fit.

4. Notes

1. Although efforts to crystallize proteins have been traditionally the domain of crystallography laboratories, the means to "grow" crystals are found in any laboratory that can produce and purify proteins. The existence of an interesting crystal of suitable diffraction properties can always be quickly followed by the development of collaboration with a protein crystallographer.

2. Protein purity is generally thought to be important for protein crystallization because it minimizes impediments to lattice formation that might arise through interactions of proteins of different shapes and atomic compositions. However, it is interesting to note that in some cases, proteins can in fact be purified by crystallization. In other undoctrinal examples, some proteins are able to crystallize in the physiological milieu. For instance, Fanconi's syndrome is a disease of the kidney involving antibody L-chain crystallization in the kidney tubules *(24)*.

   Purity involves both chemical homogeneity and conformational uniformity. Thus, denatured or partially unfolded forms of the protein can inhibit crystallization. Difficulty in crystallization might in other cases be attributed to conformational heterogeneity arising from multiple structural allomers in solution.

3. In the case of protein self-association, the interaction is revealed by the concentration dependence of the elution position of the sample. At lower concentrations, the mixture is characterized by higher relative monomer concentration and, therefore, later elution from the column.

4. This is slightly oversimplified. If the antibody affinities are low and sufficiently different from each other, an increase in rate of elution might be observed reflecting differences in composition.

5. This is true only in cases where the rate of equilibration for formation and dissociation of complexes is rapid relative to the rate of separation of complexes and free constituents.

6. Our current version of the simulation is available on request with the understanding that responsibility for results is assumed exclusively by the user.

7. These materials/protocols are only to be considered as representative examples of starting points for crystallization. The optimal protocol for any individual protein must be determined on a case-by-case basis. Also note that because of the rapidly growing activity in protein crystallography, it is now possible to obtain commercial kits (e.g., Hampton Research, Riverside, CA) that significantly facilitate the screening of potentially useful crystallization conditions.

8. Avoid over-frequent inspection. Crystal growth may be slow; manipulation required to inspect for crystal formation may generate vibrations and thermal fluctuations that could disrupt crystal formation. If containers

are opened for inspection, water vapor will be lost, and equilibria in the solution will be shifted by the ensuing increase in protein and precipitant concentrations.

9. For any quantitative interpretation of chromatography data, it is essential that fluctuations in flow rate be kept to a minimum. We typically use proteins such as chymotrypsinogen, ovalbumin, or IgG, with mol wt of approx 23,000, 45,000, and 150,000 as reference standards with the choice directed by the experimental objective. The lower-mol-wt proteins correspond to the sizes of a free L chain and an L-chain dimer/Fab. The IgG standard provides a useful reference in experiments involving MAb.

10. Ratios of antibody to antigen should be chosen such that most of the binding sites are filled by X or Y when combined separately with antigen. This assures that any apparent increase in the mol-wt distribution obtained in the three-component mixture is the result of formation of a ternary complex rather than the formation of additional binary complexes.

11. In any competition assay, the concept of "partial" overlapping epitopes is not meaningful. Whether the epitopes recognized by antibodies X and Y share 100% or 1% of the same atomic contacts, the outcome is the same in that the two antibodies cannot be concurrently bound by the antigen. However, if it can be shown that antibody X competes with Y, and Y competes with Z, but that X and Z do not compete, then it can be concluded that the three epitopes are distinct from each other.

    Competition assays cannot be used to prove that two antibodies share any overlapping surface on the antigen, even postulating the absence of induced conformational changes. The failure of an antigen to accommodate two antibodies simultaneously is assured if the relevant surfaces overlap or perhaps are even closely adjacent. However, the same result will be obtained if, because of the docking orientations of the antibodies, any portion of the remaining volume of the V domains or any other segments of the antibodies would be constrained to occupy the same space. Thus, the size of the epitopes perceived by competition experiments will be, in some cases, dependent on the size of the antibody probe used experimentally. The boundaries of an epitope determined by site-specific mutagenesis will define the contacts that are relevant for understanding the physicochemical aspects of an antigen–antibody interaction and will be smaller than that inferred from the use of competitive antibody probes. However, the latter may be more relevant for understanding the behavior of antibody mixtures in vivo, or for optimizing antibody combinations for applications, such as sandwich immunoassays.

12. A detailed description of the use of computer simulation of chromatographic data to analyze interaction is beyond the scope of this chapter. An

example of simulation used to estimate an L-chain dimerization constant may be found in Kolmar et al. *(25)*. Here we have sketched the basic experimental strategy that would be used to analyze a heterologous interaction, such as typified by an antigen interaction with an MAb.

Acknowledgments

The submitted manuscript has been authored by a contractor of the US Government under contract No. W-31-109-ENG-38. Accordingly, the US government retains a nonexclusive, royalty-free license to publish or reproduce the published form of this contribution, or allow others to do so, for US government purposes. This work was supported by the US Department of Energy, Office of Health and Environmental Research, under Contract W-31-109-ENG-38 and by US Public Health Service Grant DK43757.

References

1. Hummel, J. P. and Dreyer, W. J. (1962) Measurement of protein-binding phenomena by gel filtration. *Biochim. Biophys. Acta* **63,** 530–532.
2. Winzor, D. J. and Scheraga, H. A. (1963) Studies of chemically reacting systems on Sephadex. I. Chromatographic demonstration of the Gilbert theory. *Biochemistry* **2,** 1263–1267.
3. Ackers, G. K. (1975) Molecular sieve methods of analysis, in *The Proteins*, vol. 1 (Neurath, H. and Hill, R. L., eds.), Academic, New York, pp. 1–94.
4. McPherson, A. (1982) *Preparation and Analysis of Protein Crystals.* John Wiley, New York.
5. Chang, C.-H., Short, M. T., Westholm, F. A., Stevens, F. J., Wang, B. C., Furey, W., Solomon, A., and Schiffer, M. (1985) Novel arrangement of immunoglobulin variable domains: X-ray crystallographic analysis of the λ-chain dimer Bence Jones protein Loc. *Biochemistry* **24,** 4890–4897.
6. Schiffer, M., Ainsworth, C., Xu, Z.-B., Carperos, W., Olsen, K., Solomon, A., Stevens, F. J., and Chang, C.-H. (1989) Structure of a second crystal form of Bence Jones protein Loc: strikingly different domain associations in two crystal forms of a single protein. *Biochemistry* **2,** 4066–4072.
7. Stevens, F. J. (1986) Analysis of protein-protein interaction by simulation of small-zone size-exclusion chromatography: application to an antibody-antigen association. *Biochemistry* **25,** 981–993.
8. Stevens, F. J. (1989) Applications of size-exclusion HPLC in the analysis of protein and peptide epitopes. *Methods Enzymol.* **178,** 107–130.
9. Stevens, F. J. (1989) Analysis of protein-protein interaction by simulation of small-zone size-exclusion chromatography: stochastic formulation of kinetic rate contributions to observed high-performance liquid chromatography elution characteristics. *Biophys. J.* **55,** 1155–1167.
10. Spangler, B. D. (1991) Binding to native proteins by antipeptide monoclonal antibodies. *J. Immunol.* **146,** 1591–1595.

11. Stanfield, R. L., Fieser, T. M., Lerner, R. A., and Wilson, I. A. (1990) Crystal structures of an antibody to a peptide and its complex with peptide antigen at 2.8 Å. *Science* **248,** 712–719.

12. Stevens, F. J., Carperos, W. E., Monafo, W. J., and Greenspan, N. S. (1988) Size-exclusion HPLC analysis of epitopes. *J. Immunol. Methods* **108,** 271–278.

13. Stevens, F. J. and Schiffer, M. (1981) Computer simulation of protein self-association during small-zone gel filtration: estimation of equilibrium constants. *Biochem. J.* **195,** 213–219.

14. Stevens, F. J., Westholm, F. A., Panagiotopoulos, N., Solomon, A., and Schiffer, M. (1981) Preliminary crystallographic data on the human III Bence Jones protein dimer Cle. *J. Mol. Biol.* **147,** 179–183.

15. Ely, K. R., Herron, J. N., Harker, M., and Edmundson, A. B. (1989) Three-dimensional structure of a light chain dimer crystallized in water. Conformational flexibility of a molecule in two crystal forms. *J. Mol. Biol.* **210,** 601–615.

16. Wang, B. C, Yoo, C. S., Hwan, R. Y., Sax, M., Brown, W. E., and Michaels, M. (1977) Structure of Bence Jones protein, Pav: an initial report. *J. Mol. Biol.* **116,** 619–625.

17. Wang, B.-C. and Sax, M. (1974) Structure of a dimeric fragment related to the lambda-type Bence Jones protein: a preliminary study. *J. Mol. Biol.* **87,** 505–508.

18. Fehlhammer, H., Schiffer, M., Epp, O., Colman, P. M., Lattman, E. E., Schwager, P., Steigemann, W., and Schramm, H. J. (1975) The structure determination of the variable portion of the Bence Jones protein *Au. Biophys. Struct. Mechanism* **1,** 139–146.

19. Schiffer, M., Westholm, F. A., Panagiotopoulos, N., and Solomon, A.. (1978) Crystallographic data on a complete κ-type human Bence Jones protein. *J. Mol. Biol.* **124,** 287–290.

20. Epp, O., Lattmann, E. E., Schiffer, M., Huber, R., and Palm, W. (1975) The molecular structure of a dimer composed of the variable portions of the Bence Jones protein REI refined at 2.0-A resolution. *Biochemistry* **14,** 4943–4952.

21. Colman, P. M., Schramm, H. J., and Guss, J. M. (1977) Crystal and molecular structure of the dimer of the variable domains of the Bence Jones protein ROY. *J. Mol. Biol.* **116,** 73–79.

22. Glockshuber, R., Steipe, B., Huber, R., and Plükthun, A. (1990) Crystallization and preliminary x-ray studies of the V_L domain of the antibody McPC603 produced in *Escherichia coli. J. Mol. Biol.* **213,** 613–615.

23. Essen, L.-O. and Skerra, A. (1994) The *de novo* design of an antibody combining site. Crystallographic analysis of the V_L domain confirms the structural model. *J. Mol. Biol.* **238,** 226–244.

24. Aucouturier, P., Bauwens, M., Khamlichi, A. A., Denoroy, L., Spinelli, S., Touchard, G., Preud'homme, J.-L., and Cogne, M. (1993) Monoclonal Ig L chain and L Chain V domain fragment crystallization in myeloma-associated Fanconi's syndrome. *J. Immunol.* **150,** 3561–3568.

25. Kolmar, H., Frisch, C., Kleeman, G., Götze, K., Stevens, F. J., and Fritz, H.-J. (1994) Dimerization of Bence Jones proteins: linking the rate of transcription from an *Escherichia coli* promoter to the association constant of REI_v. *Biol. Chem. Hoppe-Seyler* **375,** 61–70.

CHAPTER 5

Detection of Human Variable Gene Family Expression at the Single-Cell Level

Moncef Zouali

1. Introduction

In mammals, the genes encoding the variable (V) domains of the immunoglobulin heavy (H) chain are assembled during lymphocyte development by rearrangements of variable (V_H), diversity (D_H), and junctional (J_H) gene segments (1). Selection of these gene elements from their corresponding libraries of germ-line genes is governed by a site-specific, developmentally ordered process. In humans, the organization of the V_H locus has been completely delineated. This cluster comprises 6 functional J_H genes, more than 30 D_H segments, and approx 100 nonallelic V_H genes that have been categorized in at least 7 families. V_H gene members within a given family are highly homologous with >80% sequence identity, whereas the degree of homology between members of distinct families is usually <70%. Human V_H families vary in size ranging from one member in the V_H6 family to over 30 in the V_H3 family (2).

Little is known concerning the cellular and molecular basis of V gene repertoire expression during differentiation along the B-lymphocyte pathway. Much of what we know about V gene utilization stems from studies of EBV lines, hybridomas, and myelomas. Previous investigations have utilized large numbers of cells to analyze V gene utilization and have not provided direct information on the frequency of lymphocytes capable of expressing these genes. To eliminate potential bias

From: *Methods in Molecular Biology, Vol. 51: Antibody Engineering Protocols*
Edited by: S. Paul Humana Press Inc., Totowa, NJ

associated with hybridomas and other B-cell derivatives, we have developed an *in situ* hybridization approach that permits analysis of V_H gene expression in primary lymphocyte populations that consist of different subsets with distinct functional potentials. This technique is sensitive enough to detect V_H gene transcripts at the single-cell level. It allows determination of the distribution of Ig gene expression in heterogenous B-cell populations. High sensitivity of detection was made possible by several improvements in methodology, including optimized hybridization conditions to prevent nonspecific binding and use of radiolabeled cloned fragments. Positive hybridization results obtained with human B-cell clones, as well as peripheral lymphocytes, indicate the general applicability of the method. *In situ* hybridization will be a useful adjunct to other methods of determining Ig gene expression. With this technique in hand, it should now be possible to address a number of important questions concerning development of the antibody repertoire.

2. Materials

2.1. Isolation and Culture of Human Lymphocytes

1. 100 mM sodium pyruvate (mol wt, 100 Daltons): 2.75 mg/mL in water.
2. Nonessential amino acids: 100X.
3. 200 mM L-glutamine: 29.426 mg/mL.
4. Antibiotics: 10 mg/mL gentamicin sulfate, 50 mg/mL kanamycin (Gibco, Grand Island, NY), 1 g/10 mL streptomycin, 5×10^6 U/10 mL benzyl penicillin.
5. RPMI-1640.
6. RPMI+: 100 mL RPMI-1640 containing 10% FCS, 100 mM sodium pyruvate, 1X nonessential amino acids, 2 mM glutamine, 20 µg/mL gentamicin sulfate, 50 µg/mL kanamycin, 50 U/mL benzyl penicillin, 50 µg/mL streptomycin.
7. Ficoll-Hypaque (Pharmacia, Uppsala, Sweden).
8. Lymphoprep (Nyegaard, Oslo, Norway).
9. Monoclonal antibodies (MAb) to CD3, CD4, and CD8 (Becton Dickinson, Mountain View, CA) and surface immunoglobulins, CD20 and CD11b/CR3 (Ortho Diagnostics, Westwood, MA).
10. Percoll (Pharmacia).
11. Neuraminidase-treated sheep red blood cells (SRBC): Suspend SRBC at 5% v/v in RPMI-1640, incubate with neuraminidase (0.01 U/mL) for 30 min at 37°C, and then wash three times in RPMI containing 10% FCS preadsorbed with SRBC.

12. Heat-inactivated fetal calf serum (FCS).
13. FCS adsorbed with SRBC: Incubate 10 vol FCS with 1 vol of SRBC pellet for 30 min at 4°C. Centrifuge 15 min at 2000 rpm. Remove the adsorbed FCS, and store frozen at –70°C.

2.2. Cell Lines and Hybridomas

A number of human B-cell hybridomas and lines of known isotype and V gene family must be used as specificity controls for *in situ* hybridization. They are cultured in RPMI+ (*see* Section 2.1.) medium.

2.3. Activation of Lymphocyte Cultures

1. Formalin-treated *Staphylococcus aureus* (Cowan I strain; Calbiochem-Behring, La Jolla, CA).
2. Pokeweed mitogen (Gibco).

2.4. Cytocentrifugation

2.4.1. Coverslips

Use 12-mm-diameter coverslips, and treat them as follows prior to use:

1. Immerse in 1*N* HCl for 30 min.
2. Wash with double-distilled water (DDW).
3. Immerse in an ethanol/acetic acid (3/1) for 30 min.
4. Wash with 70% ethanol.
5. Rinse with DDW.
6. Siliconize with 1% Aquasil (Pierce, Rockford, IL) in H_2O for 5 min.
7. Rinse extensively with DDW.
8. Bake coverslips at 180°C for 2 h.
9. Keep in a covered container.

2.4.2. Glass Slides

Use prewashed and polished glass slides. Prior to use for cytocentrifugation, process as described in Section 2.4.1., steps 1–4. Then wipe the slides individually with sterile gauze.

2.4.3. Preparation of Cytocentrifuged Cells

1. 10X phosphate-buffered saline: 1X = 10 m*M* sodium phosphate, 140 m*M* NaCl, pH 7.4.
2. 4% paraformaldehyde: For 200 mL, weigh 8 g paraformaldehyde, add 100 mL water and 25 µL 10*N* NaOH, keep at 65°C in fume hood for 5 min, filter through Whatman 3 MM, and add 20 mL 10X PBS and water to 200 mL. Check and adjust pH to 7.5 with concentrated HCl.

2.5. V$_H$ Probe Preparation

All solutions must be made with diethylpyrocarbonate-treated RNase-free water (DEPC-water), and all glassware must be baked at 200°C for a least 2 h to inactivate RNases.

1. V$_H$ gene containing DNA: These can be prepared as restriction fragments from germ-line DNA or various cell lines (*see* Section 3.4.1.). These probes can also be obtained from T. Honjo (Osaka University, Medical School, Osaka, Japan), M. P. Lefranc (University of Montpellier, France), and P. Leder (Harvard University, Boston, MA). They have been described in detail elsewhere *(3–8)*.
2. Vectors for subcloning probe DNA: pBluescript (Stratagene, La Jolla, CA) or pT$_3$-/T$_7$-18 (Pharmacia).
3. Restriction enzymes: *Eco*RI, *Sac*I, *Sph*I, *Hpa*I, *Nco*I, *Bam*HI, *Hinc*II (Stratagene, La Jolla, CA).
4. 1 mg/mL proteinase K in DEPC water.
5. TE buffer: 10 mM Tris-HCl, pH 8.0, 10 mM WaCl, 1 mM EDTA, pH 8.0.
6. Phenol.
7. Chloroform.
8. 10.5M ammonium acetate in water.
9. 50 U/mL T$_3$ RNA polymerase and T$_7$ RNA polymerase (Stratagene).
10. 5X transcription buffer (Stratagene).
11. Dithiothreitol (DTT).
12. RNasin (Promega, Madison, WI).
13. 10 mM rATC, rCTP, rGTP (Promega).
14. [^{35}S]-UTP (800 Ci/mmol; Amersham SJ40383, Bucks, UK).
15. RNase-free DNase (Boehringer Mannheim, Indianapolis, IN).
16. Phenol-extracted total yeast RNA (Sigma, St. Louis, MO).

2.6. Hybridization

1. Acetic acid/triethanolamine: For 200 mL, mix 20 mL 1M triethanolamine and 0.5 mL of acetic anhydride.
2. 2X SSC: (1 x SSC = 0.15M NaCl, 0.015M sodium citrate).
3. 0.1M Tris-HCl, 0.1M glycine, pH 7.0.
4. Ethanol solutions for dehydration: 70, 90, and 100% in water.
5. Deionized formamide (Bethesda Research Lab, Gaithersburg, MD).
6. Hybridization buffer: 50% formamide, 10 mM DTT, 1 mg/mL phenol-extracted ethanol-precipitated yeast tRNA, 1 mg/mL denatured and sheared salmon sperm DNA, 2.5 mg/mL nuclease-free bovine serum albumin.
7. RNase A (Sigma).
8. RNase T1 (Boehringer).

2.7. Autoradiography

1. NTB-2 emulsion (Eastman Kodak, Rochester, NY).
2. Light-tight slide boxes.
3. D19 developer and Unifix fixer solutions (Eastman Kodak).
4. 10% Giemsa stain.
5. Eukitt (Bender and Hobein, Munich, Germany).
6. Bright-field and dark-field illumination microscope.

3. Methods

3.1. Preparation of Peripheral Human B-Cells

3.1.1. Total Peripheral Lymphocytes

1. Collect the buffy coat from peripheral blood.
2. Dilute the cells to 20 mL in RPMI-1640 containing 0.5% heparin.
3. Gently load the diluted cells on 15-mL of Ficoll-Hypaque in a 50-mL tube.
4. Centrifuge at 8000 rpm, 20 min in a Beckman centrifuge. Do not brake.
5. Collect the ring of white cells at the interphase with a Pasteur pipet and suspend in 10 mL RPMI.
6. Centrifuge cell suspension at 1800 rpm for 15 min. Resuspend pellet in RPMI, and wash twice more with the medium.

3.1.2. Removal of Adherent Cells

1. The cell pellet is resuspended in RPMI containing 5% of FCS, at a concentration of 2×10^6 cells/mL.
2. Transfer 40 mL of the suspension to a plastic tissue-culture flask, and incubate at 37°C in 5% CO_2 for 3 h or overnight.
3. Remove nonadherent cells with a pipet, and repeat step 2 in a fresh tissue-culture flask.

3.1.3. Removal of Rosette-Forming (E⁻) Cells (see Note 1)

1. In a round-bottomed 15-mL tube, mix $8–9 \times 10^7$ cells from step 3, Section 3.1.2., 2 mL of neuraminidase-treated SRBC, and 200 mL of absorbed fetal calf serum.
2. Centrifuge for 10 min at 1000 rpm, and then incubate the cell pellet for at least 2 h at 4°C on ice.
3. Gently resuspend the cells by inverting the tube several times. Dilute 1:10 with RPMI, and check the formation of rosettes under a microscope.
4. Load 9 mL of the suspension from step 3 on 5 mL of Lymphoprep gradient in a conical 15-mL tube.
5. Centrifuge for 30 min at 500*g* in a centrifuge. Do not brake.

6. Collect the E⁻ cells at the interphase of RPMI and Lymphoprep. Wash three times in RPMI-1640, and count the cells in a hemocytometer. These cells are used as B-cell-enriched lymphocytes (*see* Note 1).

3.1.4. Preparation of Resting B-Cells

1. Resuspend the cells from step 6, section 3.1.3. in 2 mL of 60% Percoll, and apply on a discontinuous gradient composed of layers of 2 mL 50% Percoll, 2 mL 40% Percoll, 2 mL 30% Percoll gradient, and 2 mL RPMI-1640.
2. Centrifuge 12 min at 2500 rpm without brake.
3. Collect the cells banding between 50 and 60% Percoll (high-density, resting cells).
4. Wash the cells twice, and count in a hemocytometer.

3.2. Activation of Lymphocyte Cultures

1. Culture lymphocytes from step 4, Section 3.1.4. at a concentration of 10^6 cells/mL in the presence of formalin-treated *S. aureus* Cowan I (SAC, 1:10,000) and pokeweed mitogen (PWM, 1:300) at 37°C in a 5% CO_2 incubator.
2. Maintain the cultures (10^6 cells/mL) under standard conditions for 5 d, at which time cells are harvested, washed, counted, and cytocentrifuged onto slides for analysis by *in situ* hybridization.

3.3. Cytocentrifuged Cell Preparations

1. Immerse glass slides in an ethanol-acetic acid (3/1) bath for 20 min, transfer to 70% ethanol, and air-dry.
2. Wash the cultured cells from step 2, Section 3.2, twice with RPMI.
3. Resuspend cells in RPMI containing 10% FCS at $2–4 \times 10^5$ cells/mL.
4. Load 0.5 mL ($1–2 \times 10^5$ cells) onto a glass slide from step 3 by cytocentrifugation at 700 rpm for 3 min.
5. Air-dry the cell preparation, and immediately fix in freshly made 4% paraformaldehyde for 5 min at 21°C.
6. Transfer the slides immediately into ice-cold 70% ethanol, and store at 4°C until hybridization is performed.

3.4. V_H Probes

3.4.1. Background

cDNA probes do not give optimal *in situ* hybridization signals. The use of RNA probes is recommended. The human Cμ probe is derived from an *Eco*RI 1.3-kb fragment, and the Cγ probe, from an *Sac*I-*Sph*I 2-kb fragment. The V_H2 probe is from an *Sca*I-*Hha*I 369-bp fragment initially cloned from CEM-SS cell line. The V_H1 probe is derived from an

*Nco*I-*Eco*RI 0.55-kb fragment, the V_H3 probe from an *Nco*I-*Pst*I 0.55-kb fragment, and the V_H4 probe from an *Eco*RI-*Bam*HI 0.4-kb fragment, all isolated from human germ-line DNA. The V_H5 probe is from an *Hinc*II-*Pst*I 0.38-kb fragment isolated from a null acute leukemia cell line, and the V_H6 probe, from an *Eco*RI-*Stu*I 0.3-kb fragment cloned from a pre-B acute leukemia cell line.

The probes are subcloned into pBluescript or pT_3/T_7-18 phagemid vectors. These vectors provide several convenient cloning sites located between bacteriophages T_3 and T_7 RNA polymerase promoters. DNA fragments cloned into these vectors are then transcribed in vitro to produce radiolabeled single-stranded antisense RNA probes complementary to mRNA encoding V_H antibody genes.

3.4.2. Preparation of the DNA Template

1. Digest the probe-containing vector (10 μg DNA) with the appropriate restriction enzyme.
2. Digest the reaction mixture with 200 μg/μL proteinase K. Incubate 30 min at 37°C.
3. Purify the cDNA restriction fragment by two phenol extractions and two chloroform extractions. Precipitate the aqueous phase with 22 μL 10.5*M* ammonium acetate and 250 μL ethanol for 30 min at –70°C.
4. Pellet by centrifugation. Wash pellet twice with 70% ethanol, vacuum-dry, and redissolve in 10 μL TE in DEPC water to 1 μg DNA/mL.
5. Confirm template cDNA purity by standard agarose gel electrophoresis.

3.4.3. Preparation of Sense and Antisense RNA Probes
(see Note 2)

In vitro transcription reactions are carried out with T_3 or T_7 RNA polymerases (Stratagcnc, La Jolla, CA) to generate [^{35}S]-radiolabeled single-stranded RNA probes. Linearized plasmid DNA are used as template for the synthesis of radioactive antisense RNA transcripts (T_3 polymerase products). Sense-strand transcripts are also transcribed from the opposite direction and used as negative controls (T_7 polymerase products). Approximately 2×10^8 dpm are incorporated into RNA/μg of DNA template.

1. Generate the RNA probe by mixing the following reagents. The reaction volume is 20 μL. Mix 4 μL 5X transcription buffer, 2 μL 100 m*M* dithiothreitol, 0.8 μL RNasin, 1 μL 10 m*M* rATP, 1 μL 10 m*M* rCTP, 1 μL 10 m*M* rGTP, 2 μL of template (1 μg of DNA from step 4, section

3.4.2.), 3 µL DEPC water, 5 µL $^{35}[S]$-UTP (800 Ci/mmol), and 1 µL T_3 RNA polymerase (50 U/mL). Incubate 90 min at 37°C.

2. Digest the reaction mixture with 1 µL of RNase-free DNase, and incubate for 15 min at 37°C.
3. Add 6 µL of phenol-extracted total yeast RNA (10 µg/mL) and 80 µL of DEPC water.
4. Count 2 µL of the mixture in a β-counter.
5. To remove free nucleotides, precipitate the RNA probe with 22 µL 10.5M ammonium acetate and 250 µL ethanol. Keep overnight at –20°C.
6. Wash pellet twice with 70% ethanol. Vacuum-dry.
7. Redissolve RNA pellet in 10 µL of TE containing 10 µM dithiothreitol in DEPC water.
8. Count a 0.5 µL aliquot in a β-counter.

3.5. In Situ *Hybridization* (see Note 3)

The *in situ* hybridization technique of Harper et al. *(9)* can be used as modified by Pardoll et al. *(10)* and Jeong et al. *(11)*. These procedures have been modified slightly for analysis of human V_H gene expression *(12)*.

1. Remove cytocentrifuged cells on slides from the 70% ethanol bath.
2. Wash in SSC for 1 min (twice).
3. Acetylate in acetic anhydride/triethanolamine for 10 min at room temperature.
4. Rinse twice with 2X SSC (1 min each).
5. Keep slides in 0.1M Tris-HCl, 0.1M glycine, pH 7.0, for 30 min at room temperature.
6. Rinse with 2X SSC for 1 min.
7. Dehydrate in graded concentrations of ethanol (70, 95, and 100%; 1–5 min in each solution).
8. Allow the slides to air-dry.
9. Pipet 7.5 µL hybridization buffer containing 0.5–2×10^6 dpm of the $[^{35}S]$-radiolabeled probe onto the cell button on each slide.
10. Heat the slides at 90°C for 8 min, and then cool for 1 min in an ice-water bath.
11. Gently place siliconized and baked coverslips (12-mm diameter) on top of the cell buttons, and seal with rubber cement.
12. Carry out hybridization reaction at 50°C for 18 h in a humidified chamber.
13. Wash the slides by successive incubations in 2X SSC containing 50% formamide for 3 min at 54°C, 2X SSC containing 50% formamide for 5 min, 2X SSC containing 50% formamide at 54°C with shaking for 1 h, and twice with SSC at 21°C for 1 min.

14. Incubate slides in 100 µg/mL RNase A, 1 mg/mL RNase T1 in 10 mM DTT, and 2X SSC for 30 min at 37°C (30 µL/slide under coverslip in a humidified chamber).
15. Wash slides successively in 2X SSC containing 10 mM DTT, 50% formamide at 54°C for 3 min, 2X SSC containing 50% formamide at 54°C for 5 min, 2X SSC containing 10 mM DTT, 50% formamide at 54°C with shaking for 1 h, and twice with SSC for 1 min.
16. Finally, dehydrate in 70% ethanol for 1 min, 95% ethanol for 1 min, and 100% ethanol for 1 min, and allow to air-dry.

3.6. Autoradiography (see Note 4)

1. Dip slides from step 16, Section 3.5. in the nuclear track NTB-2 emulsion diluted 1:2 with 0.4M ammonium acetate at 43°C in a dark room.
2. Allow to dry vertically at room temperature for 1 h.
3. Expose slides for 3–7 d at 4°C in light-tight slide boxes containing silica gel as desiccant.
4. Develop slides in D19 developer solution for 4 min, rinse in tap water, and fix for 5 min in Unifix.
5. Wash slides with tap water for 30 min, and counterstain in 10% Giemsa stain for 5 min.
6. Wash in tap water and air-dry. Cover cells with Eukitt, and examine under the microscope.

3.7. Quantification of V_H Gene-Family Usage (see Notes 5–8)

To assess the activity of each batch of labeled probes, slides with positive and negative control cells should be included in each experiment. Discrimination of positive and negative cells on test slides is achieved by including sense-strand controls in each experiment to provide an upper limit for background hybridization. Identically prepared slides are probed with appropriate [^{35}S]-labeled antisense RNA for V_H expression, as well as for Cµ and Cγ chain expression. Slides probed with [^{35}S]-labeled sense RNA are scored as background. Because of the relative ease of discerning positively labeled cells under dark-field illumination, some of the microscopic examinations are carried out using this method. In comparative experiments, we found that there was a very close agreement between the results obtained with dark-field and light-field illuminations. For each slide, positive cells within a constant area of the slide are enumerated. Replicates are averaged, and the number of cells that are labeled with the sense RNA probe were subtracted. A V_H gene family expression percentage is calculated by dividing the number of cells hybridizing to a given V_H gene family-specific antisense RNA probe by the total number of cells hybridizing to V_H antisense RNA probes.

4. Notes

1. The cell population in Section 3.3.1., step 6 contains more than 90% B-cells and <1% T-cells and 4% monocytes, as detected by FACS analysis using MAb to CD3, CD4, and CD8, and surface immunoglobulins, CD20 and CD11b/CR3. These cell preparations show no proliferative responses to T-cell mitogens, such as phytohemagglutinin.
2. Each probe must be tested by Southern blotting of human genomic DNA from unrelated individuals. The hybridization patterns should be characteristic of the corresponding V_H family.
3. Since the degree of nucleotide homology between members of different families may reach 80%, it is critical to establish experimental conditions under which V_H probes would hybridize specifically with the cells expressing the targeted V_H gene family members. It is also important to ensure the family specificity of the various probes used for *in situ* hybridization and define stringency conditions for washing procedures. To this end, the probes can be tested first on human hybridomas and B-cell clones expressing V_H known sequences.
4. Overexposed slide preparations should show low background signals, demonstrating a high specificity of the detected Ig gene expression signal.
5. When human hybridomas and B-cell clones are used, not every cell is labeled. This results from the fact that continuous in vitro propagation of cells generates a proportion of cells that do not make antibodies. This phenomenon is observed with both constant and variable gene probes.
6. Grain numbers are not usually counted, since the positively labeled cells have too many grains (Fig. 1). With exposure times of 6–7 d, the only labeled cells are strongly labeled. This suggests that the protocol primarily permits detection of cells with high levels of message. Also, the specific grain distribution suggests clustering of message within discrete regions of the cytoplasm.
7. The total number of cells counted/slide should range between 200 and 1000, depending on the frequency of positive cells.
8. The presence of unambiguous positive and negative cells within the same field, and conversion of all positive cells to negative cells by pretreatment with RNase should help prove that the detection system picks up specific hybridization signals.

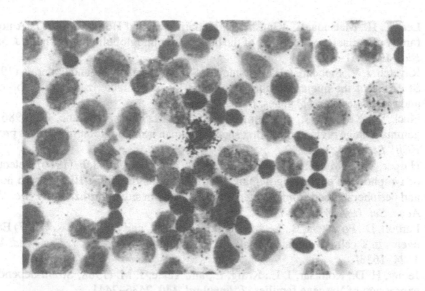

Fig. 1. Autoradiogram of Giemsa-stained cells hybridized *in situ* with a [^{35}S]-labeled V$_H$4 gene-family probe. Shown is a representative photomicrograph of in vitro activated human peripheral cells. For activation of peripheral lymphocytes, cells were cultured in the presence of PWM and *S. aureus* for 5 d. Cytocentrifuged preparations of cultured cells were hybridized with a [^{35}S]-labeled antisense single-stranded RNA probe specific for V$_H$4 transcripts. Control hybridization was performed with a sense V$_H$4-labeled probe. After a 4-d exposure, the slide was developed and counterstained with Giemsa. Note that silver grains are not positioned at the same level within the photoemulsion. Some grains are not distinctly observed and may appear out of focus in some cells.

References

1. Tonegawa, S. (1983) Somatic generation of antibody diversity. *Nature* **302,** 575–581.
2. Zouali, M. (1994) Unravelling antibody genes. *Nature Genetics* **7,** 118–120.
3. Kodaira, M., Kinashi, T., Umemura, I., Matsuda, F., Noma, T., Ono, Y., and Honjo, T. (1986) Organization and evolution of variable region genes of the human immunoglobulin heavy chain. *J. Mol. Biol.* **190,** 529–541.
4. Berman, J. E., Mellis, S. L., Pollock, R., Smith, C., Suh, H. Y., Heinke, B., Kowal, C., Surti, U., Chess, L., Cantor, C., and Alt, F. W. (1988) Content and organization of the human Ig V$_H$ locus: definition of three new V$_H$ families and linkage to the IgCH locus. *EMBO J.* **7,** 727–738.
5. Humphries, C. G., Shen, A., Kuziel, W. A., Capra, J. D., Blattner, F. R., and Tucker, P. W. (1988) Characterization of a new human immunoglobulin V$_H$ family that shows preferential rearrangement in immature B-cell tumors. *Nature* **331,** 446–449.

6. Lee, K. H., Matsuda, F., Kinashi, T., Kodaira, M., and Honjo, T. (1987) A novel family of variable region genes of the human immunoglobulin heavy chain. *J. Mol. Biol.* **195,** 761–768.

7. Ravetch, J. V., Siebentist, U., Korsmeyer, S. J., Waldmann, T., and Leder, P. (1981) Structure of the human immunoglobulin μ locus: characterization of embryonic and rearranged J and D genes. *Cell* **27,** 583–591.

8. Huck, S., Keyeux, G., Ghanem, N., Lefranc, M. P., and Lefranc, G. (1986) A gamma 3 hinge region probe: first specific human immunoglobulin subclass probe. *FEBS Lett.* **208,** 221–230.

9. Harper, M. E., Marseille, L. M., Gallo, R. C., and Wong-Staal, F. (1986) Detection of lymphocytes expressing human T-lymphotropic virus type-III in lymph nodes and peripheral blood from infected individuals by in situ hybridization. *Proc. Natl. Acad. Sci. USA.* **83,** 772–776.

10. Pardoll, D., Fowlkers, B., Lechler, R., Germain, R., and Schwartz, R. (1987) Early events in T cell development analyzed by in situ hybridization. *J. Exp. Med.* **165,** 1624–1638.

11. Jeong, H. D., Komisar, J. L., Kraig, E., and Teale, J. M. (1988) Strain-dependent expression of V_H gene families. *J. Immunol.* **140,** 2436–2441.

12. Zouali, M. and Thèze, J. (1991) Probing V_H gene family utilization in human peripheral B cells by *in situ* hybridization. *J. Immunol.* **146,** 2855–2864.

CHAPTER 6

Purification of Reduced and Alkylated Antibody Subunits

Mei Sun and Sudhir Paul

1. Introduction

Antigen-binding sites in antibodies are formed by the variable regions of light (L) and heavy (H) chains. Delineation of antigen interactions with the individual subunits of antibodies is of interest for several reasons, including:

1. Free L chains are present within B-lymphocytes and in the circulation of patients with certain types of B-lymphocyte tumors (1,2);
2. Derivation of high-affinity antibodies in vitro from randomly combined libraries of L and H chains is dependent on pairing of subunits that display appropriate interactions with each other and the antigen (3); and
3. Pairing of L and H chains from different antibodies may permit the development of new functions in the hybrid. For example, pairing of a catalytic L chain with H chains with a defined antigen-binding specificity could generate a catalyst with specificity dictated by the H chain.

Early work conducted following the definition of antibody subunit structure (4,5) showed that the individual H and L chains in antibodies can independently recognize antigens. These studies were hampered by several limitations in technologies available in the early 1960s. The development of rapid protein-purification methods, coupled with techniques to raise monoclonal antibodies (MAb) and recombinant fragments of antibodies has led to a renewed interest in the properties of the individual subunits of antibodies. Here, we describe methods to prepare pure L chains from polyclonal antibodies and MAb in a form suitable for study

From: *Methods in Molecular Biology, Vol. 51: Antibody Engineering Protocols*
Edited by: S. Paul Humana Press Inc., Totowa, NJ

of their binding and catalytic activities. Two specific examples are provided. The first deals with purification of the antibody subunits under denaturing conditions to rule out the possibility of adventitious protease contaminants *(6,7)*. The second example deals with L-chain purification from polyclonal antibodies under relatively gentle conditions, permitting retention of their native high-activity characteristics *(8)*.

H and L chains are held together by disulfide bonds and by noncovalent interactions. The disulfide bonds must be reduced, and the noncovalent interactions must be minimized in order to obtain pure antibody subunits by chromatography. The reduction should be done under gentle conditions so that intramolecular disulfide bonds are not opened. Following reduction, SH groups are alkylated to prevent reformation of disulfide bonds. The problem of noncovalent association of H and L chains during purification can be solved by use of denaturants like urea, sodium dodecyl sulfate, and guanidinium chloride, and extreme pH solvents like propionic acid. The use of denaturants is often associated with irreversible precipitation or loss of activity. However, a subpopulation of protein molecules can usually be renatured into an active conformation capable of interaction with antigen. On renaturation of resolved H- and L-chain preparations, dimers and higher-order H–H and L–L chain aggregates can be formed. These aggregation phenomena are not unique to reduced and alkylated antibody subunits. Recombinant F_v molecules also display similar intermolecular association *(9)*.

In the case of polyclonal preparations, subunits derived from different antibodies may form heterologous L–L chain and H–H chain complexes. This may lead to suppression of antigen-binding activity in incorrectly paired antibody subunits. Interesting new specificities and activities could also be generated owing to this inadvertent "hybridization" of the subunits. Notwithstanding these complexities, further studies with antibody subunits can be expected to lead to delineation of the role of the individual subunits in antibody–antigen interaction and a better understanding of the pathophysiological role of free antibody subunits found in vivo.

2. Materials

2.1. Equipment and Chemicals

1. UV/visible spectrophotometer (Ultrospec III, Pharmacia LKB, Piscataway, NJ).
2. Centrifuge (RT 6000D, Sorvall, DuPont, Boston, MA).

3. γ-Counter: 80% efficiency (COBRA™ Auto-GAMMA®, Packard, Meriden, CT).
4. Shaking water bath (American).
5. Centricon-10 or Centriprep-10 concentrators (Amicon, Beverly, MA).
6. Millex-GV4 0.22- and 0.45-μm filters (Millipore, Bedford, MA).
7. HPLC system equipped with absorbance detector (ISCO, Lincoln, NE).
8. Fraction Collector (Foxy 200, ISCO).
9. Microdialysis system and dialysis membrane (28-well, 12–14 kDa cutoff, GIBCO BRL, Gaithersburg, MD).
10. Dialysis tubing (12–14 kDa cutoff, SpectraPor, Huston, TX).
11. PhastSystem, Phast gradient gels (8–25%) and PhastGel SDS buffer strips (Pharmacia).
12. Nitrocellulose membrane (0.45 μm, Trans-Blot®, Bio-Rad, Hercules, CA).
13. Albumin, bovine (BSA) (Sigma, St. Louis, MO).
14. Ammonium sulfate (Sigma).
15. 2-mercaptoethanol (2-ME) (Sigma).
16. Iodoacetamide (Sigma).
17. Guanidine hydrochloride (GdmCl) (Sigma).
18. Bicinchoninic acid (BCA) protein assay kit (Pierce Chemical Co., Rockford, IL).
19. Sodium dodecyl sulfate (SDS) (Bio-Rad).
20. PhastGel silver-staining kit (Pharmacia).
21. PhastGel Blue R (Pharmacia).
22. Diaminobenzidine (DAB) (Sigma).
23. TRIZMA-HCl and TRIZMA-base (Sigma).

2.2. Antibodies

1. Rabbit antihuman L-chain (κ) antibody (Axèll, Westbury, NY).
2. Rabbit antihuman L-chain (λ) antibody (Axèll).
3. Rabbit antihuman H-chain (γ) antibody (Axèll).
4. Rabbit antimouse L-chain (κ) antibody (Cappel, Westchester, PA).
5. Rabbit antimouse H-chain (γ) antibody (Axèll).
6. Goat antirabbit IgG peroxidase conjugate (Cappel).

2.3. Chromatography Matrices

1. Protein-G Sepharose (Pharmacia) or FPLC protein-G Superose column (Pharmacia).
2. Superose-12 columns (Pharmacia).
3. Econo-Pac 10DG column (Bio-Rad).
4. Immobilized papain (Pierce Chemical Co.).
5. Protein-A agarose (Pierce Chemical Co.).
6. CNBr-activated Sepharose-4B (Pharmacia).

2.4. Buffers (see Notes 1 and 2)

1. Buffer A: 50 mM Tris-HCl, pH 7.3.
2. Buffer B: 0.1M glycine-HCl, pH 2.7, 0.025% Tween-20.
3. Buffer C: 50 mM Tris-HCl, pH 7.3, 0.025% Tween-20, 0.02% NaN$_3$.
4. Buffer D: 20 mM cysteine, 20 mM sodium phosphate, 10 mM EDTA, pH 7.0.
5. Buffer E: 20 mM Tris-HCl, 0.5M NaCl, 1% BSA, 0.05% Tween-20, pH 7.4.
6. Phosphate-buffered saline (PBS); 0.01M phosphate buffer, 0.0027M potassium chloride, 0.137M sodium chloride, pH 7.4 (made from Sigma tablets).

3. Methods
3.1. Preparation of MAb

1. Dilute ascites fluid containing the antibody with 1 vol of buffer A at 4°C.
2. Mix the ascites fluid slowly with an equal volume of saturated ammonium sulfate in ice, and stir for 3 h at 4°C.
3. Centrifuge (5000g, 20 min, 4°C) and decant supernatant.
4. Resuspend the pellet in ice-cold 45% saturated ammonium sulfate, and repeat step 3.
5. Dissolve the pellet in buffer A (volume equivalent to that of starting ascites fluid), and dialyze against this buffer at 4°C. Read optical density at 280 nm. An optical density reading of 1.0 (1-cm path length) corresponds to approx 0.8 mg protein/mL.
6. Wash an appropriate amount of protein-G Sepharose (the gel-binding capacity is ~20 mg IgG/mL drained gel) with 5 vol of water (three times), buffer B (twice), 1M acetic acid (once), and water (four times).
7. Pour the gel in a column, and equilibrate with buffer A (at least three column volumes). A flow rate of 1 mL/min can be used for a 1.0-cm diameter column.
8. Centrifuge the dialyzed sample at 10,000g for 10 min, filter through a 0.22-µM filter, and apply to the column.
9. Wash the column with buffer A until the optical density at 280 nm returns to baseline.
10. Elute IgG with buffer B. Collect 1-mL fraction into tubes containing of 50 µL of 1M Tris-HCl, pH 9.0. This will bring up the pH to 7.8.
11. Run buffer A until the effluent pH is neutral. Store the protein-G Sepharose gel in 20% ethanol (*see* Notes 3 and 4).

3.2. Preparation of MAb Subunits
3.2.1. Reduction and Alkylation of IgG

1. Incubate IgG (about 5 mg/mL) with 0.2M 2-mercaptoethanol in 50 mM Tris-HCl, pH 8.0, and 0.15M NaCl for 3 h at room temperature (24°C).

2. Add iodoacetamide to 0.3M, and maintain the pH at 8.0 by addition of 1M Tris base. Incubate for 15 min at room temperature.
3. Dialyze the reaction mixture against buffer C.
4. Concentrate the sample to 0.1 mL with Centricon-10 (Amicon). Mix with 0.4 mL of 6M GdmCl, pH 6.5, and concentrate again to 0.1 mL. Remove sample. Wash the ultrafiltration membrane with an additional 0.4 mL of 6M GdmCl, pH 6.5. Pool the wash with the sample and filter through a 0.22-µM filter.

3.2.2. Purification of Antibody Subunits

1. Connect two Superose-12 columns (Pharmacia) in series and equilibrate with 3 column volumes of 6M GdmCl, pH 6.5 (~100 mL).
2. Load the sample (reduced and alkylated IgG, 5 mg in 0.5 ml) on the column, and elute with 6M GdmCl, pH 6.5, at a flow rate of 0.4 mL/min.
3. Dialyze an aliquot (50 µL) of the early and late eluting protein fractions corresponding to the heavy (H)-chain and the light (L)-chain peaks, respectively, against buffer C. (Note 5). The retention times of the H and L chains in our HPLC system are 54–56 and 60–66 min, respectively (Fig. 1).
4. Analyze the fractions by SDS-electrophoresis under reducing condition to confirm purity (H-chain, ~60 kDa; L chain, ~25 kDa) (*see* Section 3.4.).
5. Pool fractions containing pure H chain and L chain.

3.2.3. Renaturation of Antibody Subunits (see Note 6)

1. Read optical density of H- and L-chain pools at 280 nm.
2. Adjust the protein concentration to 24 µM by dilution with 6M GdmCl. Then dilute 1:60-fold in dialysis buffer. The final protein concentration is 0.4 µM and the GdmCl concentration is 0.1M.
3. Incubate for 1 h at room temperature with stirring.
4. Transfer the sample into a dialysis tubing (12–14 kDa cutoff), and dialyze against the same buffer for 2 d at 4°C with three buffer changes. The final GdmCl concentration is <1µM.
5. The antibody subunits are ready for antigen-binding assay (Fig. 2) and hydrolysis assay (*see* Huang et al., this vol.).

3.3. Preparation of L-Chains
Without Denaturation (see Note 7)

The method described as follows has been used to purify polyclonal L-chains under "native conditions" *(8).* The method is based on our unpublished observations that gel filtration of Fab (~50 kDa) usually yields a small second peak, corresponding to a mixture of L-chains and half-H chains (Fd fragments). Apparently, noncovalent association of L-

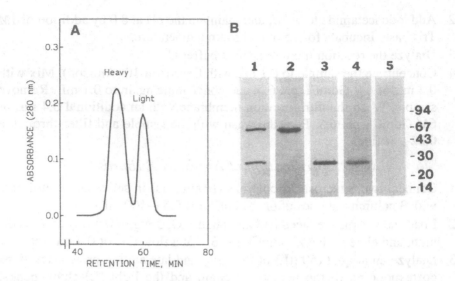

Fig. 1. Separation of the H and L chains of a monoclonal anti-VIP antibody by gel filtration. The antibody (5 mg) was reduced, alkylated, and subjected to gel filtration in 6*M* guanidinium chloride, pH 6.5, as described in the text (A). Pooled fractions corresponding to the H-chain peak (retention time: 54–56 min) and the L-chain peak (retention time: 60–66 min) were electrophoresed (8–25% polyacrylamide gels) under reducing conditions and stained with silver (lanes 2 and 3, respectively) (B). Lane 1 shows a silver-stained gel of the parent antibody electrophoresed under reducing conditions. Lanes 4 and 5 are immunoblots of the L-chain fraction stained with antibody to mouse L chain and H chain, respectively (data from ref. 6).

chains with Fd fragments is weaker than with full-length H-chains. Thus, if reduced and alkylated Fab is maintained at low protein concentrations, the subunits can be resolved by affinity chromatography.

3.3.1. Preparation of IgG from Human Plasma

This is done essentially as in Section 3.1.

3.3.2. Preparation of Fab

1. Adjust the IgG concentration to 10 mg/mL, and dialyze the IgG against 20 m*M* sodium phosphate, 10 m*M* EDTA, pH 7.0, at 4°C.
2. Wash 0.5 mL of 50% slurry of immobilized papain with 4 mL of buffer D twice. Prepare this buffer immediately before use. Cysteine in this buffer is a papain-stabilizer.

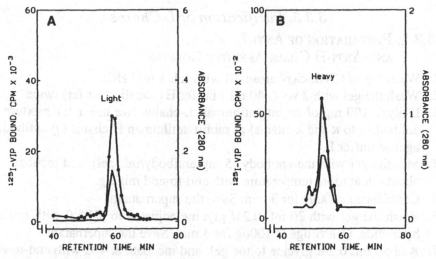

Fig. 2. Saturable binding of (tyr[10]-^{125}I)VIP by purified L chains (A) and H chains (B). Pooled L chains (500 μg) and H chains (135 μg) from Fig. 1 were rechromatographed in 6M guanidinium chloride on a gel-filtration column (Superose-12). The fractions were renatured by dialysis, and binding of (tyr[10]-^{125}I)VIP (0.1 nM) by duplicate aliquots (L chains, 20 μl; H chains, 50 μl) of the column fractions was measured (data from ref. 6).

3. Resuspend the papain gel in 0.5 mL buffer D, and mix with 0.5 mL of IgG (5 mg). The ratio is 10 mg IgG/mL settled papain gel.

4. Incubate at 37°C for 5 h in a water bath with vigorous shaking.

5. Add 1.5 mL of 10 mM Tris-HCl, pH 7.5 and centrifuge at 1000g for 5 min.

6. Remove the supernatant, and add iodoacetamide to 0.5M. This will inactivate any papain released from the gel (papain is a cysteine protease).

7. Filter the sample through a 0.22-μm filter and chromatograph on a protein-A agarose column. Run this column using the same procedures as the protein-G Sepharose column, except: (a) the protein A-agarose column is equilibrated in 10 mM Tris-HCl, pH 7.5, and (b) the gel is regenerated after each use with 0.1M of citric acid, pH 3.0, and stored in 0.05% NaN₃.

8. Collect the unretained material. This contains Fab. The retained fraction is composed of Fc fragments and undigested IgG.

9. Pool the Fab fractions from the protein-A agarose column, and concentrate to <1 mL on Centriprep-10 concentrator (Amicon).

10. Apply the protein to a Superose-12 column (0.5 mL/min). Use buffer C for elution. Fab is normally eluted at retention time 24–25 min from our HPLC system.

3.3.3. Purification of L-Chains

3.3.3.1. PREPARATION OF ANTI-L
AND ANTI-H CHAIN AFFINITY COLUMNS

1. Wash 5 g of CNBr-Sepharose 4B with 1 L 1 mM HCl.
2. Wash the gel with 2 vol (~40 mL) buffer E (coupling buffer) twice.
3. Dialyze 100 mg of rabbit antihuman L-chains (we use a 1:1 mixture of antibodies to κ and λ chains) or rabbit antihuman H-chains (γ) antibodies against buffer E.
4. Mix the gel with the antibody (5 mg antibody/mL gel), and incubate for about 4 h at room temperature with end-to-end mixing.
5. Centrifuge at 1000g for 3 min. Save the supernatant.
6. Wash the gel with 20 mL 0.2M glycine adjusted to pH 8.0 with sodium hydroxide. Centrifuge at 1000g for 3 min. Save the supernatant.
7. Add 50 mL 0.2M glycine to the gel, and incubate at 4°C with end-to-end mixing overnight (16–24 h). This saturates excess amine-reactive sites on the gel.
8. Centrifuge at 1000g for 3 min. Save the supernatant.
9. Wash the gel with 500 mL each of 0.1M NaHCO$_3$ and 0.5M NaCl, pH 8.3, followed by 500 mL of 0.1M sodium acetate, and 0.5M NaCl, pH 4.0. Repeat six times. Washing can be done rapidly using a sintered funnel.
10. Wash the gel with buffer C until the effluent pH is neutral. Store the gel in this buffer at 4°C.
11. Assay the protein concentration in aliquots of each saved supernatant and the starting antibody preparation by the bicinchoninic acid (BCA) method, using bovine serum albumin as standard.
12. Calculate coupling efficiency. This is generally >90% using this procedure.

3.3.3.2. REDUCTION AND ALKYLATION OF FAB

Do this as described in Section 3.2.1. using Fab instead of IgG as starting material.

3.3.3.3. PURIFICATION OF L-CHAINS BY AFFINITY CHROMATOGRAPHY

1. Wash the anti-L-chain Sepharose gel (5 mL) twice with 30 mL buffer C containing 0.5M NaCl.
2. Resuspend the gel in same buffer, and mix with 1 mg of the reduced and alkylated Fab. **Keep protein concentration at <30 μg/mL.**
3. Incubate at 4°C with end-to-end mixing overnight (16–24 h).
4. Centrifuge at 1000g for 5 min. Save the supernatant.
5. Resuspend the gel in buffer E containing 0.5M NaCl, and pack into column.

6. Run buffer through the gel (flow rate 0.5 mL/min) until the absorbance at 280 returns to baseline. Save the effluent. This contains mainly Fd fragments.
7. Elute bound L-chains with buffer B. Collect 1-mL fractions in tubes containing 50 µl of $1M$ Tris-HCl, pH 9.0.
8. Run buffer C through the column until the effluent pH is neutral. Store the gel in this buffer at 4°C.
9. Analyze the eluted L-chain fractions by SDS-PAGE (*see* Section 3.4.) and immunoblotting using anti-H- and anti-L-chain antibodies (*see* Section 3.5.). The L-chain should display a single band at 25 kDa, which is blotted only with anti-L-chain antibody.
10. If the L-chain preparation is still contaminated with Fd fragments (shown by immunoblotting with anti-H-chain antibody), the sample can be chromatographed further on an anti-H-chain Sepharose column using essentially the same procedures as described above. L-chains are recovered in the unbound fraction. Using this procedure, the purity of our L-chain preparations is >95%.

3.4. SDS-PAGE

1. Adjust the protein concentration to ~20 µg/mL for silver staining or to ~200 µg/mL for Coomassie blue staining.
2. Treat with 2.5% SDS with or without 20 mM 2-ME in a boiling water bath for 5 min.
3. Run electrophoresis on polyacrylamide gels using a Phastsystem or any easy-to-use electrophoresis system. Stain the gels with silver or Coomassie blue using standard protocols available in protein chemistry manuals.

3.5. Western Blotting

1. Run electrophoresis as in Section 3.4.
2. Transfer proteins to nitrocellulose (Trans-Blot®, Bio-Rad) by diffusion blotting at 50°C for 30 min (*see* Note 8).
3. Block the membrane in 20 mM Tris-HCl, 0.5M NaCl, 3% BSA, and 0.05% Tween-20, pH 7.4, for 30 min at room temperature with shaking. Then wash the membrane twice with buffer E.
4. Incubate the membrane in first antibody for 1 h at room temperature with shaking on a rocking platform. For identification of human antibody subunits, incubate with appropriately diluted rabbit antihuman L-chain (κ/λ) antibodies or rabbit antihuman H-chain (γ) antibodies. For mouse antibody subunits, use rabbit antimouse L-chain (κ) antibody and rabbit antimouse H-chain (Fc) antibody. Most commercially available antibody preparations function well at dilutions of 1:500 to 1:2000.
5. Wash three times with buffer E.

6. Incubate for 1 h with second antibody. We use a goat antirabbit IgG peroxidase conjugate (Cappel, 1:1000).
7. Wash twice with buffer E and once with PBS.
8. Develop the membrane in 0.5 mg/mL DAB and 0.03% hydrogen peroxide in PBS. Control IgG electrophoresed under reducing conditions should display two bands at 60 and 25 kDa that are blotted with anti H-chain, and anti L-chain antibodies, respectively. Fab analyzed under nonreducing conditions show a single band at 50 kDa, which is blotted with both anti-H-chain (γ) and anti-L-chain antibodies. Reducing electrophoresis of pure L-chain preparations reveals a single 25-kDa band blotted only with anti-L-chain antibody. Pure H-chains appear as a 60-kDa band blotted only with anti H-chain antibody.

4. Notes

1. Buffers are made in distilled, deionized water (Milli-Q UF plus system).
2. Buffers for chromatography are filtered through 0.22- or 0.45-μm filters and degassed before use.
3. The wash procedure in step 6 should be performed between purification of different samples to prevent possible IgG carryover.
4. Up to 10 mg IgG can be rapidly purified using an FPLC protein-G Superose column (Pharmacia). The procedure is essentially as in Section 3.1.
5. $6M$ GdmCl precipitates when mixed with the electrophoresis buffer, necessitating dialysis prior to electrophoresis. If the protein concentration is sufficiently large, the fraction can be diluted 1:100 in buffer C and electrophoresis performed directly.
6. The protein-refolding step is a sensitive procedure. Variations in experimental conditions produce major changes in antigen-binding and hydrolytic activity (Fig. 3). The important general variables are: protein concentration, constitution of the refolding buffer, pH, temperature, and presence of antigen during refolding. In our hands, the concentration at which an anti-VIP L-chain was refolded governed the magnitude of its catalytic activity *(7)*. Higher specific activity was observed at lower L-chain concentrations (0.16 μM), suggesting a negative influence of aggregation during refolding. Inclusion of excess antigen (50 μM VIP) permitted refolding of an anti-VIP L-chain at higher concentration (2 μM) with retention of hydrolytic activity.
7. The association constants for reduced and alkylated antibody subunits are usually 10^4–$10^6 M^{-1}$, but in some cases may be as high as $10^{10} M^{-1}$ *(2,10)*. To prepare L-chains and Fd fragments to satisfactory purity by affinity chromatography, it is necessary to avoid high concentration of L/Fd mixtures at all steps. This minimizes concentration-dependent aggregation effects.

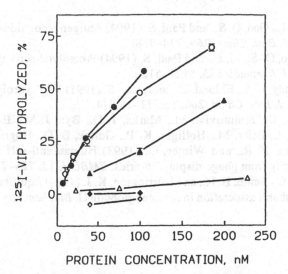

PROTEIN CONCENTRATION, nM

Fig. 3. (Y^{10}-^{125}I)VIP hydrolysis by c23.5 L-chain refolded at the following protein concentrations: (●), 0.16 μM; (▲), 0.4 μM; (△), 1.6 μM. (○) Denotes L chain refolded at 2 μM in the presence of 50 μM VIP. Refolding of c23.5 H chain (◇) and the irrelevant L chain purified from a commercially available myeloma protein (◆) was at 0.16 and 0.4 μM, respectively. Incubation of radiolabeled VIP (50 pM) with antibody subunits was for 16 h. Values are means of three replicates ± SD (data from ref. 7).

8. Greater than 50% of the proteins are blotted onto the nitrocellulose by this method, estimated from the intensity of the antibody subunit bands visualized by staining of the gels with silver.

References

1. Hopper, J. E. and Papagiannes, E. (1986) Evidence by radioimmunoassay that mitogen activated human blood mononuclear cells secrete significant amounts of light chain Ig unassociated with heavy chain. *Cell. Immunol.* **101,** 122–131.
2. Stevens, F. J., Solomon, A., and Schiffer, M. (1991) Bence Jones proteins: a powerful tool for the fundamental study of protein chemistry and pathophysiology. *Biochemistry* **30,** 6803–6805.
3. Gherardi, E. and Milstein, C. (1992) Original and artificial antibodies. *Nature* **357,** 201–202.
4. Fleischman, J. B., Porter, R. R., and Press, E. M. (1963) The arrangement of the peptide chains in γ-globulin. *Biochem. J.* **88,** 220–228.
5. Edelman, G. M., Olins, D. E., Gally, J. A., and Zinder, N. D. (1963) Reconstitution of immunologic activity by interaction of polypeptide chains of antibodies. *Proc. Natl. Acad. Sci. USA* **50,** 753–761.

6. Sun, M., Li, L., Gao, Q. S., and Paul, S. (1994) Antigen recognition by an antibody light chain. *J. Biol. Chem.* **269,** 734–738.
7. Sun, M., Gao, Q.-S., Li, L., and Paul, S. (1994) Proteolytic activity of an antibody light chain. *J. Immunol.* **153,** 5121–5126.
8. Sun, M., Mody, B. S., Eklund, H., and Paul, S. (1991) VIP hydrolysis by antibody light chains. *J. Biol. Chem.* **266,** 15,571–15,574.
9. Griffiths, A. D., Malmqvist, M., Marks, J. D., Bye, J. M., Embleton, M. J., McCafferty, J., Baier, M., Holliger, K. P., Gorick, B. D., Hughes-Jones, N. C., Hoogenboom, H. R., and Winter, G. (1993) Human anti-self antibodies with high\specificity from phage display libraries. *EMBO J.* **12,** 725–734.
10. Bigelow, C. C., Smith, B. R., and Dorrington, K. J. (1974) Equilibrium and kinetic aspects of subunit association in immunoglobulin G. *Biochemistry* **13,** 4602–4608.

CHAPTER 7

Murine Monoclonal Antibody Development

Donald R. Johnson

1. Introduction

Major advances in the analysis of biomolecular structure have emerged from the development of highly specific monoclonal antibodies (MAb) by Köhler and Milstein in 1975 *(1)*. MAb are produced from hybridoma cell lines that secrete a single species of antibody to a unique antigen. The advantages of MAb as reagents for antibody engineering are:

1. They are extremely pure immunological reagents that can be produced by immunization with a heterogenous antigenic preparation;
2. They are homogenous with respect to affinity and specificity;
3. The specificity of the antibody is directed to a single epitope;
4. The desired MAb can be selected for activity, affinity, and subclass by applying appropriate screening methods; and
5. Virtually unlimited quantities of MAb can be produced.

1.1. Antigens and Immunization Protocols

The procedure for induction of MAb is similar to the production of polyclonal antibodies. The ability to generate high titers of circulating antibodies varies with the chemical nature of the antigen, the animal used, and the immunization protocol. The use of a purified antigen for immunization increases the probability of obtaining hybridomas producing specific antibodies. Whole cells, membrane-enriched fractions, purified receptors, protein antigens produced by expression in prokaryotic or eukaryotic cells, and synthetic peptides have been successfully used as

From: *Methods in Molecular Biology, Vol. 51: Antibody Engineering Protocols*
Edited by: S. Paul Humana Press Inc., Totowa, NJ

immunogens. Immunization with impure antigens creates antibodies to contaminants that must be selected against during clonal screening. The antigen must be of sufficient molecular weight (>1000 Dalton) and be recognized as a foreign molecule by the host. This is because the antigen must be recognized by both T-and B-cells cooperatively in order to stimulate B-cell differentiation and antibody production. Molecules too small to stimulate an immune response can be conjugated to larger carrier proteins. Such hapten molecules are coupled to the carrier proteins (often serum albumin or keyhole limpet hemocyanin [KLH]) via N-terminal and lysine amino groups, C-terminal carboxyl groups, or cysteine sulfhydryl groups. Tramontano et al. and others have used the conjugation of enzymatic transition-state analogs with KLH to create an immunogen to induce antibodies that displayed enzymatic properties *(2)*.

Balb/c mice are the most common hosts for immunization, since many of the myeloma cell lines available for fusion are of Balb/c origin *(3)*. Young adult (8–12 wk) females are generally used and consistently produce a vigorous immune response to most antigens. Other strains of mice or even rats may be used if Balb/c mice do not produce the antibodies of interest.

Adjuvants activate the immune response and act as a depot for slow release of antigen. Thus, successful immunization occurs in the presence of adjuvant using smaller amounts of immunogens or with poorly immunogenic substances. Traditionally, complete Freund's adjuvant has been used with the primary immunization, but the side effects of this potent adjuvant are severe and its use is becoming restricted. Two synthetic adjuvants that have been used with equal success without the severe side effects of Freund's adjuvant are RIBI Adjuvant System and TiterMax™.

The immunization protocol most commonly used involves a primary ip injection of antigen with adjuvant and a secondary boost 3 wk later to induce a high-affinity IgG response. For protein antigens, 50–100 µg/ mouse are recommended for the preliminary injections. Shortly afterward (7–10 d), the immunized mice can be bled from the retro-bulbar plexus to measure antibody levels against the antigen and determine if further booster injections are necessary. A final booster challenge is then administered to induce activated B-cells, which preferentially fuse to the myeloma partners. This final boost is usually given intravenously without adjuvant. Intrasplenic injection is also highly effective in that antigen is delivered directly to splenic B-cells. The spleen is removed

3–4 d later when it appears to contain the greatest number of antibody-producing cells.

1.2. Fusion and Cloning

Also critical for MAb development is an appropriate myeloma fusion partner to provide the genetic information for continued cell division in culture. The myeloma cell lines arose from mineral oil-induced mouse plasmacytomas and have been selected for growth in tissue culture, inability to secrete or synthesize immunoglobulins, and possession of a selectable marker that is reconstituted following fusion with the plasma cell partner. The selectable marker most commonly used in the myeloma cells is a deficiency for the enzyme hypoxanthine-phosphoribosyl-transferase (HGPRT), which is involved in the salvage pathway for purine synthesis. HGPRT-deficient myeloma cells die in medium containing hypoxanthine, aminopterin, and thymidine (HAT). It is advisable to monitor the myeloma cells for possible reversion by determining sensitivity to HAT-containing medium. In addition to HAT sensitivity, it is important to use myeloma cells that are free of mycoplasma, since infected cells have lower hybridization frequency and the hybrid cells often die following fusion. Best fusion frequency occurs with myeloma cells in a logarithmic growth phase. These are usually expanded by a daily 1:2 split for 3 d before cell fusion. Two commonly used myeloma cell line partners for hybridoma formation are P3/NS-1/1-Ag4-1 (NS-1) and Sp2/0-Ag14 (Sp2/0). NS-1 *(4)* is a very efficient fusion partner that secretes κ light (L) chain following lymphocyte hybridization. Sp2/0 *(5)* does not constitutively secrete either heavy or light chains, but displays a more variable efficiency of fusion. Both of these cell lines will also form stable hybridomas with mouse, rat, and hamster B-cells.

Fusion of splenic B-lymphocytes from an immunized host and a myeloma cell line partner results in a somatic hybrid with the properties of both parent cells. The optimal conditions for fusion require an efficient cell fusogen and a selection system for hybrid cells. High-molecular-weight polymers of polyethylene glycol (PEG) are potent fusing agents for most cell types and are relatively nontoxic. PEG induces cell membrane fusion by formation of aggregates in which extensive areas of membrane are brought in close approximation. Fusions occur via lipid–lipid interaction with the formation of small cytoplasmic bridges. PEG also induces changes in membrane permeability, resulting in cell swelling and the formation of spherical fused cells with two or more nuclei. PEG-induced fusion is most efficiently performed at 37°C, pH 8, at a concentration of 50% (w/v) PEG of mol wt 1500–4000 at a myeloma to spleen cell ratio of 1:4. These conditions favor maximal fusion frequencies with minimal PEG toxicity.

A strong selection system for hybrid fused cells depends on the drug selection marker, HGPRT deficiency, which is present in the myeloma fusion partner. Culture in HAT medium will only allow growth of the heterokaryons consisting of myeloma cells fused with normal spleen cells (hybridomas), since unfused myeloma cells are lethally sensitive to aminopterin and unfused spleen cells survive only a few days in culture. To increase the outgrowth of viable hybridomas, thymocyte feeder suspensions or a source of hybridoma growth factors can be added to the fusion mixture. Hybridomas are apparent usually within 5 d, and by 10–14 d postfusion, antibody secretion can be detected.

1.3. Selection of Antibody-Producing Clones

Screening for specific antibody-producing hybridomas is the most critical step in the production of MAb. The purpose of the screening is to identify the wells containing hybrids secreting the desired antibodies out of millions of irrelevant hybrids generated by the fusion. The procedure employed to screen the hybrid cells for antibody production determines the properties of the selected MAb-producing hybridoma. The screening procedure used depends on the eventual use of the MAb. It should be sufficiently sensitive, easily reproducible, and able to process several hundred samples at one time, with the results available as rapidly as possible. The wells with viable fused cells are initially screened for antibody production when they are 1/3–1/2 confluent in the microtiter plate, usually at 10–14 d postfusion. Supernatant fluids from the 96-well culture plates can be efficiently tested for antibody activity using a solid-phase immunoassay by antibody or antigen capture in a 96-well microtiter plate. Detection of positive antibody binding is often by enzyme-linked immunoassay (ELISA). Preliminary selection for Ig producers can be done using enzyme- or [125]iodine-labeled antimouse immunoglobulin. Antibodies to be used for binding assays can be screened by ELISA. Functional assays may be required for antibodies with a desired biological activity. Immunoblotting screening is performed for antibodies to be used as probes in immunoelectrophoresis.

When positive wells are identified, the cells must be subcloned to select for the single hybridoma (clone) producing antibody against the desired antigen. The clones are assayed for antibody activity when 50% confluent. Clones secreting the highest amount of antibody with the appropriate specificity are selected. The purpose of cloning is to isolate single antibody-producing cells to obtain monoclonality. Cloning by limiting dilution takes advantage of Poisson statistics in that the hybrids are first cloned at 3–5 cells/well (miniclones), and then cells from positive wells are cloned at a dilution of 1/3 cell/well. The most positive wells from this cloning are selected and recloned at 1/3 cell/well to ensure monoclonality. The final clone should display the desired antibody specificity in each of the microtiter wells. The heavy- (H) and L-chain isotypes of the mouse immunoglobulin are determined from the final clones to assure monoclonality. The cloned hybridomas then can be expanded for antibody production and storage by freezing.

1.4. Large-Scale Production

1.4.1. Ascites Production

A major reason for preparing hybridomas is to provide a virtually unlimited source of MAb. Hybridoma clones can be grown in tissue culture or as a tumor line as ascites. Growth of the hybridoma cells intraperitoneally in syngeneic mice results in a 100- to 1000-fold greater concentration of the MAb compared to the concentration achieved in tissue culture. Balb/c mice (or a mouse strain syngeneic to myeloma cell line fusion partner) must be primed by intraperitoneal inoculation with pristane (2,6,10,14-tetramethyl pentadecane) 10 d prior to injection of the hybridoma cells. Five million hybridoma cells are inoculated intraperitoneally into each mouse, and the resultant ascitic fluid (5–10 mL/mouse) is harvested at 1–3 wk postinoculation. It is possible to achieve levels of 1–10 mg/mL of antibody in ascitic fluid. A disadvantage of in vivo production of MAb is the contamination of the preparation with endogenous mouse immunoglobulins.

1.4.2. In Vitro Production Methods

Useful amounts of MAb may be obtained by propagation of the hybridoma clones in vitro and collection of the cell-culture fluid. The yield of antibody in the cell-culture supernatant ranges from 5–50 μg/mL. Hybridoma clones should be routinely screened for the levels of antibody production, especially before large-scale propagation is attempted. It is possible to reclone the hybridoma for high antibody-producing clones. Several aliquots of the cells should be frozen for future use. Hybridoma cell lines that grow in suspension can be adapted to continuous culture in spinner flasks or roller bottles. Adherent cell lines can be cultured in large tissue-culture flasks or attached to dextran microcarriers. Higher levels of antibody yields can be obtained by culture in a hollow-fiber reactor that increases the surface area of culture and perfusion with culture medium. The culture supernatant contains large amounts of fetal bovine serum, which is expensive and is precipitated during protein concentration. Affinity purifications of the culture supernate can be designed to obtain concentrated MAb. Alternatively, the hybridoma can be adapted to culture in low or serum-free medium. This can, however, result in decreased yields of antibody. Other problems with large-scale culture of hybridomas include possible loss of secretor phenotype, poor adaptation to spinner flasks or roller bottles, and the expense of and contamination with fetal bovine serum proteins.

1.5. Antibody Purification

The choice of immunoglobulin purification technique depends on the intended use, the degree of purity required, the need to preserve antibody activity, the amount of material required, and the expense. Classical immunoglobulin purification by salt fractionation, followed by ion exchange- and molecular-sieving chromatography, have been used successfully. Affinity chromatography is used to purify and concentrate MAb in a simple one-step procedure. Immobilized antigen-attached Sepharose beads can be used to bind antibody. Bacterial protein A or protein G attached to Sepharose beads can bind antibody mainly via the Fc portion of the immunoglobulin. The bound antibody is released by decreasing the pH to <3. The binding affinity of protein A and protein G for each immunoglobulin subclass is different and is species- and pH-dependent. Different immunoglobulins from different species can be eluted from protein A- or protein G-Sepharose by altering the pH and other elution conditions.

2. Materials

2.1. Immunization

1. Antigen (50–100 µg) in isotonic solution.
2. Pathogen-free Balb/C female mice 8–12 wk of age.

3. RAS adjuvant: Each vial of MPL + TDM lyophilized product contains: 0.5 mg monophosphoryl lipid A (MPL), 0.5 mg trehalose dimycolate (TDM), 0.04 mL squalene (hexamethyl-tetracosahexane), and 0.004 mL monooleate (Tween 80) (RIBI ImmunoChem Research, Inc., Hamilton, MT).
4. 1.0-mL syringes.
5. Sterile 22–23-gage needles.
6. 100-µL Hamilton syringe.

2.2. Fusion

1. Culture medium RPMI+: RPMI 1640 with 50 U/mL penicillin G, 50 µg/mL streptomycin sulfate, 2 mM L-glutamine, 100 mM HEPES, and 1 mM sodium pyruvate, and 500 mL (Gibco/BRL Life Technologies, Grand Island, NY).
2. Fusion medium: RPMI+ with 10% fetal bovine serum (FBS).
3. Growth medium: RPMI+ with 10% FBS and 1% ORIGEN hybridoma cloning factor (IGEN, Inc., Rockville, MD).
4. 2X HAT medium: RPMI+ with 10% FBS, 1% ORIGEN, and 100 µM hypoxanthine, 0.4 µM aminopterin, and 16 µM thymidine (Gibco/BRL Life Technologies).
5. HT medium: RPMI+ with 10% FBS, 100 µM hypoxanthine, and 16 µM thymidine (Gibco/BRL Life Technologies).
6. 50% PEG: 1500 mol wt (Boehringer-Mannheim, Indianapolis, IN) in HEPES.
7. 37°C water bath.
8. 50-mL sterile conical tubes, 12 × 75 mm tubes, pipet tips, and 20-µL pipetter.
9. Sterile 1-, 10-, and 25-mL pipets, and Pasteur pipets.
10. Hemacytometer.
11. Sterile flat-bottomed microtiter plates.
12. Spleen cells from antigen-primed mouse, syngeneic to the myeloma cells used (usually Balb/c mice).
13. P3-NS1 or Sp2/O myeloma cell line (ATCC, Rockville, MD).

2.3. Cloning

1. RPMI growth medium.
2. HAT medium (Gibco/BRL Life Technologies).
3. Flat-bottomed sterile microtiter plates.
4. Sterile 1.0-mL pipets.

2.4. Ascites Production

1. Syngeneic mice (Balb/c female, retired breeders or 64 d old, 22–24 g).
2. Hybridoma cells, 5 × 10^6/mouse.

3. Pristane (2,4,10,14-tetramethyl pentadecane; ICN Biochemicals, Costa Mesa, CA), 0.5 mL/mouse.
4. Syringes, 1 and 3 mL.
5. 20- and 22–25-gage needles.
6. 75% Isopropanol.
7. Centrifuge tubes, sterile.
8. Phosphate-buffered saline (PBS): 10 m*M* sodium phosphate, pH 7.2, and 0.14*M* NaCl.

2.5. Antibody Purification

1. Protein A-Sepharose 4 Fast Flow (Pharmacia Biotech, Piscataway, NJ).
2. Binding buffer: 20 m*M* sodium phosphate buffer, pH 7.0.
3. Protein A-elution buffer: 100 m*M* citric acid, pH 3.0.
4. Chromatography column, Pharmacia K9 series (Pharmacia Biotech).

3. Methods (*see* Fig. 1)

3.1. Immunization (see Notes 1–7)

For mice, the suggested dose of antigen in MPL + TDM adjuvant emulsion is 0.2 mL/ip injection. Boost on d 21 or 28, and then bleed 10–14 d after the booster injection to check for the production of antibody titers. Boost every 3–4 wk, using the same protocol for each injection. An example of a protocol for immunizing mice prior to spleen removal is to inject on day 0, boost on d 21, and trial bleed on d 26. If the titers are adequate, boost on d 35, sacrifice the mouse, and remove the spleen for fusion 3 d after the boost.

1. Prior to reconstituting the adjuvant emulsion, place vial in a water bath at 40–45°C for 5–10 min.
2. Reconstitute each vial with 2.0 mL of sterile saline containing the desired amount of antigen at a concentration range of 0.05–0.25 mg/mL of saline (100–5000 μg of antigen for 2-mL vol) (*see* Notes 1 and 2).
3. The final antigen preparation using MPL + TDM will contain 50 μg of each adjuvant (MPL and TDM)/0.2 mL.
4. Immunization protocol for raising antibodies in mice:
   Day 1:   First injection, ip with RIBI adjuvant; 22- or 23-gage needle, 0.5 mL or less antigen emulsion, 100 μg/mouse.
   Day 21:   Second injection, ip with RIBI adjuvant; 22- or 23-gage needle, 0.5 mL or less antigen emulsion, 100 μg/mouse.
   Days 28–31: Eyebleed to measure serum antibody levels against antigen (*see* Note 3).

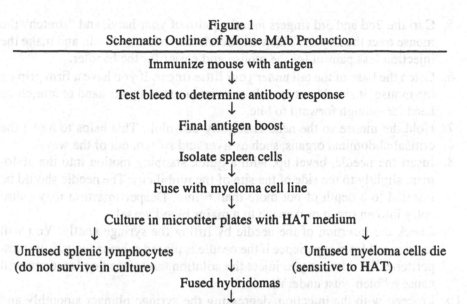

Figure 1
Schematic Outline of Mouse MAb Production

Immunize mouse with antigen
↓
Test bleed to determine antibody response
↓
Final antigen boost
↓
Isolate spleen cells
↓
Fuse with myeloma cell line
↓
Culture in microtiter plates with HAT medium
↓   ↓
Unfused splenic lymphocytes   Unfused myeloma cells die
(do not survive in culture)   ↓   (sensitive to HAT)
Fused hybridomas
↓
a. Screen wells for specific antibody production
b. Clone positive wells by limiting dilution
c. Rescreen clones for specific antibody production
d. Reclone positive wells
e. Confirm specific MAb production
f. Expand in culture and induce ascites production

Day 35: Last injection, iv or intrasplenic; 27- or 30-gage needle and
Hamilton syringe, 0.1-mL maximum vol 50–100 µg/
mouse, without adjuvant; the timing of this injection is
flexible and is determined by achievement of the desired
serum antibody.

Day 38: Animal sacrifice, with spleen recovery and fusion (3 d following final injection).

3.1.1. Intraperitoneal Injections

1. Prepare antigen/adjuvant suspensions as aseptically as possible, and eliminate air bubbles near the needle end of the syringe (*see* Note 4).
2. Grasp a mouse by the tail, and place it on the wire lid of the animal box.
3. Allow the mouse to grasp the wires, and pull gently on the tail to extend
the animal's body.
4. Pick the mouse up by holding the scruff of the neck between the thumb and
forefinger of the left hand.

5. Curl the 2nd and 3rd fingers into the palm of your hand, and "stretch" the mouse over the fingers. This will stretch the abdominal wall, and make the injection less painful for the mouse and easier for the handler.
6. Catch the base of the tail under your little finger. If you have a firm grip on the mouse, it should not be able to twist around in your hand or stretch its head far enough forward to bite.
7. Hold the mouse so the head is slightly downhill. This helps to move the critical abdominal organs, such as liver and spleen, out of the way.
8. Insert the needle, bevel up, with a quick stabbing motion into the abdomen, slightly to the side of the site of the umbilicus. The needle should be inserted to a depth of not more than 6 mm. Deeper insertion may cause entry into an organ or damage to a major blood vessel.
9. Check the insertion of the needle by lifting the syringe gently. You will learn to tell from experience if the needle is placed subcutaneously or intraperitoneally. Also, as you inject the solution, an sc needle placement will cause a "bleb" just under the skin.
10. Proceed with the injection, depressing the syringe plunger smoothly and not too fast, watching for bleeding or "bleb" formation. Occasionally the mouse will contract the abdominal muscles and cause ejection of the inoculum through the needle hole following the removal of the needle.

3.1.2. Intravenous Injections

1. Prepare antigen suspension aseptically.
   a. Draw the fluid into the Hamilton syringe using a 22–23-gage needle.
   b. Change the needle to 30 gage and eliminate **all** air bubbles at the needle end of the syringe. Air injected intravenously will cause sudden death.
   c. The bevel of the needle should be on the same side as the graduations on the barrel.
2. Remove the mouse from the box by grasping the tail, and lifting the animal out of the plastic box and onto the wire lid (*see* Note 5).
3. Locate the tail veins. Using hot water, saturate some gauze pads and warm the tail (1–2 min).
4. Remove the gauze pad, and observe the dilated veins in the tail. Choose a vein that is placed uppermost for injection, and clean with alcohol.
5. Hold the tail with the left hand, drape it over the forefinger, and secure it with the thumb.
6. Bring the syringe, with needle bevel uppermost, up to the tail so that it is in line with the part of the tail lying over the forefinger, but is slightly below its surface.
7. Insert the needle, bevel up, so that it follows directly along the line of the vein and comes to lie within its lumen.

8. Gently press on the plunger of the syringe; if the needle is in the vein, there should be no resistance and the inoculation will be easily made (*see* Notes 6 and 7).
9. After inoculation, blot any blood leakage with the gauze pads, and return the mouse to the box.

3.2. Fusion

3.2.1. Cell Preparation

1. Grow myeloma cells (NS-1) to log phase. Start growth 5 d prior to fusion. Initiate the culture at 5×10^4 cells/mL in RPMI+ and 10% FBS. Feed for three consecutive days.
2. On the day of fusion, spin down myeloma cells in sterile 50-mL conical tubes, and wash twice with RPMI (no FBS) at 800 rpm for 5 min.
3. After the second wash, resuspend cells in RPMI and count. Determine cell concentration and total cell count.
4. Prepare the spleen cells by gentle disruption using sterile needles to obtain a single-cell suspension. Be sure to wash the spleen cells twice with RPMI (no serum). Then resuspend and count cells.
5. Combine the cells in a 1:4 ratio of myeloma:spleen cells into one 50-mL conical tube, and centrifuge at 800 rpm for 5 min.
6. Remove **all** of the medium from the pellet, using pipet and Pasteur pipet, so that the cell pellet is dry.

3.2.2. Fusion with PEG

1. Begin by using a 1-mL pipet. With a slow circular motion and without the pipet touching the inside surface of the centrifuge tube, add 1 mL of 50% PEG in HEPES over 1 min. Do not add too fast, since the PEG is toxic and the membranes become very fragile as the cells are exposed to it.
2. Stir very gently for 1 min using the same pipet.
3. Rapidly change to a 10-mL pipet, and fill with 10 mL of RPMI+ containing 10% FBS.
4. Add 1 mL over 1 min, and then the second milliliter over another minute (total of 2 mL over 2 min). These dilution steps are critical. If the fusion medium is added too quickly, the barely fused hybrids will break apart and membranes will be sheared, leading to cell death and unsuccessful fusion. If added too slowly, the PEG may become too toxic for the cells.
5. Add the remaining 8 mL over 2 min, using the same gentle mixing motion throughout.
6. Cap the 50-mL centrifuge tube, and spin at 800 rpm for 5 min, with **no brake engagement**.

7. Remove most of the medium using a pipet. Add enough growth medium to make a 5×10^5 or 5×10^4 cells/mL concentration (cell number corresponds to splenocytes). Again, be sure to add the dilution medium gently without creating a vortex. Pipet up and down once or twice to resuspend the cells evenly.

8. Distribute the cell suspension into 96-well flat-bottom tissue-culture plates (0.1 mL/well; 2 drops from a 10-mL pipet).

9. Check the wells using the inverted microscope. You should see fusions of large myeloma cells with smaller spleen cells. Incubate overnight at 37°C in 5% CO_2.

10. Feed the next day with HAT medium, and examine daily for signs of hybrid outgrowth. Cultures should remain on HAT medium for 14 d to ensure myeloma cell death and **no regrowth** of the myeloma cell line.

11. Production of antibody will be detectable when the wells show 1/3 to 1/2 confluent growth of hybridoma cells. This may occur within 1 wk, depending on the concentration and health of the cells (*see* Note 8).

12. Culture wells should be refed either when medium is removed for assay, when cell growth is confluent, or when the medium in the wells turns yellow (up to 14 d with HAT).

13. Follow within growth for 1–2 wk (two to four feedings) HT medium to ensure successful transfer of hybridomas from HAT-selective medium to standard growth medium.

3.3. Cloning
3.3.1. Minicloning Procedure

1. Count the number of cells in the well positive for the desired antibody.

2. Determine the number of plates to be used for this step (usually 1–5 plates/positive well). The number of plates depends on the number of wells that can be screened at one time and the number of positive wells you plan to miniclone.

3. Aliquot the cells so there will be 5 cells/well of the 96-well plate (480 cells/plate).

4. Resuspend the cells in 14 mL of growth medium/plate and distribute 2 drops/well from a 10-mL pipet (~100 μL).

5. Add an additional 100 μL of medium/well, and incubate the plates at 37°C.

6. Save the remaining cells to grow to at least 10^7 cells/line. These should be frozen with DMSO as the "back-up" parent lines.

7. Check by visual screening for evidence of growth (7–9 d) to judge when you can retest for immunoglobulin production.

8. Refeed cells when you remove supernatant for testing.

3.3.2. Formal Cloning

1. Select a limited number of positive wells for formal cloning. Plan on setting up 6–10 plates/positive well.
2. Calculate the number of cells needed to set up limiting dilution cloning (1 cell/3 wells of 96-well plate = 32 cells/plate). This is a very small number of cells. To be accurate, do serial dilutions so the volume of cell suspension you add to the dilution medium is at least 0.5 mL or more.
3. Dilute the cells to 14 mL of growth medium for each plate, and distribute at 2 drops/well from a 10-mL pipet.
4. Add an additional 100 µL of medium/well.
5. As in the minicloning step, grow up any remaining cells to be frozen as the parent "back-up" lines at this step.
6. Incubate the plates at 37°C. Check visually for signs of growth at 7–10 d to determine when retesting should take place.
7. Remove 100 µL from growing wells for screening, and refeed the cultures.
8. Select the single best well per formal clone, and repeat the formal cloning to ensure that the cell line is monoclonal (steps 1–7).
9. Once the final cells lines are selected, grow them up to be frozen. Freeze 6–10 vials/line. At this point, you can produce more supernatant for recovery of immunoglobulin or grow cells for ascites production.

3.4. Ascites Production

1. Prime the mice by ip inoculation with 0.5 mL of pristane 7–10 d prior to injection of the hybridoma cells.
2. Remove the hybridoma cells from culture, and wash 1X with PBS to remove FBS.
3. Adjust the cells to 5×10^6/mL in sterile PBS.
4. Inject 0.5 mL of the cell suspension intraperitoneally into the mouse using a 22–25-gage needle.
5. After 7–14 d, the abdomen of the inoculated mouse will be swollen, indicating ascites production. The growth rate depends on the growth characteristics of the hybridoma cells.
6. The ascitic fluid is removed using a 20-gage needle (*see* Note 9).
7. When the animal is ready to be retapped (2 d later), it is euthanized using CO_2 and/or cervical dislocation prior to removal of ascitic fluid.
8. Cells and fibrin clots are sedimented by centrifugation at 200g for 15 min. The clear ascitic fluid is frozen at –20°C.
9. Cells recovered from step 8 can be cultured if collection of ascites fluid is done under sterile conditions.

10. Titer the ascitic fluid for production of antibody. The antibody content can vary from 1–10 mg/mL.

3.5. Antibody Purification

Protein A and protein G bind mainly to the Fc region of immunoglobulins through interactions with the H chain. Protein A and protein G have different immunoglobulin binding specificities depending on the source of antibody. They can be used to isolate and purify immunoglobulins from ascites fluid or cell-culture medium. An example of a purification protocol using protein A-Sepharose Fast Flow follows:

1. Wash the column with 3 column volumes of binding buffer.
2. Filter sample through a 0.22-μm filter and apply to the column.
3. Wash the column with binding buffer until baseline returns to zero. Monitor protein elution at 280 nm.
4. Elute bound fraction with 100 mM sodium citrate–citric acid, pH 3.0.
5. Wash with 3 column volumes of pH 3.0 buffer or until the baseline returns to zero (*see* Note 10).
6. Fractions should be adjusted to pH 7 immediately (400 μL 1M Tris-HCl, pH 9, will raise the pH of a 2-mL fraction to pH 7.0).

4. Notes

1. Remove cap seal and rubber stopper of vial, and pipet a 2-mL vol of saline containing antigen directly into the vial. Replace rubber stopper, and vortex vial vigorously for 2–3 min to form emulsion if adding antigen/saline solution by pipet. When using a syringe, form an emulsion by drawing the material back into the syringe and reinjecting it forcibly back into the vial. Repeat the process five to six times or until an emulsion is obtained. The emulsion can be briefly vortexed prior to animal inoculation.
2. If the entire contents of the vial are not used up, it can be stored at 4°C (up to 60 d).
3. Try out iv injection of buffer in which antigen is to be dissolved using a nonimmunized mouse. EDTA, CHAPS, or other chemicals may be toxic and can cause internal bleeding.
4. Have ready an extra box for separating the injected mouse from noninjected mice. Wear latex gloves for mouse procedures. This protects the mouse from random contaminants on your skin and also makes it harder for the mouse to get a firm grip on your hand, should it decide to bite you. Many mice will urinate or defecate when they are captured.
5. Set the mouse down on the bench, hold it by the tail, and use a 1-L beaker as the restrainer. Turn the beaker upside down, and position it over the

mouse, with the pouring lip over the tail. Place an appropriate object under the opposite edge of the beaker to provide for air circulation.

6. As the inoculum enters the vein, it should be visible. Signs of incorrect inoculation are: the need to exert pressure on the plunger, swelling and opaque appearance of the tail over the vein, and, usually, the absence of a slight blood leak after the needle is withdrawn.

7. If the iv inoculation is not achieved in the first attempt, the other tail veins can be tried after rewarming. It is best to initiate attempts some way down the tail, later working upward.

8. Antibody assay should begin when microscopic examination indicates growth. By identifying antibody-producing hybrids at this stage, clones may be recovered before becoming overgrown with nonantibody-producing cells.

9. Insert the needle no more than 1 cm into the abdomen and allow the fluid to collect in a sterile tube. Gently massage the abdomen and manipulate the needle to maintain a good flow of ascitic fluid.

10. If a new sample is to be purified, the column should be equilibrated with binding buffer (3 column volumes). If the column is to be stored, it should be placed into the binding buffer containing either 20% ethanol or 0.05% sodium azide.

References

1. Köhler, G. and Milstein, C. (1975) Continuous cultures of fused cells secreting antibody of predefined specificity. *Nature* **256**, 495–497.
2. Tramontano, A., Janda, K. D., and Lerner, R. A. Catalytic antibodies. *Science* **234**, 1566–1573.
3. Potter, M. and Boyce, C. R., (1962) Induction of plasma cell neoplasms in strain Balb/c mice with mineral oil adjuvants. *Nature* **193**, 1086,1087.
4. Kohler, G. and Milstein, C. (1976) Derivation of specific antibody-producing tissue culture and tumor lines by cell fusion. *Eur. J. Immunol.* **6**, 511–519.
5. Shulman, M., Wilde, C. D., and Kohler, G. (1978) A better cell line for making hybridomas secreting antibodies. *Nature* **276**, 269,270.

CHAPTER 8

Comparative Properties of Polyclonal and Monoclonal Antibodies

L. Scott Rodkey

1. Introduction

This chapter was written with the express goal of introducing several basic concepts involved when antigens and antibodies interact in vitro to the novice reader and to serve as a review of these concepts to the more advanced reader. Most of these concepts also apply to in vivo reactivity. Antigen–antibody reactions in vivo frequently involve subsequent reactions of the complexes with complement, but these reactions will be largely ignored for the purpose of this chapter. Reactivity properties of antibodies are determined by several important structural features of the antigens and antibody preparations used. Major properties of antigens that influence their reactivities with antibodies include structural features such as whether individual epitopes are repeated on the molecule, the relative proportion of sequential and conformational epitopes, and the degree of purity of the antigen preparation. For purposes of this chapter, it will be assumed that the antigens used as examples arc purc, but thc knowledgeable reader will understand that this is almost never the case.

The development of monoclonal antibody (MAb) production technologies provided experimental scientists with a reagent that could behave quite differently from the classic polyclonal antibody reagent, depending on the application and the type of assay being used. The widespread use of MAb has been facilitated by the assumption that these reagents are more specific than classic polyclonal preparations. This is certainly true in some applications, but not in others. The use of either IgG or IgM

From: *Methods in Molecular Biology, Vol. 51: Antibody Engineering Protocols*
Edited by: S. Paul Humana Press Inc., Totowa, NJ

MAb can pose additional questions depending on the format of the assay being contemplated.

This chapter will focus on several specific examples of antigen–antibody reactions and the use of either polyclonal antibodies or MAb. The reactions will be illustrated with cartoon examples when appropriate.

2. Antigens

2.1. Epitopes

The word "epitope" is now universally accepted as the descriptive noun that defines a physical site on an antigen molecule bound to a generally complementary structure on the antibody called the "paratope." Studies of the epitope–paratope interaction were pioneered by Landsteiner (1). His extensive studies of interactions of chemically defined haptens with polyclonal antibodies laid the groundwork for virtually all our current concepts dealing with immunological specificity and antigen–antibody interactions. The biochemical form of the antigen-carrying epitopes of immunological interest varies greatly and can include proteins, carbohydrates, lipids, and nucleic acids. Metals, small peptides, and numerous organic chemicals can serve as epitopes under controlled conditions, generally when they are appropriately coupled to carrier antigens for immunization.

There are two clearly definable subclasses of epitopes that have been studied over the years. The distinctions between the two are on the one hand simplistic, and on the other hand, highly significant in understanding epitope–paratope interactions in different formats, particularly when using MAb. Sela (2) was the first to recognize that epitopes could be subdivided into two distinct subclasses. His basis for subdividing them depended on whether the amino acid sequence alone was sufficient to define epitope–paratope binding or whether a specific three-dimensional stereoconformation of the particular sequence was also critical in defining the binding with antibody. He called these two epitope subclasses sequential and conformational, respectively.

2.1.1. Sequential Epitopes

Sequential epitopes are generally defined as requiring only a specific sequence of amino acids to bind successfully to the complementary paratope. Studies defining sequential epitopes generally are done by injecting the animal with intact antigen and measuring the ability of short synthetic peptides to inhibit the reaction between antigens and antibodies. When relatively low concentrations of peptide can successfully inhibit the reaction, a sequential epitope has been defined. It should be noted that paratope sites are thought to be rather rigid and inflexible, and that free peptides have high flexibility. Therefore, free peptides must conform to the shape of the paratope. This situation can make for significant crossreactivity in these kinds of studies, and rigid definitions of specificity with free peptides are sometimes difficult.

2.1.2. Conformational Epitopes

Conformational epitopes are defined as requiring a specific rigid three-dimensional stereoconformation of a given amino acid sequence on a molecule for successful paratope recognition. These epitopes frequently consist of amino acids from different parts of the amino acid sequence of a protein antigen that are brought in close proximity by the precise folding of the chain. Studies of epitopes of myoglobin as well as of other protein antigens have shown that these assembled topographic sites are major epitopes (3).

2.2. Antigens with Nonrepeating Epitopes

Many small molecules that typically exist in solution in a monomeric molecular form will exhibit only one copy of each epitope on its surface. Antigens that have been widely used in immunological investigations and have no repeating epitopes in the monomeric form include myoglobin, various serum albumins, and hen ovalbumin. These molecules are synthesized as single-chain polypeptides and behave as monomers in solution. Each antigen of this type will have no two equal areas on its surface with the same topology, although many distinct epitopes may possess areas similar to each other. In practice, it must be emphasized that purification techniques frequently yield antigen preparations with small but significant portions of dimers, trimers, and higher order polymers. Indeed, rigorous purification protocols must be used to minimize the presence of these aggregates. Clearly, if the molecules are aggregated, each dimer could have two copies of each epitope. As will be seen below in Section 2.3., these molecules would behave quite differently in some assays as compared to monomers.

2.3. Antigens with Repeating Epitopes

Antigen molecules that display repeating epitopes are best exemplified by carbohydrate antigens. Long-chain carbohydrates, such as pneumococcal polysaccharides, dextrans, and streptococcal group-specific carbohydrate antigens, are some of the best examples of antigens with repeating epitopes. The ingenious studies of Kabat, which determined that the largest epitope that could be accommodated by a paratope was of the size of a hexasaccharide, were done using dextran for immunization and short segments to inhibit the antigen–antibody reaction. Since dextran consists of long chains of glucose units, oligosaccharides of glucose ranging from the disaccharide (isomaltose) to the heptasaccharide (isomaltoheptose) could be used as inhibitors in precipitation reactions *(4)*. Such inhibition studies showed that the upper limit of oligosaccharide that was accommodated in the paratope was a hexasaccharide. However, the parent antigen, dextran, could bear hundreds of identical hexasaccharide unit sites on each molecule, depending on the molecular weight of the dextran preparation used. Various lipopolysaccharides and protein antigens can exhibit the same type of multiepitope structures. Several types of isoenzymes are made up of two or more identical units that are held noncovalently in dimers or tetramers to form the intact enzyme. These are conceptually equivalent to making dimers or tetramers of molecules, like myoglobin, in that each would have two or four epitopes of each kind that were found on the monomer (*see* Section 2.2. above). A tetrameric isoenzyme, for example, would have four copies of each individual epitope available. It is possible that some of the epitopes in the tetramer would be functionally unavailable owing to the interaction between the monomeric units. However, many epitopes would be functionally repeated.

3. Antibody Affinity and Avidity

The behavior of antibodies in polyclonal mixtures or of MAb preparations is frequently misunderstood because of a misconception about the definitions of antibody affinity and antibody avidity.

3.1. Antibody Affinity

Antibody affinity is defined based on the law of mass action. Association constants derived from equilibrium dialysis studies or other studies that measure only primary binding properties of antibodies can be used to compare one antibody preparation with another preparation for strength of interaction with antigen. Such measurements typically measure only the strength of interaction of a single paratope with a single

Table 1
Binding Avidity Advantage of Multivalent Paratopes[a]

	Fab	IgG	IgM
Effective valence	1	2	10
Ag valence	1	Multiple	Multiple
Association constant	10^4	10^7	10^{11}
Advantage of multivalence	—	10^3-fold	10^7-fold

[a]Binding of Fab with an association constant of 10^4 is substantially enhanced when divalent IgG binds the multivalent antigen and is dramatically higher when the decavalent IgM binds. The resulting advantage of binding as a result of multivalence is 10^3 and 10^7, respectively, for IgG and IgM.

epitope. For this reason, the results of affinity measurements obtained with intact antibodies of the IgG class are identical with those Fab or $F(ab')_2$ fragments. Valence of the antibody being measured does not affect the association constant or the affinity.

3.2. Antibody Avidity

Antibody avidity is contrasted with antibody affinity in that the valence of the antibody plays a major role in avidity measurements, and the use of multivalent antigens also enhances avidity. As shown in Table 1, the valence of the antibody increases its functional affinity or avidity by a substantial amount. When IgG bearing two Fab arms that have intrinsic affinities of 10^4 interacts with a multivalent antigen in a form such that both Fab arms can bind simultaneously, the effective affinity can rise by as much as 10^3 to a value of 10^7. When the same Fab paratopes are on an IgM molecule with 10 paratope sites/molecule, the effective affinity can be as high as 10^{11} or 10^7 higher than the individual Fab affinity. This enhanced binding, which is really a function of valence of both the antibodies and the antigen, is the avidity value.

4. Polyclonal Antibodies

In the intact, immunocompetent vertebrate, polyclonal antibody responses are the routine way for the animal to respond to an antigenic challenge. Most antigens can be recognized by several different B-cells when appropriately presented to these cells. Since it is clear that the immunoglobulin receptor on each B-cell recognizes only a single epitope on the antigen molecule, it follows that each antigen may be capable of triggering many B-cells to respond. The epitopes may be somewhat overlapping on the surface of protein antigens *(3)*. If overlap of epitopes is taken into account, a single small protein antigen could then elicit the production of scores of different antibodies, each from a separate B-cell progenitor. This was clear very early in the history of immunology when it became evident that a wide range of binding constants was present in antibodies specific for small haptens. Even immunization with small chemically defined organic molecules coupled to carrier proteins elicited very heterogeneous mixtures of antibodies with a wide range of binding constants for the same small haptenic group.

5. MAb

The Köhler and Milstein method for producing MAb *(5)* revolutionized many immunological investigations by making available homogeneous reagents for numerous applications. The essence of the methodology was to immortalize normal antibody-producing cells and select only one progenitor cell to expand in vitro, so that all daughter cells were making the same product. The antibodies isolated from such cultures were shown to be biochemically homogeneous and functionally monospecific in antigen binding. As opposed to purified polyclonal antibodies, MAb have homogeneous binding constants. In essence, polyclonal antibodies are best visualized as being similar to cocktails of several MAb, each of which is specific for an epitope on the same antigen molecule.

6. Comparative Properties of Monoclonal and Polyclonal Antibodies

Rigorous comparisons of the behavior and properties of monoclonal and polyclonal antibodies in the published literature are sparse. For this reason, illustrative comparisons will be made using simple diagrams.

6.1. Polyclonal Antibodies–Liquid-Phase Reactions

For purposes of discussion, precipitation reactions will be used to illustrate liquid-phase reactions. There will be no attempt here to go into great detail about the kinetics of reactions or methods of calculation of molar ratios of reagents.

A diagrammatic illustration of a model antigen with nonrepetitive epitopes and the polyclonal antibody populations it could elicit is shown in Fig. 1. This antigen has four distinct epitopes that are each unique and

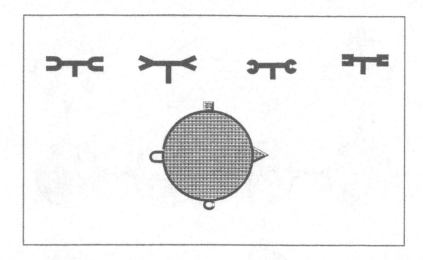

Fig. 1. Diagram of an antigen molecule with four distinct, nonrepeating epitopes (below) and the four populations of IgG antibody specificities elicited by the antigen (above).

nonoverlapping; antibodies reactive with one epitope will not react with any of the other three epitopes. During polyclonal responses, the respective concentrations of each of the antibody subsets will never be known for certain. One may predominate, all may be present in equal concentrations, two may predominate, or three may predominate. The relative ratios of the four specificities will dictate the extent to which the fluid phase antigen–antibody reaction will be detectable. If all four were equally represented, an optimal precipitation reaction would likely proceed. The complex that might be formed under these conditions is shown in Fig. 2. An antibody specific for one epitope will link two antigen molecules, whereas yet another antibody specific for a second epitope on the first antigen molecule will link it with another antigen molecule. The lattice-like polymer of antigen and antibodies that eventually builds up was first envisioned by Marrack *(6)* and has been verified using electron microscopy. It is clear that the polyclonal mixture of antibodies provides links between individual molecules, with alternating specificities of antibodies and epitopes appearing as one traces the length of the polymer complex. In the zone of antibody excess, a situation encountered by an infectious agent such as a virus on entering the bloodstream of an animal that has been previously vaccinated, each of these antigen molecules

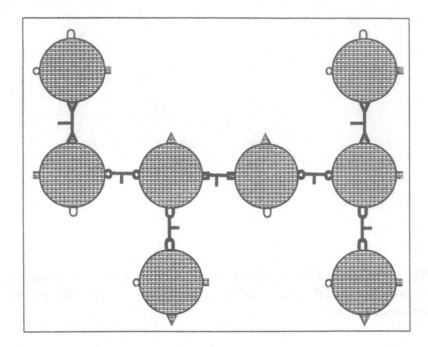

Fig. 2. Diagram of fluid-phase antigen–antibody complex with a monomeric antigen preparation with four nonrepetitive epitopes on its surface reacting with a polyclonal IgG antibody preparation.

would be covered by four antibody molecules, with one Fab arm of each of the four antibodies dangling free. In the zone of antigen excess, one antibody would exist with two antigen molecules bound to each antibody, and one antigen bound to each Fab arm.

The reactivity patterns of polyclonal antibodies with antigens bearing multiple copies of the same epitope are similar to that of an antigen with nonrepetitive epitopes. The significant difference is that the molar ratios of Ab:Ag required for precipitation are reduced when the Ag contains multiple copies of an epitope. This was shown dramatically by Porter in his seminal study of papain cleavage of antibodies *(7)*. He showed that Fab fragments of antipneumococcal antibodies had to be added to free antigen in concentrations as high as 180 mg/mL to inhibit precipitation of the antigen with the intact antibodies, but Fab fragments of antihuman serum albumin antibodies would inhibit an equivalent precipitation reaction completely at a concentration of 8–10 mg/mL.

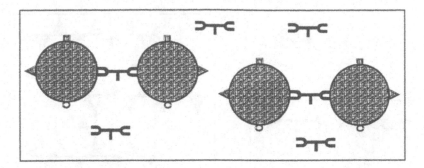

Fig. 3. Diagram of a reaction of an antigen with four nonrepetitive epitopes after interaction with an excess of IgG MAb specific for only one epitope.

6.2. MAb—Liquid-Phase Reactions

As compared to polyclonal antibodies, MAb can behave quite differently in liquid-phase reactions. The presence of only a single specificity of antibody eliminates all except single crosslinks.

MAb reacting with antigens with no repeating epitopes will not function in precipitation reactions. Mixing of an MAb with these molecules at any ratio can have only one of two possible outcomes: formation of a complex composed of one antigen molecule and one antibody molecule, or a complex of two antigen molecules and one antibody molecule. Neither of these complexes will precipitate out of solution under normal circumstances. The reason for this is readily apparent in Fig. 3. The MAb has no opportunity to crosslink more than two antigen molecules, and so a lattice structure cannot be formed. After the two antigen molecules interact with the MAb, no other epitopes are available on the two antigen molecules that can be recognized by the MAb remaining.

MAb will react as well as polyclonal antibodies do in reactions with antigens that have multiple identical epitopes in liquid-phase reactions. Since these kinds of antigens are multivalent with respect to one epitope, a MAb specific for that epitope is very efficient at crosslinking these kinds of molecules, and, consequently, lattices are made very efficiently and precipitation occurs routinely from liquid phase. Such a reaction is diagrammed in Fig. 4.

6.3. ELISA and RIA Format Reactions

The prevalence of ELISA and RIA formats for immunoassays demands a clear understanding of the conditions involved in order that

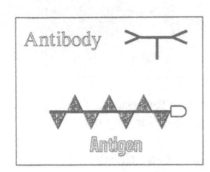

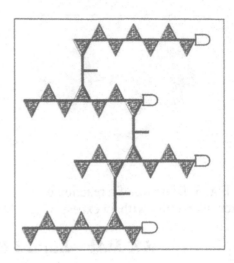

Fig. 4. Diagram of an antigen containing repetitive identical epitopes and a monoclonal IgG antibody specific for the repetitive epitope (left). After reaction in solution, crosslinking can occur to form lattice-like polymeric complexes (right).

informed decisions can be made in interpreting the results obtained. There are many variants in the basic technique that are related to the properties of particular antigens, antibodies, blocking agents, buffers, and enzymes. Only a few common concepts related to the use of either monoclonal or polyclonal reagents are discussed here.

In the basic ELISA or RIA format, plates are normally incubated with an antigen, rinsed, and then blocked with an unrelated protein. This format has been described as using a "carpet of denatured protein." Numerous studies suggest that some degree of denaturation of antigen occurs when it sticks to the plastic surface. For some antigens, the denaturation may be negligible, and for others, it can be significant. For the present discussion, the concept of an "antigen carpet" is useful. In fluid-phase antigen–antibody reactions, one can readily calculate the mean distance between antigen molecules at any given timepoint, and this is usually a large value. When these antigens are immobilized in a plastic well, the distance between molecules can be negligible, with the entire surface of the plastic covered, much like a carpet. This has one important effect on both polyclonal antibody and MAb reactions used in the assays. A monoclonal IgG antibody with a low affinity for its epitope will exhibit a very high avidity owing to divalent binding (*see* Table 1), when the epitopes are close enough together to engage both binding sites of the same molecule simultaneously. This will usually be possible with the "carpet" arrangement of antigens coating the plastic plate. Likewise, even polyclonal antibodies with low average affinities will bind very efficiently under these conditions. When antibodies are used for other purposes after selection on ELISA or RIA plates, the modest affinities of the antibodies may not allow efficient binding to, for example, a tissue antigen or tumor antigen.

6.4. Western Blot Format

Western blot assays are common formats for studying antigens using an MAb for subsequent identification. Typically, a Western blot is done by separating a mixture of antigens in an SDS gel after denaturation. The separated proteins are then transferred to a nitrocellulose membrane by capillary action or by electrophoretic transfer, so that the membrane receives the separated proteins in their separated pattern. SDS is displaced from the protein during the transfer and washing process, and native epitopes are often regained as a result. The degree of reacquisition of native structure is highly variable from protein to protein, and must be checked for every antibody and every protein. Some epitopes can partially refold, and some can never recover from SDS denaturation. Conformational epitopes, of course, are most sensitive to proper refolding.

Partially refolded epitopes can frequently be successfully identified in Western blots because of presentation of the "carpet" format. Once again, the close juxtaposition of the proteins on the nitrocellulose membrane promotes divalent binding of antibody molecules. Thus, even if affinity is lower owing to partial denaturation of the transferred antigen, binding avidity may remain high enough for a positive signal.

7. Concluding Comments

The principal distinction in immunoassay of polyclonal antibodies and MAb involves the question of assay format. Spacing of the antigen targets is a major variable in the assay format. Close proximity of epitopes favors reaction with MAb because of the enhanced avidity of antibodies for closely spaced antibodies. Solution-phase reactions, such as might be encountered in vivo, tend to favor polyclonal antibodies owing to multiple specificities being present for different epitopes on the same antigen. Application of immunoassays with due attention to these considerations can significantly enhance the likelihood of success in finding the desired antibody specificities.

References

1. Landsteiner, K. (1962) *The Specificity of Serological Seactions.* Dover Publications, New York.
2. Sela, M. (1969) Antigenicity: some molecular aspects. *Science* **166,** 1365–1374.
3. Benjamin, D. C., Berzofsky, J. A., East, I. J., Gurd, F. R. N., Hannum, C., Leach, S. J., Margoliash, E., Michael, J. G., Miller, A., Prager, E. M., Reichlin, M., Sercarz, E. E., Smith-Gill, S. J., Todd, P. E., and Wilson, A. C. (1984) The antigenic structure of proteins: a reappraisal. (1984) *Ann. Rev. Immunol.* **2,** 67–101.
4. Kabat, E. A. (1976) *Structural Concepts in Immunology and Immunochemistry,* 2nd ed. Holt, Rinehart and Winston, New York.
5. Köhler, G. and Milstein, C. (1975) Continuous cultures of fused cells secreting antibody of predefined specificity. *Nature* **256,** 495–497.
6. Marrack, J. R. (1938) The chemistry of antigens and antibodies, in *Medical Research Council Special Report,* Series no. 230. H. M. Stationery Office, London.
7. Porter, R. R. (1959) The hydrolysis of rabbit γ-globulin and antibodies with crystalline papain. *Biochem. J.* **73,** 119–126.

CHAPTER 9

Evaluation of Antibody Clonality

L. Scott Rodkey

1. Introduction

The seminal development shaping our current understanding of the immune system was the formulation of the concept of clonal selection by Sir Macfarlane Burnet *(1)*. This idea revolutionized the approach to formulation of experimental design in immunology. At the heart of clonal selection was the idea that antibody specificity preexisted before antigen arrival and that the antigen triggered the system by selecting only cells preprogrammed to make antibody molecules with significant affinity for that particular antigen. The former instructional theories of antibody formation clearly were rendered obsolete by this concept. Many scholars attribute the subsequent formal proof of clonal selection to Raff et al. *(2)*.

Once clonal selection became the accepted paradigm, questions arose about the extent of heterogeneity of the B-cell repertoire for various antigens. Various approaches to this problem were confounded by features of antibody heterogeneity that were unrelated to the central question of variability. Differences in molecular weights of different classes of Ig and differences in valence for antigen binding between different Ig classes were initial complicating factors that had to be resolved. Once the molecular approaches of the 1970s and 1980s were applied to the problem, many of these complications were clarified. However, the established molecular approaches are not yet capable of quantitatively defining antibody clonality expression in vivo.

It is often important to define the allotype and class of Ig synthesized in response to antigen preparations. Further, it is often critical to be able

From: *Methods in Molecular Biology, Vol. 51: Antibody Engineering Protocols*
Edited by: S. Paul Humana Press Inc., Totowa, NJ

to track the earliest appearance during immunization of a specific clonal product and the time of its disappearance. This can be critical for understanding and defining idiotype network participation in immune responses, since network functionality is clonal, unlike some other immune regulatory mechanisms. Several important questions in bone marrow transplantation and in autoimmunity require clonal quantitation.

2. Quantitative Cell Analysis

The original methodology for quantitative cell analysis was published first in 1963 by Jerne and Nordin *(3)*. Spleen cells from mice immunized with sheep red blood cells (SRBC) were mixed with SRBC in agar with guinea pig complement added. Wherever a spleen cell was located that synthesized antibodies specific for SRBC, lysis of the SRBC in the neighborhood of that cell could be seen as a clear plaque in the SRBC lawn, much like clear spaces in lawns of bacteria seen when bacteriophage is applied to the lawn. This method ushered in the era of cellular immunology and made possible quantitative studies of cells participating in immune responses. The original method detects primarily IgM antibody. Later modifications by Dresser and Wortis *(4)* were introduced to detect "indirect plaques," which generally are attributed to IgG antibodies.

These approaches only detected the total number of cells synthesizing antibodies to the antigen at a given point in time. The problem of clonal dynamics in individuals at different points in time cannot be addressed with this approach. Direct measurement and identification of individual clonal products at different points in time in the same individual must be done to answer many questions about the clonal dynamics of the immune response.

3. Isoelectric Focusing Methods
of Protein Separation

Isoelectric focusing (IEF) finally became a routine laboratory tool after Vesterberg *(5)* developed reliable zwitterion mixtures, which would give stepless pH gradients. These were made available commercially initially from LKB in Sweden under the trade name of Ampholine. These reagents were first used in a preparative liquid media format, using a jacketed column that was also commercially available from LKB. This column was available in two sizes: a 110-mL and a 440-mL version. Attempts to use the columns as analytical tools instead of the preparative format for which they were intended were quite successful, but large quantities of proteins had to be focused, since analysis after electrophoretic separation was usually carried out by reading the optical density of collected fractions at 280 nm. Therefore, formats for doing analytical IEF using very small quantities of sample were sought.

Polyacrylamide gel formats for IEF were eventually developed, and the advantages of this method over the liquid media format in the LKB column were described in a sudden flood of papers published independently and almost simultaneously by several labs *(6–11)*. Shortly following the publication of the methodology, numerous application papers verified the utility of this method of protein analysis.

4. Antibody Analysis by IEF

Awdeh et al. *(12)* used IEF in acrylamide gels to study a myeloma protein. This is a homogeneous form of Ig in which a plasma cell undergoes transformation to a plasmacytoma and millions of daughter cells are produced, all synthesizing the same molecular form of Ig. These myeloma proteins accumulate in the serum and urine. The myeloma proteins from patients with multiple myeloma provided the homogeneous Ig used for many of the early studies of immunoglobulin amino acid sequence. Although these proteins are homogeneous, the specificity of the paratope is usually not known. Transplantable plasmacytomas in Balb/c mice provided important reagents for numerous immunological investigations in the early 1970s.

The paper by Awdeh et al. *(12)* showed that the myeloma protein was synthesized as a population of Ig with homogeneous IEF properties. The newly synthesized Ig focused as a single band on IEF, and electrophoretic microheterogeneity developed with time. This study clearly showed that IEF can be used as a measure of Ig heterogeneity. Although the myeloma proteins were shown to have microheterogeneity, this approach suggested that good estimates of clonal heterogeneity might be obtained using this method, particularly if large numbers of clonal products were not present.

Further work by Askonas and her coworkers *(13)* showed that induced antibodies could also be studied by IEF. This paper showed that a wide electrophoretic spectrum of antihapten antibodies were detected when they allowed radioactive hapten to diffuse into the gel and then precipitated the antibodies *in situ* with sodium sulfate. Radioautography of the washed gels showed localization of radioactive hapten in antibody-containing bands in the gels.

5. Keck Modification

Keck et al. *(14)* modified this IEF methodology by first precipitating the focused antibodies *in situ* in the gel with sodium sulfate immediately upon completion of the focusing run and subsequently crosslinking the precipitated molecules with glutaraldehyde, covalently locking the Ig into the gel matrix. Radioactive soluble antigen was then diffused into the gel, eliminating the concern that antibodies would leach out of the gels during incubation with the ligand. Following additional washing to remove unbound antigen, the gels were dried and radioautographed either after or before staining the dried gel for total protein.

This method was applied successfully to a variety of studies of antibodies specific for streptococcal-group-specific antigens by Braun and coworkers. Braun et al. *(15)* showed the utility of the Keck modification for studying human, mouse, and rabbit antistreptococcal antibody responses.

In further studies, Braun's group developed methodology for preparative IEF to purify monoclonal subsets of antistreptococcal group A-variant antibodies directly from whole serum of hyperimmunized rabbits *(16)*. Antibodies purified using this approach were shown to be isoelectrically homogeneous by analytical IEF after developing bands with radioactive A-variant carbohydrate. Such preparations were shown to be as electrophoretically homogeneous as myeloma proteins. Studies of numerous homogeneous antibodies purified by this group *(17)* showed that:

1. Each preparation showed clear epitope specificity for either internal repeating epitopes in the streptococcal carbohydrate-group-specific antigen or for the nonreducing terminal disaccharide on group A-variant carbohydrate;
2. Epitope specificity of the purified antibodies was directly predictive for binding affinity, with antibodies specific for internal repeating epitopes displaying high affinity and those specific for the nonreducing terminal disaccharide displaying low binding affinity; and
3. Epitope specificity was predictive for the functional properties of the antibodies, such as complement fixation and precipitation reactions done in liquid phase.

These studies showed the power of IEF clonotype analysis for study of antibody properties in the intact animal during immunization.

The Keck modification was also used successfully to assess the functional effects of idiotype network regulation during normal immune responses. Brown and Rodkey *(18)* showed that nearly all antibody clones that were present in the primary response of one rabbit to *Micrococcus lysodeikticus* cell-wall carbohydrate antigen disappeared and were replaced with a completely new set of antibodies with a totally different IEF pattern after a second round of immunization, when auto-anti-idiotype antibodies specific for first-round antibody idiotypes were detected. Sera from a third round of immunizations were analyzed by IEF, and all the first-round clones were shown to be expressed again in the absence of regulatory auto-anti-idiotype antibodies.

The Keck modification was also used by Binion et al. *(19)* to analyze the fractions of antibodies isolated by recycling isoelectric focusing. These studies showed that polyclonal antibodies could be fractionated to single-band purity in large quantity using recycling IEF technology. Other IEF studies *(20)* of serum of rabbits immunized by multiple rounds of *Micrococcus lysodeikticus* vaccine administration revealed that significant variations in clonal expression of small subsets of antibodies are a routine occurrence during immunization.

Several other research groups have adopted the Keck modification for analysis of antibody clonal patterns. Insel et al. *(21)* studied clonal responses of humans to the *Hemophilus influenza* b capsular polysaccharide and showed highly restricted isoelectric patterns of antibody binding, which sometimes showed patterns similar to monoclonal antibodies (MAb). D'Amelio et al. *(22)* found wide variations in the antibody clonotype patterns in the 13 human hydatidosis patients. Le Moli et al. *(23)* analyzed clonotype patterns in human antibodies specific for *Neisseria meningitidis* antigens and showed that most patients responded to vaccination by enhanced expression of preimmunization clones, but in approx 1/3 of the patients, completely new basic antibodies were elicited that appeared to mature into clones with neutral and/or acidic charge.

6. Western Blot Format Analyses

Studies have shown the utility of a Western blot format for analysis of antibody clonality. The general approach was to separate immune serum samples on PAGE-IEF gels, transfer the separated serum proteins passively or electrophoretically to nitrocellulose membranes, and identify antibody bands in most cases using radioactive antigen probes.

Roos et al. *(24)* studied responses to murine encephalomyelitis virus with the Western format. Most antibodies specific for the virus were synthesized locally in the CNS and had moderate clonal restriction. Stott et al. *(25)* studied IEF patterns of thyroglobulin autoantibodies in rat models of autoimmune thyroiditis. They showed dramatically different clonal responses in two rat strains; the AUG strain responded with oligoclonal or polyclonal responses, similar to the responses seen in humans with Hashimoto's disease, and the PBG/c rat displayed highly restricted IEF clonal patterns that varied over time. Muryoi et al. *(26)* studied anti-DNA antibody clonal expression in immune complexes isolated from lupus patients. Electrophoretically restricted clonality of the antibodies found in immune complexes in lupus patients was observed, compared to heterogeneity of clones found free in circulation. Similar studies by Stott *(27)* observed substantial clonal restriction of serum anti-DNA antibodies and stable expression of antibodies by these clones, with some clonal products remaining detectable as long as 6 yr.

One study using the Western format employed nonradioactive antigen to detect antibodies. D'Amelio et al. *(28)* used chemiluminescence to detect bands corresponding to anti-gp120 antibodies in HIV disease. They found clonal patterns to be stable over long periods. The patterns were oligoclonal, suggesting some degree of clonal restriction.

7. Affinity Immunoblotting

The affinity immunoblotting method for studying antibodies *(29)* was developed because of certain unsatisfactory characteristics of the Keck modification and the Western-format-type blots. The Keck method suffers from several technically undesirable features. First, very high specific activities of radioactive antigens are necessary to ensure radioautographic detection of weak antibody bands. Second, the efficiency of Ig precipitation by sodium sulfate is highly dependent on the concentration of the Ig. Therefore, bands corresponding to very low concentrations of IgG are not precipitated efficiently *in situ* and will wash out of the gels during the antigen-binding step. Further, only one concentration of glutaraldehyde can be used for the entire gel, and this concentration may be nonideal for many of the bands in the gel. Studies in our laboratory showed that efficiency of glutaraldehyde crosslinking of several different proteins is quite variable and depends on the concentration of protein. Thus, many bands are likely to be missed owing to problems in sodium sulfate precipitation and glutaraldehyde crosslinking. The Western format also suffers from the drawback of potential antibody denaturationon binding of transferred antibodies to the nitrocellulose membrane. We felt that a method relying exclusively on the antigen-binding properties of the antibodies would be most suited for clonotype analysis. Further, we felt that elimination of the radioactive probes was desirable.

The affinity immunoblotting method that was developed has a number of positive features and only one disadvantage: substantial amounts of antigen must be available. For most antigens, this is really not a problem. Optimal antigen concentrations are approx 5–10 μg/mL for most antigens and approx 5–10 mL of antigen solution are needed, depending on the size of the nitrocellulose sheet. The specific methodology of the affinity immunoblotting method is presented in the accompanying chapter by Knisley and Rodkey (Chapter 10).

This method has been exploited by several groups to study clonotypic properties in several different experimental systems. Knisley and Rodkey *(30)* adapted the affinity immunoblot method to analyze immune sera using immobilized pH gradients for the initial antibody separation. This report reconfirmed earlier studies *(20)* in which individual antibody bands were shown to disappear rapidly or suddenly appear during the course of the response. Mehrazar et al. *(31)* used affinity immunoblotting methods to compare the antibody responses of piglets deprived of maternal colostrum and raised in germ-free conditions with immune responses of conventionally reared piglets. The antibodies elicited to the arsonate hapten were more heterogeneous in the conventionally reared piglets than in germ-free colostrum-deprived piglets, indicating that transferred maternal antibodies can influence the expressed B-cell repertoire in the offspring.

Affinity immunoblotting techniques have been successfully used in bone marrow transplantation studies to follow the clonal origin of antibody responses in recipients of bone marrow grafts. Seferian et al. *(32)* studied a rabbit model of bone marrow transplantation using affinity immunoblotting. Cells were transplanted into recipients from a rabbit matched for histocompatibility antigens coded at the RLA locus, but differing in Ig allotype. An affinity immunoblot analysis was done. The response to antigen was monitored by specific detection of the Ig allotype, which was bound to the antigen on the nitrocellulose, as a means of distinguishing between donor and recipient responses. This study showed that recipients of cells from antigen-primed donors responded to antigen challenge with antibody of donor cell origin. Thus, the transplanted cells were effectively triggered into antibody production in the recipient. The responding B-cell clonotype repertoire remained virtually unchanged throughout the extensive cell-transfer protocol used in this study. Adler et al. (33) also used a rabbit model of B-cell transplantation. This study showed that the induction of effective memory in cells from naive donors can be achieved by in vitro exposure to antigen prior to donor cell transfer to the recipient. In vivo antigen challenge of the recipient enhanced the expression of the transferred immune response and resulted in the preservation of a larger diversity of donor clones. Labadie et al. (34) used affinity immunoblotting to demonstrate rapid recovery of specific humoral immunity in a human recipient of an allogeneic bone marrow transplant from an immunized donor.

The three transplantation studies cited above took advantage of the allotypic variants of Ig heavy chains to follow the fate of the transplanted cells. The affinity immunoblotting technique can be used to distinguish between allotypic Ig variants in the immunized animal and, thus, independently monitor each allelic type of Ig in heterozygotes. To do this, the blots are usually developed using biotinylated antiallotype antibodies followed by avidin-peroxidase. This extends the utility of the affinity immunoblot method, permitting simultaneous analysis of clonality and allelic variation.

Hamilton's group (35) used affinity immunoblotting to study the microheterogeneity of murine MAb. Several murine MAb specific for epitopes on the four subclasses of human IgG were studied. The MAb displayed pIs ranging from 6.1–7.8, with the pH spreads of the minor bands from 0.1–0.6 pH unit. One to five major dense bands flanked by up to four minor fainter bands were observed. The clonotype patterns were unique for each antibody. In further work, Hamilton et al. (36) showed that affinity immunoblotting could be successfully used for quality control in hybridoma production facilities. These studies showed that batches of ascites obtained years apart gave identical immunoblot patterns, confirming constant antibody production and stability of the hybridoma clones. The microheterogeneity IEF patterns of each hybridoma cell line were individually characteristic, and the blots were like fingerprints of individual clones.

Rieben's group used affinity immunoblotting to study several interesting properties of natural human anti-A and anti-B blood group antibodies. Their first study *(37)* was directed at studying anti-A antibodies. Clonotype banding patterns of anti-A antibodies in sera from 18 blood donors were individually distinct, showing oligoclonal patterns of <15 bands. Time-course studies showed that the banding patterns in two individuals stayed stable over the observation period of 167 and 82 d, respectively. In a followup report *(38)*, antibody clonotype patterns of ABO antibodies in paired samples of sera and breast milk of postpartum young mothers were examined. The banding patterns of anti-A/B IgG were individually distinct, but shared clonotypes were documented for IgM and IgA. Identical IEF bands detected for IgA in breast milk and serum were shown to be of clonally related origin.

Krolick has exploited the affinity immunoblot method very effectively in his studies of autoimmune myasthenia gravis. In his first study *(39)*, it was shown that rat antiacetylcholine receptor antibodies were oligoclonal, and IgG2a dominated both the primary and secondary responses. In further work *(40)*, affinity immunoblot analyses of antibodies elicited with denatured acetylcholine receptor expressed the same clonotypic heterogeneity and isotype distribution as antibodies elicited by the native acetylcholine receptor. However, an apparent shift was deduced in the preferred clonotypes expressed in response to the denatured receptor; the antibodies were of lower binding affinities than those elicited by the normal receptor. Individual clonotypes were then identified by affinity immunoblotting of preparative IEF fractions corresponding to antibodies capable of passive transfer of the disease *(41)*. The pI of the pathologic antibodies was not confined to one part of the pH gradient, but was spread throughout the gradient, suggesting that many different clonal products were involved in the pathology. Additional studies showed that antibodies in myasthenia gravis patient sera crossreactive with myosin were of restricted clonotype, implying that crossreactivity was not a universal property of all antiacetylcholine receptor antibodies *(42)*.

8. Concluding Remarks

At this time, clonal analysis of antibody responses as a function of time in the intact animal can be studied only by some form of IEF methodology of serum antibodies. Since the only differences in different antibodies of the same class and allotype are differences in V region amino acid sequences, IEF is the only separation method capable of making these fine distinctions. The remaining drawback of this method is that microheterogeneity can cause some clonal products to overlap on the gel. However, for relatively oligoclonal or clonally restricted responses, such as the anticarbohydrate antibodies, the method can be highly informative for detecting sudden appearance or disappearance of individual clones. These types of clonal changes elude detection by simple titration of the antibody mixtures. The titer determinations of the antibodies reactive with a specific antigen in serum will not generally yield information about the clonal composition of the antibodies.

The IEF analysis method of Askonas was improved markedly by Keck, but the drawbacks related to the chemistry used for band immobilization and polymerization were significant. The affinity immunoblot method appears at this point the best method of approximating clonal stability and appearance or disappearance of various antibody clones. The successful application of affinity immunoblotting for studies of clonal responses and clonal fluctuation in intact animals, autoimmune diseases, like lupus and myasthenia gravis, natural blood group antibodies, and bone marrow transplantation suggests that other applications might benefit greatly from adoption of this analytical method.

Acknowledgments

The work done in the author's laboratory that is cited in this chapter was supported by NIH grant AI-20590, NSF grant PCM79-2110, and by NASA contract NAS 9-17403.

References

1. Burnet, F. M. (1959) The clonal selection theory of acquired immunity. Cambridge University Press. London, England.
2. Raff, M., Feldmann, M., and de Petris, S. (1973) Monospecificity of bone marrow derived lymphocytes. *J. Exp. Med.* **137**, 1024–1030.
3. Jerne, N. K. and Nordin, A. A. (1963) Plaque formation in agar by single antibody-producing cells. *Science* **140**, 405.
4. Dresser, D. W. and Wortis, H. H. (1965) Use of an antiglobulin serum to detect cells producing antibody with low haemolytic efficiency. *Nature* **208**, 859–861.
5. Vesterberg, O. (1969) Synthesis and isoelectric fractionation of carrier ampholytes. *Acta Chem. Scand.* **23**, 2653–2666.
6. Awdeh, Z. L., Williamson, A. R., and Askonas, B. A. (1968) Isoelectric focusing in polyacrylamide gel and its application to immunoglobulins. *Nature* **219**, 66,67.
7. Dale, G. and Latner, A. L. (1968) Isoelectric focusing of serum proteins in acrylamide gels followed by electrophoresis. *Clin. Chim. Acta* **24**, 61–68.

8. Fawcett, J. S. (1968) Isoelectric fractionation of proteins on polyacrylamide gels. *FEBS Lett.* **1**, 81,82.

9. Leaback, D. H. and Rutter, A. C. (1968) Polyacrylamide-isoelectric-focusing. A new technique for the electrophoresis of proteins. *Biochem. Biophys. Res. Commun.* **32**, 447–453.

10. Riley, R. F. and Coleman, M. K. (1968) Isoelectric fractionation of proteins on a microscale in polyacrylamide and agarose matrices. *J. Lab. Clin. Med.* **72**, 714–720.

11. Wrigley, C. W. (1968) Analytical fractionation of plant and animal proteins by gel electrofocusing. *J. Chromatogr.* **36**, 362–365.

12. Awdeh, Z. L., Williamson, A. R., and Askonas, B. A. (1970) One cell-one immunoglobulin. Origin of limited heterogeneity of myeloma proteins. *Biochem. J.* **116**, 241–248.

13. Askonas, B. A., Williamson, A. R., and Wright, B. E. G. (1970) Selection of a single antibody-forming cell clone and its propagation in syngeneic mice. *Proc. Natl. Acad. Sci. USA* **67**, 1398–1403.

14. Keck, K., Grossberg, A. L., and Pressman, D. (1973) Specific characterization of isoelectrofocused immunoglobulins in polyacrylamide gel by reaction with ^{125}I-labeled protein antigens or antibodies. *Eur. J. Immunol.* **3**, 99–102.

15. Braun, D. G., Hild, K., and Ziegler, A. (1979) Isoelectric focusing of immunoglobulins, in *Immunological Methods* (Lefkovits, I. and Pernis, B., eds.), Academic, New York, pp. 107–121.

16. Schalch, W. and Braun, D. (1979) Isolation of monoclonal antibody by preparative isoelectric focusing in horizontal layers of Sephadex G-75, in *Immunological Methods* (Lefkovits, I. and Pernis, B., eds.), Academic, New York, pp. 123–130.

17. Schalch, W., Wright, J. K., Rodkey, L. S., and Braun, D. G. (1979) Distinct functions of monoclonal IgG antibody depend on antigen site specificities. *J. Exp. Med.* **149**, 923–937.

18. Brown, J. C. and Rodkey, L. S. (1979) Autoregulation of an antibody response via network-induced auto–anti–idiotype. *J. Exp. Med.* **150**, 67–85.

19. Binion, S. B., Rodkey L. S., Egen, N. B., and Bier, M. (1982) Rapid purification of antibodies to single band purity using recycling isoelectric focusing. *Electrophoresis* **3**, 284–288.

20. Binion, S. B. and Rodkey, L. S. (1982) Isoelectric focusing studies of antibody clonotype patterns in outbred rabbits during prolonged immunization. *Electrophoresis* **3**, 289–293.

21. Insel, R. A., Kittelberger, A., and Anderson, P. (1985) Isoelectric focusing of human antibody to the Haemophilus influenza b capsular polysaccharide: restricted and Identical spectrotypes in adults. *J. Immunol.* **135**, 2810–2816.

22. D'Amelio, R., Del Guidice, G., De Rosa, F., Brighouse, G., Teggi, T., and Lambert, P. H. (1986) Spectrotypic analysis of humoral response in human hydatidosis. *Clin. Exp. Immunol.* **76**, 117–120.

23. Le Moli, S, Matricardi, P. M., Quinti, I., Stroffolini, T., and D'Amelio, R. (1991) Clonotypic analysis of human antibodies specific for Neisseria meningitidis polysaccharides A and C in adults. *Clin. Exp. Immunol.* **83**, 460–465.

24. Roos, R. P., Nalefski, E. A., Nitayaphan, S., Variakijis, R., and Singh, K. K. (1987) An isoelectric focusing overlay study of the humoral immune response in Theiler's virus demyelinating disease. *J. Neuroimmunol.* **13**, 305–314.
25. Stott, D. I., Hassman, R., Neilson, L., and McGregor, A. M. (1988) Analysis of the spectrotypes of autoantibodies against thyroglobulin in two rat models of autoimmune thyroiditis. *Clin. Exp. Immunol.* **73**, 269–275.
26. Muryoi, T., Sasaki, T., Hatakeyama, A., Shibata, S., Suzuki, M., Seino, J., and Yoshinaga, K. (1990) Clonotypes of anti-DNA antibodies expressing specific idiotypes in immune complexes of patients with active Lupus nephritis. *J. Immunol.* **144**, 3856–3861.
27. Stott, D. I. (1992) Spectrotypes of anti-DNA antibodies show that anti-DNA-secreting B-cell clones of SLE patients are restricted in number, stable and long lived. *Autoimmunity* **12**, 249–258.
28. D'Amelio, R., Biselli, R., Nisini, R., Matricardi, P. M., Aiuti, A., Mezzaroma, I., Pinter, E., Pontesilli, O., and Aiuti, F. (1992) Spectrotype of anti-gp120 antibodies remains stable during the course of HIV disease. *J. Acquired Immune Deficiency Syndromes* **5**, 930–935.
29. Knisley, K. A. and Rodkey, L. S. (1986) Affinity Immunoblotting. High resolution isoelectric focusing analysis of antibody clonotype distribution. *J. Immunol. Methods* **95**, 79–87.
30. Knisley, K. A. and Rodkey, L. S. (1988) Isoelectric focusing analysis of antibody clonotype changes occurring during immune responses using immobilized pH gradients. *Electrophoresis* **9**, 183–186.
31. Mehrazar, K., Gilman-Sachs, A., Knisley, K. A., Rodkey, L. S., and Kim, Y. B. (1993) Comparison of the immune response to ARS-BGG in germfree or conventional piglets. *Dev. Compar. Immunol.* **17**, 459–464.
32. Seferian, P. G., Rodkey, L. S., and Adler, F. L. (1987) Selective survival and expression of B-lymphocyte memory cells during long–term serial transplantation. *Cell. Immunol.* **110**, 226–232.
33. Adler, F. L., Adler, L. T., Seferian, P. G., and Rodkey, L. S. (1989) Adoptive immunity transferred by naive donor cells immunized in vitro. *Bone Marrow Transplant* **4**, 663–668.
34. Labadie, J., van Tol, M. J. D., Dijkstra, N. H., van der Kaaden, M., Jol-van der Zijde, C. M., de Lange, G. G., Zwaan, F. E., and Vossen, J. M. (1992) Transfer of specific immunity from donor to recipient of an allogeneic bone marrow graft: evidence for donor origin of the antibody producing cells. *B. J. Hematol.* **82**, 437–444.
35. Hamilton, R. G., Roebber, M., Reimer, C. B., and Rodkey, L. S. (1987) Isoelectric focusing-affinity immunoblot analysis of mouse monoclonal antibodies to the four human IgG subclasses. *Electrophoresis* **8**, 127–134.
36. Hamilton, R. G., Roebber, M., Reimer, C. B., and Rodkey, L. S. (1987) Quality control of murine monoclonal antibodies using isoelectric focusing affinity immunoblot analysis. *Hybridoma* **6**, 205–217.
37. Rieben, R., Fraunfelder, A., and Nydegger, U. E. (1992) Naturally occurring ABO antibodies: long-term stable, individually distinct anti-A IgG spectrotypes. *Eur. J. Immunol.* **22**, 2129–2133.

38. Rieben, R., Frauenfelder, A., and Nydegger, U. E. (1994) Clonality of naturally occurring antibodies to histo-blood group substances A and B from human serum and breast milk revealed by spectrotype analysis. *Blood*, in press.
39. Brown, R. M. and Krolick, K. A. (1988) Clonotypic analysis of the antibody response to the acetylcholine receptor in experimental autoimmune myasthenia gravis. *J. Neuroimmunol.* **19**, 205–222.
40. Yeh, T. M. and Krolick, K. A. (1989) Clonotypic analysis of anti-acetylcholine receptor antibodies produced against native and denatured antigen. *J. Neuroimmunol.* **24**, 133–142.
41. Thompson, P. A. and Krolick, K. A. (1992) Acetylcholine receptor-reactive antibodies in experimental autoimmune myasthenia gravis differing in disease-causing potential: subsetting of serum antibodies by preparative isoelectric focusing. *Clin. Immunol. Immunopathol.* **62**, 199–209.
42. Mohan, S., Barohn, R. J., and Krolick, K. A. (1992) Unexpected cross-reactivity between myosin and a main immunogenic region (MIR) of the acetylcholine receptor by antisera obtained from myasthenia gravis patients. *Clin. Immunol. Immunopathol.* **64**, 218–226.

CHAPTER 10

Affinity Immunoblotting

Keith A. Knisley and L. Scott Rodkey

1. Introduction

Chapter 9 developed the concept of antibody clonality and described several methods that have been used to define antibody clonality in polyclonal sera. Affinity immunoblotting *(1)* has proven to be a powerful and high-resolution method for estimating clonality of immune responses to a variety of antigens. This chapter describes the affinity immunoblotting method in detail.

2. Materials

1. Multiphor or Multiphor II (Pharmacia Biotech Inc., Piscataway, NJ) isoelectric focusing unit with a recirculating refrigerated cooling unit.
2. 125 × 250 mm, 0.5 mm U-frame gel cassette (Pharmacia Biotech) consisting of 125 × 250 mm, 0.5 mm U-frame plate (#80-1106-89); 125 × 250 × 3 mm glass plate (#80-1106-99); flexi clamps 6/pk (#18-1013-73).
3. Reciprocal rocking platform.
4. Sealable plastic containers.
5. Repel Silane (#17-1331-01, Pharmacia Biotech).
6. 124 × 248 mm Acrylamide Gelbond (FMC Bioproducts, Rockland, ME).
7. Electrofocusing electrode strips (#18-1004-40, Pharmacia Biotech).
8. 1*M* sodium hydroxide.
9. 1*M* phosphoric acid.
10. Acrylamide:bis-acrylamide solution (29.1 g acrylamide, 0.9 g bis-acrylamide in 100 mL).
11. TEMED.
12. Silicone rubber surface applicator (#18-1002-26, Pharmacia Biotech).
13. 10% ammonium persulfate.
14. Nitrocellulose (0.45 µm).

From: *Methods in Molecular Biology, Vol. 51: Antibody Engineering Protocols*
Edited by: S. Paul Humana Press Inc., Totowa, NJ

15. Absorbent paper (e.g., #903, Schleicher & Schuell, Keene, NH).
16. Antigen solution in 0.5M sodium bicarbonate.
17. Immune and preimmune serum.
18. Phosphate-buffered saline (PBS): 10 mM sodium phosphate in 0.14M sodium chloride, pH 7.4.
19. Tween-20.
20. Peroxidase conjugated anti-immunoglobulin.
21. Substrates: 30 mg diaminobenzidine and 20 µL hydrogen peroxide in 50 mL PBS.

3. Methods

3.1. Summary of Affinity Immunoblotting Protocol

Approximate time required for each step is shown in parentheses.

Day 1
1. Prepare the gel (15 min). Polymerize overnight.
2. Coat nitrocellulose with antigen overnight.

Day 2
1. Isoelectric focusing (2.5 h).
2. Block nonspecific sites on antigen-coated nitrocellulose (15 min).
3. Immunoblot the gel surface (15 min).
4. Develop the blot (2.5 h).

3.2. Preparation of Polyacrylamide Gel

1. Assemble a 0.5-mm gel cassette. Apply a liberal amount of 70% ethanol to a clean 125 × 250 mm glass plate. Place a piece of acrylamide Gelbond (FMC Bioproducts, Rockland ME) onto the ethanol-covered plate with the hydrophilic side of the Gelbond up. The ethanol reduces surface tension, and helps prevent the entrapment of air bubbles between the Gelbond and the glass plate. The ethanol layer also assures efficient heat transfer between the gel and the cooling plate. Stand the Gelbond-covered plate on edge horizontally on a stack of paper towels and allow the excess ethanol to drain until the Gelbond no longer slides on the plate. Place the U-frame gasket plate over the Gelbond, and clamp it into place. Treat the U-frame gasket plate before use with Repel Silane to reduce adherence of the gel to the plate. (This treatment should be repeated periodically as needed.) Stand the assembled cassette up so that the open end of the U-frame gasket is up. Gently pry the cassette open slightly with a microtip spatula, and insert two bent paper clips at the top of the cassette to permit a slightly wider space at the top of the cassette. This will reduce the chance of air bubble entrapment in the gel during pouring.

2. Mix the acrylamide reagents. Add 2.5 mL of the acrylamide:bis-solution, 1.12 mL 40% ampholyte, and 0.15 mL 10% Tween-20. Bring to a final volume of 15 mL with water.
3. Immediately prior to pouring the gel, add 75 μL 10% ammonium persulfate and 7.5 μL TEMED to the solution in step 3, and mix thoroughly. Add the solution to the cassette with a pipet or a 20-cc syringe. Remove the paper clips, and clamp the top of the cassette. Cover the top of the cassette with Parafilm or Saran Wrap and allow the gel to polymerize overnight at room temperature.

3.3. Coating of Nitrocellulose with Antigen (see Notes 1 and 2)

1. Hydrate a piece of nitrocellulose that is at least large enough to cover the number of lanes of focused antibody. Hydrate for 5 min in water, and then rinse several times with water.
2. Dissolve the antigen solution in 0.5M NaHCO₃. Slowly remove the water from the hydrated nitrocellulose. Replace with the antigen solution. There should be enough antigen solution to cover the nitrocellulose completely when the container is on a flat surface. Place the container with the nitrocellulose and antigen on a reciprocal rocker platform, and rock at room temperature (or at 4°C if desired) overnight.

3.4. Isoelectric Focusing (see Note 3)

1. Precool the flat-bed focusing unit to 8–10°C.
2. Remove the polymerized gel from the cassette. Place a small amount of 70% ethanol (EtOH) on the cooling plate and carefully roll the gel onto the cooling plate, making every attempt to exclude all air bubbles under the Gelbond. If excess EtOH is present around the gel, place a Kimwipe or other absorbent material on the cooling plate for a few minutes to prevent excess liquid from running onto the gel surface.
3. Cut two electrode wicks, each approx 0.5 cm shorter than the length of the gel. Place each on separate pieces of Parafilm. Saturate one wick with 1M phosphoric acid (anode) and the other with 1M sodium hydroxide (cathode). Wicks should be saturated, but not dripping. If they are too wet, carefully touch a paper towel or Kimwipe to them just enough to absorb the sheen from their surface. Place the anode and cathode wicks onto the gel.
4. Place a sample applicator approximately one-third of the distance to the cathode on the anode side of the gel. Gently press down on the applicator to ensure that it has good contact with the gel surface. The surface of the gel must be free of excess fluid, or the sample applicator will not seat properly.

5. Carefully apply the sample to the wells of the applicator. Avoid touching the applicator with the pipet tip, and carefully pipet the samples directly onto the gel surface.
6. Position the electrode cover and close the lid of the IEF unit.
7. Focus at the following settings: 100 V for 15 min; 200 V for 15 min; 5 W for 90 min; and 8 W for 30 min.

3.5. Blocking Nonspecific Nitrocellulose-Binding Sites

About 15 min prior to completion of the IEF run, rinse the antigen-coated nitrocellulose six times with PBS, and then rock in PBS containing 1% Tween-20 for 10-15 min to block nonspecific sites on the membrane.

3.6. Immunoblotting

1. On completion of the run, turn off the power and open the IEF unit. Remove the electrode wicks and sample applicator. Place the gel on a glass plate, and place on a tray that has been covered with wet paper towels.
2. Fully saturate a sheet of absorbent paper (Schleicher & Schuell #903 works well) with PBS-1% Tween. Place the saturated paper onto a clean glass plate. Drain off the excess liquid, and blot the edge with dry paper towels until the sheen is removed and the blot again has the capacity for absorbing more liquid.
3. Remove the nitrocellulose sheet from the 1% Tween-20, and place it onto the moistened absorbent paper long enough for all of the excess liquid to be absorbed from the nitrocellulose. This process is an easy and reproducible way to ensure that excess liquid is removed from the blot without excessive drying.
4. Carefully roll the antigen-coated nitrocellulose onto the gel surface, taking care to not trap any air bubbles between the nitrocellulose and the acrylamide gel. Place an air-tight cover on the tray to form a humidity chamber. Place the chamber into a 37°C incubator for 15 min.

3.7. Blot Development (see Note 4)

1. Carefully peel the nitrocellulose from the gel surface, and place immediately into PBS-0.05% Tween-20. Rinse four times, then rock for 15 min, rinse four more times, rock for 15 min, and finally rinse four more times.
2. After the last rinse, add peroxidase-conjugated antibody specific for IgG (preferably F_c-specific) for the animal species that was used. Rock at room temperature for 45 min, then rinse as in step 1 with PBS-0.05% Tween, and finally pour off the residual liquid.
3. Develop the blot with peroxidase substrates. Band development is usually complete within 5–10 min.

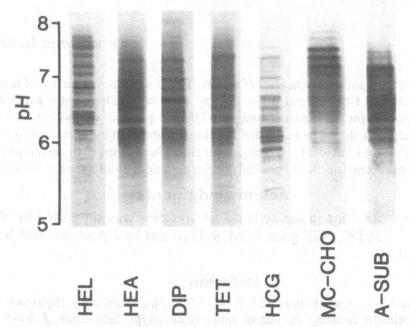

Fig. 1. Affinity immunoblot analysis of antisera specific for different protein and carbohydrate antigens. HEL, hen egg lysozyme; HEA, hen egg albumin; DIP, diphtheria toxoid; TET, tetanus toxoid; HCG, human chorionic gonadotropin; MC-CHO, Micrococcus cell-wall carbohydrate; A-SUB, human blood group A substance derived from porcine gastric mucosa. From *(2)*, with permission.

4. Rinse the nitrocellulose sheet several times with distilled water, rock for 15 min, and then rinse again to remove unreacted substrate. Place the blot on dry paper towels to remove excess liquid, then transfer it to another paper towel, and allow to dry completely. Protect the blot from bright light. Take care when handling the wet nitrocellulose, since it can be easily torn.

4. Notes

1. A concentration of 10 µg/mL works well for most protein antigens, but some standardization may be needed to determine the optimal coating concentration for different antigens. Most antigens bind directly to nitrocellulose under these conditions. However, some antigens (e.g., carbohydrates) may require modification to enhance their binding to nitrocellulose *(1)*.
2. Rotator platforms often coat the outer edges of the nitrocellulose more than the inner surface and are therefore less desirable than a reciprocal rocker platform for this purpose.
3. The affinity immunoblotting can also be done in immobilized pH gradients *(2)*. Gradients are prepared according to the manufacturer (Pharmacia Biotech) with the exception that each gradient chamber contains 1% carrier ampholyte and 0.1% Tween-20. Typical run conditions are 3000 V, 4 mA, and 10 W for at least 6 h. All other manipulations are done as described in Sections 3.5–3.7.

4. Figure 1 shows a typical set of results. This is a composite picture of results obtained from several different sera, each of which contains antibodies specific for the indicated antigens. Distinct patterns are evident for each serum. It should be noted that the clonal patterns in the sera derived from the same individual can change over time. Such changes in clonotype pattern permit detection of naturally occurring auto-anti-idiotype antibodies (3).

Acknowledgments

The work done in the authors' laboratories was supported by NIH grant AI-20590, NSF grant PCM79-2110 and by NASA contract NAS 9-17403.

References

1. Knisley, K. A. and Rodkey, L. S. (1986) Affinity immunoblotting. High resolution isoelectric focusing analysis of antibody clonotype distribution. *J. Immunol. Methods* **95,** 79–87.
2. Knisley, K. A. and Rodkey, L. S. (1988) Isoelectric focusing analysis of antibody clonotype changes occurring during immune responses using immobilized pH gradients. *Electrophoresis* **9,** 183–186.
3. Brown, J. C. and Rodkey, L. S. (1979) Autoregulation of an antibody response via network-induced auto-anti-idiotype. *J. Exp. Med.* **150,** 67–85.

CHAPTER 11

Epitope and Idiotope Mapping Using Monoclonal Antibodies

Srinivas Kaveri

1. Introduction

Serum from normal individuals contains a repertoire of antibodies even in the absence of apparent immunization. The B-cell compartment of the immune system can recognize not only the antigens of the external environment, but also internal or self-antigens. Normal serum contains natural autoantibodies of the IgM and IgG classes that recognize a wide range of self-antigens, including nuclear antigens, intracellular and membrane components, and circulating plasma proteins *(1,2)*. Some of the antigens recognized by natural autoantibodies are also the targets of autoantibodies in autoimmune diseases, e.g., thyroglobulin (Tg), neutrophil cytoplasmic antigens, glomerular basement membrane antigens, intrinsic factor, and factor VIII. Despite the presence of autoreactive B- and T-cells in the normal available immune repertoire, autoimmune disease remains a relatively rare event. Autoimmune diseases cannot be diagnosed by the mere finding of increased titers of autoantibodies in serum. The question arises whether the structure, specificity, affinity, idiotypy, and genetics of autoantibodies in healthy subjects differ from those of pathological autoimmunity *(3,4)*. Determining the fine specificity of autoantibodies may lead to a means of distinguishing natural vs disease-associated autoantibodies.

The use of monoclonal antibodies (MAb) directed against a series of self-antigens has allowed the revelation of the fine specificity of certain disease-associated autoantibodies. MAb have also proven to be advanta-

From: *Methods in Molecular Biology, Vol. 51: Antibody Engineering Protocols*
Edited by: S. Paul Humana Press Inc., Totowa, NJ

geous in the dissection of the interactions between pathogens and host cells. It is reasonable to expect that accurate definitions of the autoantibody combining sites and antigenic determinants in key autoantigens will lead to better understanding of the pathophysiology of autoimmune diseases and to the development of immunotherapeutic strategies. Topographic analysis of polypeptide ligands using MAb can aid in identification of the specific binding site(s) responsible for binding to receptors and the regions involved in activation of receptors *(5)*. These analyses can then be applied toward development of improved pharmaceutical agents and design of novel molecules with agonist or antagonist activity. The binding site (or paratope) of antibodies interacts with a particular region on antigen molecules, termed antigenic determinants or epitopes. The interface between the antibody paratope and antigen epitope can involve about 15–20 amino acid residues. An epitope in polypeptide antigens is not necessarily contiguous in the primary linear sequence. The shape of the epitope is often established by the folding of the protein, e.g., by juxtaposition of two distinct chains of polypeptides *(6)*. One can thus distinguish between: (1) linear, continuous determinants that depend solely on the amino acid sequence of the peptide antigen, and (2) conformational or discontinuous determinants that depend on the native, spatial orientation.

Epitope mapping consists of the topographic analysis of antigens. The binding of a large panel of radiolabeled or enzyme-labeled MAb to the antigen is measured. Inhibition of the binding of individual labeled antibodies by other unlabeled antibodies is then determined. This permits designation of unique and shared antigenic determinants recognized by these antibodies. This approach is discussed below in the context of mapping of human Tg, which is the target for disease-associated autoantibodies in autoimmune thyroditis. Another approach is to use peptide fragments obtained by digestion of protein antigens by enzymes or chemicals. Similarly, the use of synthetic peptides and antibodies to the synthetic peptides has facilitated progress in epitope mapping of proteins.

Thus, antibodies directed to the first 16 amino acid residues of the LDL receptor in fibroblasts have been used to demonstrate that the N-terminus of the receptor is exposed on the external surface of the plasma membrane *(7)*. Competitive inhibition of antibody binding to proteins by various synthetic peptides allows definition of the antigenic determinants.

Analysis of human chorionic gonadotrophin (hCG) reactivity with antipeptide antibodies and monoclonal antinative hCG antibodies has permitted elucidation of the surface topology of this protein *(5)*. The primary immunogenic region of the acetylcholine receptor, which is the target of pathogenic autoantibodies in myasthenia gravis, has been localized by measuring binding of antibodies to recombinant or synthetic peptides, and competition between autoantibodies and MAb for binding to the native receptor *(8)*. Site-directed mutagenesis of the sequences encoding a protein is another powerful approach to map nonoverlapping epitopes recognized by MAb *(9)*. Substitutions of critical amino acids in the epitope results in profound changes in the binding strength of MAb. Recently, surface plasmon resonance to investigate real-time antibody–antigen interactions has provided a simple method for epitope mapping and affinity determination, since this method does not require purification or labeling of antibodies *(10)*.

1.1. Epitope Mapping of Human Tg

Sera from patients with Hashimoto's thyroiditis contain IgG autoantibodies to one or more thyroid antigens including Tg. The level of anti-Tg autoantibodies fluctuates with the course of the disease, and the autoantibodies, together with autoreactive T-cells, are believed to be involved in the pathogenesis of autoimmune thyroiditis *(11)*.

However, autoantibodies to Tg are also frequently observed in the sera of healthy subjects. Several attempts have been made to distinguish the nature of these autoantibodies between healthy and diseased individuals. Tg is an iodinated glycoprotein with a mol wt of 660,000 and a sedimentation coefficient of 19S. It is composed of two identical 12S subunits. Tg plays a crucial role in the biosynthesis and secretion of the thyroid hormones T3 and T4. The epitopes in the primary structure of human Tg responsible for reactions have been localized *(12)*. The epitope mapping of Tg using a battery of MAb is described here.

1.2. Idiotope Mapping Using MAb

An antibody molecule has dual functional characteristics. It can recognize antigens and be recognized by other antibodies. Each unique antigenic determinant in the antibody binding site is an idiotope, with the ensemble of idiotopes referred to as the idiotype. The role of idiotypy in immune regulation has been widely studied. Some anti-idiotypic antibodies (anti-ids) can recognize the same site in the primary antibody as the antigen. These anti-ids are called "internal images" (or Ab2β), and can be used as tools for various biochemical and immunochemical studies. The existence of antibodies that serve as internal images also forms the conceptual backbone of anti-idiotype-based therapy and vaccination. The dissection of the nature of idiotope- anti-idiotype interaction is thus of considerable importance. Here, a common technique for idiotope mapping using monoclonal anti-ids is described using the example of human anti-Tg autoantibodies.

2. Materials

2.1. Coupling MAb to Alkaline Phosphatase (*According to Avrameas and Ternynck* [13])

1. Alkaline phosphatase (AP).
2. 100 mM Sodium phosphate buffer, pH 6.8.
3. Glutaraldehyde.
4. Sephadex G-25.
5. MAb (IgG, 5 mg) or F(ab')$_2$ fragments of IgG (2.5 mg).
6. 500 mM sodium carbonate–bicarbonate buffer, pH 9.5.
7. 1M lysine monochlorohydrate in PBS. Adjust pH to 7.0 using sodium hydroxide.
8. Amicon or Centricon microseparation filters for concentration (exclusion limits, 20,000–50,000 Dalton).
9. PBS: 10 mM sodium phosphate, pH 7.4, 0.15M sodium chloride.

2.2. Human Tg Reactivity with MAb by ELISA

1. PBS.
2. 1% BSA in PBS (PBS-BSA).
3. Polystyrene microtitration plate (Nunc, Roskilde, Denmark).
4. Human Tg (UCB Bioproducts, Belgium).
5. Murine monoclonal anti-Tg antibodies.
6. Peroxidase-labeled goat antimouse Ig.
7. Peroxidase substrate solution: Dissolve 6 mg o-phenylenediamine in 10 mL of 0.05M sodium citrate, and 0.15M sodium phosphate, pH 4.6. Add 20 μL of H$_2$O$_2$. Prepare fresh before use.
8. 3N HCl.
9. Alkaline phosphatase substrate solution: Dissolve 10 mg p-nitrophenyl phosphate in 10 mL 10 mM diethanolamine, pH 9.5, containing 0.5 mM MgCl$_2$.
10. ELISA plate reader.

2.3. Idiotope Mapping by Radioimmunoassay

2.3.1. ^{125}I-Labeling of Anti-Idiotypic Antibodies

1. Iodogen (Pierce).
2. Dichloromethane.
3. Conical capped polypropylene tubes (Eppendorf).
4. 0.25M sodium phosphate buffer, pH 7.5.
5. Monoclonal anti-ids: 1 mg/mL.
7. Na^{125}I (Amersham, les Ulis, France): 200 µCi.
7. Sephadex G-50 desalting column equilibrated with PBS containing 1% BSA.
8. Polystyrene tubes.
9. γ-counter.

2.3.2. Radioimmunoassay

1. Flexible microtiter plates (Falcon Microtest III).
2. Affinity-purified human anti-Tg antibodies.
3. Radioiodinated antibodies.
4. 1% PBS-BSA.
5. γ-counter.

3. Methods

3 1. Coupling of MAb to Alkaline Phosphatase (AP)

1. To 10 mg AP in 200 µL of 100 mM sodium phosphate buffer, pH 6.8, add 2 mL glutaraldehyde (*see* Note 1). Mix and incubate for 18 h at room temperature.
2. Remove unreacted glutaraldehyde by passage of the reaction mixture through a Sephadex G-25 column equilibrated with PBS. Collect protein eluting at the void volume.
3. Reduce the volume of the protein to 1 mL using the concentrating ultrafilter device.
4. Add 5 mg of IgG or 2.5 mg F(ab')$_2$ fragments and 200 µL of 500 mM carbonate-bicarbonate buffer, pH 9.5. Incubate overnight at 4°C.
5. Block the remaining activated groups on AP with 100 µL 1M lysine, pH 7.0, for 2 h.
6. Dialyze overnight against PBS. Store the enzyme–antibody conjugate at –20°C after filter sterilization.

3.2. Human Tg Reactivity with MAb by ELISA

Murine anti-hTg MAb are raised by standard hybridoma techniques (*see* Johnson, Chapter 7). The standard curves for binding of unlabeled MAb to hTg are first established by ELISA (Voller et al. *[14]*).

1. Coat 96-well polystyrene microtitration plates with 100 µL/well of a 10 µg/mL solution of human Tg in PBS. Incubate overnight at 4°C.
2. Remove human Tg solution. Saturate remaining protein binding sites with PBS-BSA for 1 h at room temperature. Wash four times with PBS.
3. Dispense 100 µL/well of MAb over a concentration range of 50– 0.05 µg/mL diluted in PBS-BSA. Incubate for 2 h at room temperature.
4. Remove MAb solution. Wash four times with PBS.
5. Incubate with 100 µL/well of peroxidase labeled goat antimouse Ig antibodies diluted in PBS-BSA for 1 h at room temperature.
6. Remove antibody. Wash at least five times with PBS.
7. Add 100 µL/well of substrate solution.
8. Stop the reaction with 25 µL of 3N HCl.
9. Read the optical density at 495 nm using a plate reader.

3.3. Epitope Mapping by Competitive Inhibition ELISA (see Notes 2 and 3)

The topological relationship of the different antigenic determinants of human Tg are determined by measurement of inhibition of binding of enzyme-labeled MAb by competitor unlabeled MAb.

1. Prepare a 96-well polystyrene microtitration plate coated with human Tg as described in Section 3.2., steps 1 and 2.
2. Mix 100 µL of AP-MAb with 100 µL of unlabeled MAb. The latter can be either the same MAb as the enzyme-labeled MAb or one of a panel of different MAb. The concentration of AP-MAb is chosen to yield binding corresponding to an OD value of about 1.0 at 405 nm in step 7, this section. This can be determined by performing preliminary experiments at varying AP-MAb concentrations. Use unlabeled MAb at an excess concentration, corresponding to plateau values of OD in step 9, Section 3.2.
3. Add 100 µL of the MAb:unlabeled MAb mixture to each human Tg-coated well. Incubate for 1 h at 37°C.
4. Wash the plates five times with PBS.
5. Add 100 µL of AP substrate solution. Incubate for 10–30 min at room temperature.
6. Stop the reaction with 50 µL/well 0.1M EDTA.
7. Measure the OD at 405 nm using a plate reader.
8. Calculate percent inhibition as

$$1 - [(\text{OD with inhibitor MAb present})/(\text{OD with inhibitor MAb absent})] \times 100$$

9. Construct a checkerboard schematic to deduce antigenic clusters (Fig. 1) from the competitive inhibition data. If the unlabeled MAb inhibits the

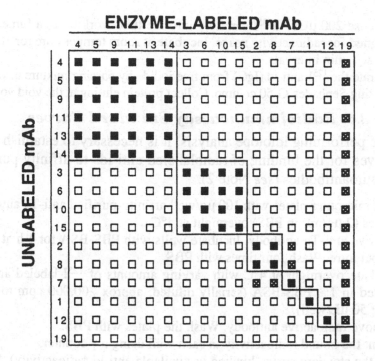

Fig. 1. Antigenic clusters deduced from the schematic representation of competitive inhibition of a panel of 16 enzyme-labeled MAb by the unlabeled MAb. Filled squares, complete inhibition; crossed squares, partial inhibition; open squares, no inhibition (reproduced with permission from ref. *15*).

binding of labeled MAb, the appropriate box is filled in. After all boxes are designated as complete, partial, or no inhibition, the columns and rows are organized to gather together similarly designated boxes *(15,16)*. The antigenic clusters are then deduced. For example, Fig. 1 suggests the presence of seven determinants.

3.4. Labeling of Anti-Idiotypic Antibodies with 125I (see Note 4)

1. Dissolve 1 mg Iodogen in 1 mL dichloromethane. Dispense 20 μL of this solution into polypropylene tubes. Allow the solution to evaporate at room temperature leaving a thin film of Iodogen at the bottom of the tube. The tubes can be stored desiccated for several weeks at −20°C.
2. Add 10 μL 0.2*M* phosphate buffer, pH 7.5, and 10 μL of anti-id solution to an Iodogen-coated tube. Mix.

3. Dispense 200 μCi Na^{125}I carefully into the tube working in a fume hood designed for radioactivity usage. Incubate at room temperature for 10 min. Mix at 1-min intervals.
4. Separate the ^{125}I-anti-id (IgG) from free iodide by passing mixture through a desalting Sephadex G-50 column. Collect protein eluting at the void volume.

3.5. Radioimmunoassay Standard Curves

Before performing idiotope analysis, it is necessary to establish standard curves for the binding of radiolabeled anti-ids to affinity-purified anti-Tg autoantibodies *(see* Note 2).

1. Coat microtiter plates with 100 μg/well affinity-purified anti-Tg autoantibodies (2 μg/mL in PBS) overnight at 4°C.
2. Remove anti-Tg antibody. Incubate wells with PBS-BSA for 1 h at room temperature. Wash four times with PBS.
3. Incubate overnight at 4°C with varying amounts of ^{125}I-labeled anti-ids diluted in 1% PBS-BSA (serially diluted, approx 200,000 cpm to 3000 cpm; 50 μL/well).
4. Remove radioactive antibody. Wash the plates with PBS.
5. Count the bound radioactivity in each well using a γ-counter.
6. Plot the standard curve (binding vs available anti-id radioactivity). Select the concentration of radiolabeled antibody displaying 50–80% binding for idiotope mapping.

3.6. Idiotope Mapping by Competitive Radioimmunoassay

1. Coincubate 50-μL mixtures of increasing concentrations of different anti-ids with individual ^{125}I-labeled anti-id antibodies (at a concentration giving a 50–80% binding) in plates coated with autoantibody to Tg (overnight, 4°C; *see* step 1, Section 3.5.). Make antibody dilutions in PBS-BSA.
2. Remove fluid. Wash the plates with PBS.
3. Count the bound radioactivity in the wells using a gamma counter.
4. Calculate the percent inhibition as:

$$1 - [(\text{CPM with inhibitor anti-id present}/(\text{CPM with inhibitor anti-id absent})] \times 100$$

5. Tabulate results and classify the idiotopes as shown in Table 1 (ref. *17*).

4. Notes

1. In place of AP, antibodies may be coupled with indicators, such as horseradish peroxidase, β-galactosidase or biotin.
2. Epitopes recognized by anti-Tg autoantibodies from patients can be identified by similar competitive inhibition assays. In this case, the ability of the

Table 1
Inhibition of Binding of Radiolabeled Anti-ids
to Tg Autoantibodies by Unlabeled Anti-ids

	1C2	1B1	2B3	1B4	2D2	1E3	1C2	1B1
1C2	100	0	66	100	5	25	+	−
1B1	0	48	0	26	0	90	−	+
2B3	42	0	100	60	0	18	+	−
1B4	100	0	95	100	10	20	+	−
2D2	0	23	6	20	85	30	−	−
1E3	4	57	0	30	7	90	−	+

Values are percent inhibition of the binding. The last two columns show the classification of anti-idis into 1C2 or lB1 idiotope clusters (reproduced from ref. *17*).

Fig. 2. Specificity of anti-Tg autoantibodies from seven patients with Hashimoto's disease. The epitopes on human Tg (I–VI) recognized by autoantibodies (identified by three-letter codes) are deduced using a competitive inhibition assay. Enzyme-labeled anti-Tg MAb are identified by arabic numerals below the epitope designation. Filled squares, >25% inhibition; crossed squares, 25–20% inhibition; open squares, <20% inhibition (reproduced with permission from ref. *17*).

anti-Tg autoantibodies to inhibit binding enzyme-labeled MAb is measured. Results of a typical experiment are shown in Fig. 2. Anti-Tg autoantibodies are purified from the 50% ammonium sulfate cut of sera of patients with Hashimoto's thyroiditis by affinity chromatography on human Tg covalently bound to Sepharose. Bound antibodies are eluted from the column with $0.1M$ glycine-HCl, pH 2.8. The eluted fractions are immediately brought to pH 7.0 using $2.0M$ Tris base and assessed for anti-Tg binding activity by an ELISA.

3. Since the assay system consists of competitive inhibitions using enzyme-labeled MAb, it is necessary to use purified MAb. The MAb can be purified from either culture supernatant or ascitic fluid by appropriate procedures, depending on the isotype of the MAb.
4. Monoclonal anti-ids against anti-Tg autoantibodies are generated in Balb/c mice by injecting F(ab')$_2$ fragments of affinity-purified anti-Tg antibodies from a patient *(17)*. The fusion of splenocytes from mice with the nonsecreting mouse myeloma cell line SP2/0 is performed as previously described (*18* and Chapter 7, this vol.). Clones secreting antibodies reactive with the patient's anti-Tg antibody fraction, but not with the effluent of the Tg-Sepharose affinity column are selected for further characterization.

References

1. Avrameas, S. (1991) Natural autoantibodies: from "horror autotoxicus" to "gnothi seauton." *Immunol. Today* **12,** 154–159.
2. Hurez, V., Kaveri, S. V., and Kazatchkine, M. D. (1993) Expression and control of the natural autoreactive IgG repertoire in normal human serum. *Eur. J. Immunol.* **23,** 783–789.
3. Hurez, V., Dietrich, G., Kaveri, S. V., and Kazatchkine, M. D. (1993) Polyreactivity is a property of natural and disease-associated human autoantibodies. *Scand. J. Immunol.* **38,** 190–196.
4. Dietrich, G. and Kazatchkine, M. D. (1994) *Human Natural Self-Reactive Antibodies. Autoimmunity: Physiology and Disease* (Coutinho, A. and Kazatchkine, M., eds.), Wiley-Liss, New York, pp. 107–128.
5. Bidart, J. M., Troalen, F., Salesse, R., Bousfeld, G. R., Bouhoun, C., and Bellet, D. (1987) Immunochemical mapping of a specific domain on human chorionic gonadotropin using anti-protein and anti-peptide MAb. *J. Biol. Chem.* **262,** 8551–8556.
6. Amit, A. G., Mariuzza, R. A., Phillips, S. E. V., and Poljak, R. J. (1985) Three-dimensional structure of an antigen-antibody complex at 6 A resolution. *Nature* **313,** 156–158.
7. Schneider, W., Slaughter, C. J., Goldstein, J. L., Anderson, R. G. W., Capra, J. D., and Brown, M. S. (1983) Use of anti-peptide antibodies to determine external orientation of the NH2-terminus of the low density lipoprotein receptor in the plasma membrane of fibroblasts. *J. Cell Biol.* **97,** 1635–1640.
8. Harcourt, G. and Jermy, A. (1987) Mapping the autoimmunizing epitopes on acetylcholine receptors. *Immunol. Today* **8,** 319–321.
9. Smith, A. and Benjamin, D. C. (1991) The antigenic surface of staphylococcal nuclease. *J. Immunol.* **146,** 1259–1264.
10. Dubs, M. C., Atschuh, D., and Reggenmortel, M. H. V. (1991) Interaction between viruses and monoclonal antibodies studied by surface plasmon resonance. *Immunol. Lett.* **31,** 59–64.
11. Charreire, J. (1989) Immune mechanisms in autoimmune thyroiditis. *Adv. Immunol.* **46,** 263–284.

12. Henry, M., Malthiery, Y., Zanelli, E., and Charvet, B. (1990) Epitope mapping of human thyroglobulin. Heterogeneous recognition by thyroid pathologic sera. *J. Immunol.* 145, 3692–3698.

13. Avrameas, S. and Ternynck, T. (1969) The cross-linking of proteins with glutaraldehyde and its use for the preparation of immunoadsorbents. *Immunochemistry* 6, 53–66.

14. Voller, A., Bidwell, D. E., and Burek, C. L. (1980) An enzyme linked immunosorbent assay (ELISA) for antibodies to thyroglobulin. *Proc. Soc. Exp. Biol. Med.* 163, 402–405.

15. Piechaczyk, M., Chardes, T., Cot, M. C., Pau, B., and Bastide, J. M. (1985) Production and characterization of MAb against human thyroglobulin. *Hybridoma* 4, 361–367.

16. Bresler, H. S., Burek, L. C., Hoffman, W., and Rose, N. R. (1990) Autoantigenic determinants on human thyroglobulin: determinants recognized by autoantibodies from patients with chronic autoimmune thyroiditis compared to auto-antibodies from healthy subjects. *Clin. Immunol. Immunopathol.* 54, 76–86.

17. Kaveri, S. V., Wang, H. T., Rowen, D., Kazatchkine, M. D., and Kohler, H. (1993) Monoclonal anti-idiotypic antibodies against human anti-thyroglobulin autoantibodies recognize idiotopes shared by disease-associated and natural anti-thyroglobulin autoantibodies. *Clin. Immunol. Immunopathol.* 69, 333–340.

18. Galfre, G., Howe, S. C., Milstein, C., Butcher, G. W., and Howard, J. C. (1977) Antibodies to major histocompatibility antigens produced by hybrid cell lines. *Nature* 266, 550–552.

CHAPTER 12

Anti-Idiotypic Antibodies That Mimic Opioids

Jay A. Glasel and Dianne Agarwal

1. Introduction

The existence of opioid receptors as "narcotic analgesic binding components" in mammalian brain was first documented in the early 1970s (1–3). Shortly thereafter, endogenous opioid peptides (endorphins) that also bound to these receptors were found in mammalian brain tissue. Subsequent pharmacological work revealed the existence of three main subclasses of receptors designated μ, δ, and κ. This work was confirmed by the recent cloning of these three subclasses (4–8) that bear sequence homologies to each other and to the G-protein-coupled receptor superfamily. Before the successes in cloning the subclasses, several investigators seeking to answer questions about the molecular basis of the different opioid-receptor classes prepared anti-idiotypic antibodies to the opioid receptors. This approach was taken because unsuccessful experiments showed that antiopioid-receptor antibodies could not be prepared by immunization with cells expressing the receptors. The general experimental approach has been to use subclass-selective ligands as immunogens to raise antihapten antibodies (Id[+], AB1), which in turn are used as immunogens to prepare anti-idiotypic antibodies (AB2). Anti-idiotypic antibodies have been described in theory as containing an "internal image" of the ligand at their binding site (9,10). This implies that portions of the binding region of the anti-idiotypic antibody can demonstrate binding properties and, in some cases, pharmacological properties similar to the original ligand. In accordance with this view, the resulting anti-idiotypic antiopioid receptor antibodies have been shown to mimic their respective agonists both kinetically and pharmacologically (11–13).

From: *Methods in Molecular Biology, Vol. 51: Antibody Engineering Protocols*
Edited by: S. Paul Humana Press Inc., Totowa, NJ

Thus, antiopioid receptor antibodies have proven to be important tools for studying the functionality and localization of receptors within their native environment *(12,14)*. A significant advantage to using AB2s as probes for membrane-bound receptors is that they can be fluorescently labeled at sites distant from their receptor-binding site, whereas this cannot be done with the much smaller opioid ligands. Furthermore, fluorescently labeled AB2s can be used to monitor binding to individual cells within a large total population of cells, whereas more commonly used radioreceptor-binding assays can only address the average binding properties of an entire cell population *(15)*.

1.1. Receptor-Binding Portions of Opioid Ligands

Two types of ligands are known to interact specifically with neuronal opioid receptors. Those of type I are quite rigid polycyclic organic structures based on the structure of morphine, the archetypal opioid derived from plants. All of the biologically active compounds of this type contain the tertiary nitrogen and the aromatic ring. The absolute stereochemistry of the asymmetric carbon atoms in the structures is very important for both binding and biological action. The type II opioid structures consist of single-chain polypeptides that have lengths of from 5 to more than 30 residues *(16)*. Invariably the N-terminus of the polypeptide is a tyrosyl residue. Extensive structure–activity studies done on opioids show that the receptor-binding sites specifically recognize the tertiary nitrogen/aromatic (tyramine) ring system.

1.2. Conjugation of Opioid Ligands to Immunogenic Proteins

The specific succinylation of the 6-hydroxyl group of morphine results in a derivative useful for the coupling of morphine to proteins for the preparation of Abs. Morphine linked to bovine serum albumin (BSA) is very immunogenic, and high titers are achieved very rapidly in all animals. Coupling is done via the 6-hydroxyl group, which is unnecessary for pharmacological activity.

2. Materials

2.1. Ligand-Carrier Conjugation

1. Succinic anhydride.
2. Morphine as the free-base (may be prepared from soluble morphine salts by precipitation from neutralized aqueous solution).

3. Benzene.
4. Sintered glass filter.
5. 1M HCl.
6. Concentrated NaOH.
7. Ethanol.
8. Vacuum oven.
9. Deionized H_2O.
10. Two small beakers (5 mL).
11. Tetrahydrofuran.
12. BSA (Sigma, St. Louis, MO, "essentially fat free").
13. **Fresh** carbodiimide.
14. 0.1M ammonium bicarbonate.
15. Trifluoroacetic acid.
16. 30% Acetic acid.

2.2. Purification of Monoclonal Idiotypic Antibodies

2.2.1. Column Preparation

1. Sepharose CL4 or CL4B packing: 100 g washed and filtered but still wet, in 100 mL H_2O.
2. CNBr: 5 g in 25 mL acetonitrile. (Danger: work in a well-ventilated fume hood.)
3. 0.5N NaOH.
4. 0.1M NaHCO$_3$.
5. 1,6-Hexanediamine: 1.16 g, dissolved in 100 mL cold NaHCO$_3$ (0.1 M).
6. Deionized H_2O.
7. 0.5M NaCl.
8. Sodium azide.
9. Methanol.
10. Acetone.
11. Filter paper.
12. Ninhydrin/cadmium acetate solution.
13. 50, 25, and 10% dioxane.
14. Refrigerator.
15. Tributylamine.
16. Tributylchloroformate.
17. t-Butylamine.
18. Phosphate-buffered saline (PBS): 0.01M sodium phosphate, 0.15M sodium chloride, pH 7.4; PBS-azide, PBS containing 0.1% sodium azide.
19. Morphine-6-hemisuccinate (MHS), 2X recrystallized.

2.2.2. Affinity Purification

1. PBS.
2. 0.22 μM Millipore GV syringe filter.

3. Fluorescence or absorption spectrophotometer.
4. Econo-column (Bio-Rad, Hercules, CA).

2.2.3. Column Elution

1. PBS-azide, *see* Section 2.2.1.
2. 0.05M citrate, pH 5.5.
3. 0.1M glycine, pH 2.8.
4. 2M Tris base, pH 10.
5. 6M guanidine hydrochloride, neutralized to pH 7.

2.3. Binding Assay

1. 1-mL plastic syringe barrels fitted with round polyethylene fritted disks at their base to form small chromatography columns.
2. 13 × 100 mm test tubes.
3. Sephadex G-25F.
4. Centrifuge.
5. Test tube rack.
6. Scintillation counting vials (plastic, 7 mL).
7. Liquid scintillation counter.
8. Aqueous scintillation cocktail.
9. PBS (*see* Section 2.2.1.).
10. BSA in PBS, 10 mg/mL (1%).
11. Id$^+$, affinity-purified, 2 mg/mL, preserved with 1% sodium azide.
12. 2 μM [^{3}H]morphine (3–4 Ci/mol) made up to 500 μM with PBS.
13. 1000 μg **crude** anti-Id or 20 μg affinity-purified anti-Id made up to 500 μL with PBS.

2.4. Preparation
of Polyclonal Anti-Idiotypic Antibodies

1. Fab fragments (*see* Note 1).
2. Complete Freund's adjuvant (CFA).
3. PBS (*see* Section 2.2.1.).
4. 20- or 21-gage needle.
5. Sodium azide.
6. Sorvall SS-34 rotor.
7. Phenylmethylsulfonyl fluoride (PMSF, dissolved in acetone at 100X working concentration, 10^{-4}M).
8. 70% (w/v) saturated ammonium sulfate (freshly made up, pH 7.4).

2.5. Preparation of Monoclonal Anti-Idiotypic Antibodies

1. Fab fragments.
2. PBS (*see* Section 2.2.1.).

3. *Bordella pertussis* bacteria (Difco, Detroit, MI).
4. 5- to 6-wk-old mice.
5. Freund's incomplete adjuvant.
6. SP2/0 myeloma cells.
7. Soft agar.

2.6. Purification and Analysis of Anti-Idiotypic Antibodies

2.6.1. Column Preparation

1. Swelled, wet-filtered, matrix (Sepharose CL4B).
2. Deionized H_2O.
3. 200-mL beaker.
4. 0.5M NaOH.
5. CNBr.
6. Dimethylformamide.
7. Pasteur pipet.
8. 0.1M and 0.2M $NaHCO_3$.
9. Id^+ (58 mg, determined spectrophotometrically [17]).
10. 1M acetic acid.
11. Cold room.
12. PBS and PBS-azide (*see* Section 2.2.1).

2.6.2. Affinity Purification

1. Silanized glassware and columns.
2. Small columns with bed sizes of the order of 15 mL.
3. Dialysis tubing.
4. Refrigerator.

2.6.3. Column Elution

1. PBS.
2. NaSCN, pH 8.1.
3. Guanidine hydrochloride, pH 7.
4. Small test tubes.
5. Fluorescence detector.
6. Millipore CX-10 ultrafiltration tips.
7. Individual small MHS affinity columns (*see* Section 2.6.1. *above*).

2.6.4. Radioimmunoassay

This protocol pertains to mouse Id^+. Appropriate antibody should be used for other species.

1. 96-well ELISA plate.
2. Goat antimouse antibody (commercially available from several sources, 50 µg/mL).

3. Refrigerator or 37°C incubator.
4. 1% BSA in PBS-azide.
5. 100 µL hybridoma cell supernatant.
6. PBS-azide (*see* Section 2.2.1.).
7. 0.05% (v/v) Tween-20.
8. Putative active protein in PBS solution.
9. 0.5*M* HCl.
10. Aqueous scintillation cocktail.
11. Scintillation counting vials.
12. Liquid scintillation counter.

2.7. Conjugation of Immunoglobulin to Reporter Molecules

1. Immunoglobulin in form of affinity-purified antibody or IgG fraction of antiserum.
2. Biotin hydrazide (powder) higher than 99% purity (Sigma).
3. Sodium metaperiodate, $NaIO_4$, analytical-grade.
4. Sephadex G25 equilibrated in PBS.
5. Sodium cyanoborohydride, $NaCNBH_3$, analytical-grade.
6. 1*M* HCl solution
7. PBS-azide.

3. Methods

3.1. Preparation of MHS and Conjugation to BSA

1. In a round-bottom flask, mix 2.4 g succinic anhydride, 2.2 g morphine free-base, and 40 mL benzene. (The cold starting material may be doped with ^{3}H-morphine for certain applications in order to trace yield. However, this should **not** be done for samples destined to be used as immunogens.)
2. Stir with refluxing for 2 h. Add further 2 g of succinic anhydride and 20 mL benzene. Continue refluxing for 1 h more. Cool mixture and filter through a medium sintered glass filter. Discard the filtrate.
3. Scrape the material off the filter and into a beaker, add 20 mL H_2O in two portions, and bring to pH 2 with 1*M* HCl. Filter off any undissolved solids. Bring to pH 9 with NaOH (the solution may pass through a precipitation step as the pH increases). Let stand 15 min or longer, and filter off any precipitate. Bring back down to pH 5 with 1*M* HCl, and let stand overnight in a refrigerator. Crude MHS will precipitate.
4. Filter out the precipitate, and wash with 96% ethanol. Dissolve in minimal hot 60% ethanol, and reduce volume by 60%. Allow to crystallize on cooling. For every 0.25 g of morphine, about 60 mL of 60% ethanol are needed to dissolve the crude mixture. Repeat this crystallization once more.

5. Dry recrystallized materials at 75°C overnight in vacuum oven.
6. Place 28 mg of MHS derivative in 1 mL of water in a small reaction vessel. Add tetrahydrofuran dropwise with stirring and gentle heating to bring into solution.
7. In a separate vessel, dissolve 20 mg Sigma "essentially fat-free" BSA and 38 mg **fresh** carbodiimide in 2 mL H_2O. Bring to pH 3 with 0.1 and 1.0M HCl.
8. Ice all solutions. When cold, mix together, and place on ice. Stir for 1 h. Solutions turn cloudy within a short time.
9. Dialyze the suspension against 0.1M ammonium bicarbonate (some fluffy precipitate may remain). Lyophilize.
10. Add 5 mL trifluoroacetic acid (TFA) to the white lyophilized powder from above. Stir for 15 min. Pump off the TFA leaving a wet white precipitate. Add 10 mL 30% acetic acid in small amounts. Dialyze against 0.1M ammonium bicarbonate. Yield = 9 mg (*see* Note 2).

3.2. Production of Idiotypic (Id⁺) Antibodies

We immunized female Balb/c strain mice with MHS conjugated to BSA. The standard procedure for deriving hybridomas is described by Johnson (Chapter 7). Briefly:

1. Mouse spleen cells were fused with SP2/O myeloma cells.
2. Hybrid colonies appeared at 17–21 d following fusion. Antiligand screening assays were performed via the column method described below (*see* Section 3.4.).
3. The second recloning resulted in 100% positive colonies for surviving lines.
4. Cells from these colonies were used to produce large quantities of monoclonal Abs via the ascites tumor technique (*18*).

3.3. Purification of Id⁺ Antibodies
3.3.1. Column Preparation

1. Add CNBr solution to gel packing dropwise at first after bringing gel to pH 11.0 ± 0.2. Cool and stir mixture maintaining the pH at 11 with NaOH. Wash gel with 0.1M NaHCO$_3$ after pH stabilizes.
2. Immediately add hexanediamine solution to the activated gel and couple for 6 h at room temperature in a shaking flask. Wash with: 0.1M NaHCO$_3$, H_2O, 0.5M NaCl, H_2O.
3. Store at 4°C with addition of sodium azide. Check qualitatively for coupling by washing a sample with methanol and acetone, and drying on filter paper. Spray a dried aliquot of beads with ninhydrin/cadmium acetate solution. Brown color indicates coupling has been achieved.

4. The following proportions are for 30 mL of wet sucked gel. Wash hexanediamine-Sepharose with ≈500 mL 50% dioxane. Add 10 mL of 50% dioxane, cover, and refrigerate until use.

5. Add 12 mg MHS to 15 mL **dry** (molecular sieved) dioxane. MHS dissolves slowly with heat and stirring. Cool to room temperature, and cover until use.

6. Add 14.5 µL of tributylamine to the MHS solution, and place on an ice bath. Add 9 µL of tributylchloroformate, and stir with cooling for 20 min. Keep the reaction mixture unfrozen by taking it out of the ice bath briefly when it starts to freeze up.

7. Bring the gel slurry to apparent pH 10.5. Add the MHS solution from above dropwise with cooling and stirring. Keep pH at 10.5 with NaOH. The pH should begin to drop immediately when the MHS is added.

8. Wash the gel with: 200 mL 50% dioxane, 200 mL 25% dioxane, 200 mL 10% dioxane with 1 drop of *t*-butylamine added, and 200 mL PBS-azide.

9. Check for coupling using the ninhydrin method. Properly coupled gel will be pink with ninhydrin, whereas unreacted hexanediamine-gel will be brown (as above). Store in cold with azide. Coupling yield is ≈75% as determined by subtraction. Couplings ranging from 30 to 390 µg MHS/mL gel are common.

3.3.2. Affinity Purification (see Note 3)

1. MHS column (MHS coupled to Sepharose 4B-CL via a 1,6-hexanediamine spacer). For 100–150 mg of crude ascites proteins, a 15-mL Econo-column will suffice.

2. Wash column with at least 3 column volumes of PBS.

3. Sample should be dialyzed against PBS. Volume should be ≈2 mL. Filter with GV filter if any debris is present. Obtain an optical density (OD) reading at 280 nm.

4. Load sample onto column. After the entire sample has entered the packing, begin PBS elution. Monitor the eluant fluorescence or A_{280}. When the signal just begins to be observable, shut off the column valve and allow the column to absorb at room temperature for at least 45 min.

3.3.3. Column Elution

1. Begin PBS elution into tubes, and continue until monitor returns to baseline. Pool peak fractions, and obtain an A_{280} reading.

2. Begin elution with citrate buffer. Monitor A_{280} and monitor and collect fractions. Obtain an OD reading on pooled peak fractions.

3. Begin elution with glycine buffer. Collect fractions in tubes containing $2M$ Tris base in the proportion 60 µL of Tris/1 mL fraction. Place fractions on ice as soon as possible. Pool peak fractions, and begin dialysis of the pool

against PBS. Protein concentrations obtained at this stage are approximate because of the mixed composition of the buffer.

4. Wash the column with PBS-azide. Complete cleaning can be done by washing the column with $6M$ guanidine-HCl until column turns opalescent, and then washing exhaustively with PBS-azide. Store column in refrigerator in PBS-azide.

5. After dialysis (at least three changes of dialysis buffer), obtain an A_{280} reading vs the buffer. Precipitate the dialysate with 50% ammonium sulfate overnight in a refrigerator. Pellet the suspension, and store in 50% ammonium sulfate-azide in the refrigerator. In this form, the antibodies are stable for longer than a year.

6. Quality control: Perform centrifugal column assay (described below) and polyacrylamide gel electrophoresis on the batch to assure activity and purity.

3.4. Determination of Idiotypic Specificity and Crossreactivity

3.4.1. Centrifugal Column Assay
(Assay for Antimorphine Activity; see Note 4)

1. Sample preparation (*see* Note 5): Incubate the following for 30 min at room temperature; 2 μg Id$^+$, 40 μL BSA-PBS, 2 μM [^{3}H]morphine (3-4 Ci/mol) made up to 500 μL with PBS.

2. Column preparation: While samples are incubating, fit each 1-mL plastic syringe barrel with a fritted disk. Place the syringe barrels in 13 × 100 mm test tubes. Prepare 3 barrels/incubation mixture. Fill each barrel with a suspension of Sephadex G-25F taken from a continuously agitated vessel. This last step should be done no more than 15 min before the end of incubation. Just before loading samples onto columns, centrifuge the barrels in the test tubes at a setting of 500g for 3 s (counted out from the start of acceleration). Remove the barrels from the test tubes and put the tubes in a rack. Place the barrels in 7-mL scintillation counting vials.

3. Assay: Carefully load 150 μL of each incubation mixture onto the top of each of three dried columns. When all of the mixtures have been loaded, place the columns and the vials into the centrifuge. Accelerate to 500g, immediately starting a timer when the speed rheostat is turned on. After 1.5 min, turn the rheostat to zero, and allow the rotor to slow down by itself. Remove columns from the scintillation vials, tapping the last drops from the tip of each barrel. Add 150 μL of water to each vial and 4.5 mL of aqueous scintillation cocktail to each. Vortex and count after capping.

4. Tritiated morphine (*see* Note 6): The molecular mass of (morphine)$_2$ sulfate (assume the pentahydrate) being 758.8 Dalton, 10 mg dissolved in 250 mL H_2O gives 100 μM morphine. Mix 7 μL [^{3}H]morphine (SA 50–60 Ci/

mmol), 18 µL 100 µM morphine (M), and 975 µL H_2O to give [M] = 1800 nM, [^{3}H-M] = 122 nM, and [M]$_{tot}$ = 1922 nM. A 50-µL aliquot of this stock mixture should give 200,000+ cpm with a typical liquid scintillation counter.

3.5. Preparation of Polyclonal Anti-idiotypic Antibodies (see Note 7)

3.5.1. Immunization Schedule

1. Primary immunization is with 300–800 µg Fab fragments (*see* Note 8) emulsified in CFA and administered intramuscularly (im) in four to eight sites.
2. This is followed after a 1-mo interval with a duplicate secondary immunization.
3. A tertiary immunization is done after a month. This consists of an iv injection of 1 mg Fab in PBS. Thereafter, the animals are reimmunized every month with the same procedure.
4. The animals are bled just prior to reimmunizations beginning with the quaternary immunization, and 2 wk later. We find that we can keep an animal producing titer over a long period of time. However, we observed that titers of individual animals are highly variable and aperiodic in the production of antimorphine monoclonal antibodies (MAb). None of the rabbits exhibited any extraordinary physiological behavior during the postimmunization period. Titers are monitored by the column assay or the radioimmunoassay.

3.5.2. Bleeding and Crude Antibody Preparation

1. The animals are bled via the large ear vein using a 20- or 21-gage needle, with a 30–40 mL whole blood being collected each time.
2. Sodium azide is added to a concentration of 0.01% and PMSF, to $10^{-4}M$. The blood is allowed to sit overnight in the refrigerator.
3. On the next day, the coagulated blood is centrifuged twice at 11,000 rpm for 30 min in a Sorvall SS-34 rotor to remove blood cells and other debris.
4. A crude antibody fraction is precipitated using an "optimal" procedure previously reported *(19)*. An equal volume of 70% (w/v) saturated ammonium sulfate (freshly made up, pH 7.4) is slowly mixed with the serum. This is allowed to sit at room temperature for 4 h, followed by centrifugation as above, and the supernatant is discarded.
5. The pellet is redissolved in deionized water to the same volume as the original serum and then slowly mixed with another equal volume of 70% saturated ammonium sulfate. This is immediately centrifuged again and the supernatant discarded.

6. Step 5 is repeated. The final crude pellet is stored refrigerated in 70% ammonium sulfate with added azide and PMSF. The antibodies stored in this way are stable for longer than a year.

3.6. Preparation of Monoclonal Anti-idiotypic Antibodies

3.6.1. Immunization Schedule

1. Primary immunization of 5- to 6-wk-old mice is with 100–200 µg of Fab fragments (125 µL aqueous PBS solution **without** azide) supplemented with 10^9 *Bordella pertussis* bacteria (Difco) and emulsified with 125 µL CFA (*see* Note 9). Immunization is at four subcutaneous sites on the ventral surface and one intraperitoneal (ip) site with 50 µL each.
2. Secondary immunization (ip) 1 mo later is with the same amount of Fab in 100 µL of emulsion prepared from equal volumes of aqueous antigen solution and incomplete Freund's adjuvant (IFA).
3. Further immunizations are at 1-mo intervals using whole IgG in the same amount as the secondary immunization. Boost responding mice with 100 µg IgG in IFA emulsion 3 d before cell fusion. Contrary to expectation, antimorphine MAb derived from mice are immunogenic in syngeneic mice. Titers are monitored by the column assay or radioimmunoassay.

3.6.2. Fusion

The fusion protocol is a standard one using SP2/O or NSO myeloma cells. The ratio of spleen to myeloma cells is 10:1. Subsequent cloning is performed in soft agar. Screening of wells is performed using the solid-state radioimmunoassay described below (*see* Note 10).

3.7. Purification and Analysis of Anti-Idiotypic Antibodies

3.7.1. Antimorphine Affinity-Column Preparation

1. Operations are performed in a hood. Thirty milliliters of swelled, wet-filtered packing are washed with 600 mL of deionized water. This is then placed in a 100-mL beaker with addition of 30 mL of water. Using 0.5 NaOH, the pH is adjusted to 11.
2. Two grams of CNBr dissolved in 2 mL of dimethylformamide are added dropwise from a Pasteur pipet. The pH is maintained with 0.5 and 0.1 $NaHCO_3$. Id$^+$ IgG (58 mg, determined spectrophotometrically) previously dialyzed against $0.2M$ $NaHCO_3$ and diluted to 60 mL with the bicarbonate solution is added to 50 mL of the slurry, and the mixture is stirred in a cold room for 16 h.

3. After filtering, about 1% of IgG remains in solution. The column material is washed successively with 1 L water, 1 L 1M acetic acid, 500 mL water, and 500 mL PBS.
4. The slurry is stored in the refrigerator in PBS-azide. Routine coupling achieved is 1.5-2 mg IgG/mL packing, and therefore a column containing 10 mg IgG has an upper limit of 14×10^{-8} mol of available morphine-binding sites.

3.7.2. Affinity Purification

For affinity purification of anti-idiotypic antibodies all glassware and columns are silanized before use. Small columns with bed sizes on the order of 15 mL are convenient. The crude antibody preparations are dialyzed against PBS and loaded on the columns in amounts of 20–50 mg of protein (crude preparations are assumed to have an extinction coefficient of 1.4 at 280 nm) and allowed to incubate overnight in a refrigerator after washing the adsorbed material with PBS.

3.7.3. Column Elution (see Note 11)

1. The columns are eluted discontinuously with PBS, 3.5M NaSCN (pH 8.1), 3M guanidine-HCl (pH 7), and either 4.5 or 6M guanidine-HCl (pH 7). The reason for the different guanidine concentrations is that elution efficiency is a function of the affinity of the anti-idiotypic antibody for the Id^+.
2. The thiocyanate and guanidine fractions are collected in vials containing enough water to dilute the fractions to 0.15M guanidine-HCl and immediately placed on ice. Determination of peaks is best done using a fluorescence detector with excitation at 289 nm and emission at 340 nm.
3. Peak fractions are pooled and dialyzed in the cold against PBS.
4. When purifying polyclonal anti-idiotypic antibodies, it has been found that morphine-binding material is present in pooled elution fractions from some preparations. Hence, an additional purification step is used. The dialyzed pools are concentrated using Millipore CX-10 ultrafiltration tips. The resulting samples are then passed through individual small MHS affinity columns before use in competition assays. The PBS void volume pools contain the desired active material.

3.7.4. Solid-State Radioimmunoassay (see Notes 12 and 13)

1. Coat wells in a 96-well ELISA plate with goat antimouse antibody (50 µg/mL, 100 µL/well, and incubate overnight in the refrigerator or 2 h at 37°C).
2. Block wells with 1% BSA in PBS-azide overnight in the refrigerator or 1 h at room temperature.
3. Flick dry without washing.

4. Add 100 µL mouse antimorphine hybridoma (or polyclonal antimorphine antibodies) cell supernatant, and incubate at room temperature for 2 h or keep overnight in the refrigerator. For control wells, add fresh medium in PBS-azide, and for blanks, add only PBS-azide.
5. Aspirate and wash twice with PBS plus 0.05% (v/v) Tween-20.
6. Add putative active protein in PBS solution, 100 µL, to duplicate wells. Incubate 2 h at room temperature.
7. Aspirate and wash three times with PBS-Tween-20.
8. Add [^{3}H]morphine in 0.01% BSA-PBS, 100 µL/well. The radioligand should be carrier-free and should give about 10,000 cpm/100 µL. Incubate in the dark for 1 h.
9. Aspirate and wash three times with PBS-Tween-20.
10. Add 100 µL/well of 0.5M HCl to release bound radioligand. Incubate <5 min. Remove 75 µL from each well, and count with the aqueous scintillation cocktail system (*see* Note 13). For polyclonal anti-idiotypic serum monitoring, several hundred cpm should be recovered from wells not containing anti-idiotypic antibodies. Wells containing anti-idiotypic antibodies display radioactivity at near-background levels.

3.8. Conjugation of Immunoglobulin to Reporter Molecules

1. Prepare the immunoglobulin solution in PBS, and adjust protein concentration to 1.0 mg/mL.
2. Add NaIO$_4$ to a final concentration of 1 mM. Incubate for 30 min at 0°C.
3. Separate protein from inorganic salts on Sephadex G25. Pool protein peak.
4. Add 7.5 mg biotin hydrazide/1.0 mg immunoglobulin in a 1-mL vol. Incubate for 30 min at room temperature.
5. Adjust pH of reaction mixture to pH 6.9 by adding 1M HCl.
6. Add NaCNBH$_3$ to a final concentration of 1 mM. Incubate for 16 h at 4°C.
7. Separate on Sephadex G25, and pool protein peak.
8. Mix 1 mL of 0.53 mg/mL biotinylated IgG with 0.5 mL of 8.8 µM fluorophore (avidin). Stir for 1 h at room temperature. Store at 4°C. Since the labeled antibody is often used with live cells or animals, it cannot be kept sterile with azide. It may be filtered into a sterile vial using a low protein-binding filter with some loss of material.

4. Notes

1. Crude fragments are prepared from the affinity-purified *(20)* antibodies using an unmodified classical protocol *(21)*. The binding fragments are then repurified using the same affinity packing. An overall yield of 40–60% is expected from these procedures. Immunizing with only the Fab

region of the monoclonal antimorphine antibody should stimulate a poly-clonal antibody response predominantly directed against the antigen-binding fragment of the antibody.

2. Quality control is done by TLC using dioxane-benzene-ethanol-ammonium hydroxide (5:50:40:5) and staining with I_2 vapor. The hemisuccinate has an R_f value of 0.13, whereas morphine runs at R_f 0.69. Yield is 25%.

3. Monitor column effluent via fluorescence with excitation at 280 nm and emission at 340 nm for greatest sensitivity. Absorption spectroscopy at 280 nm is also possible, but is less sensitive.

4. Screening for an MAb with ligand-binding properties similar to those of the receptor is done by measuring binding activity of competitor molecules that are structurally related to the hapten and display a high affinity for the receptor.

5. For Id$^+$ activity, incubate for 30 min at room temperature. Perform the centrifugal assay as described in triplicate. For anti-idiotypic activity, incubate **without** the anti-idiotypic antibodies for 30 min at room temperature, add the anti-idiotypic antibodies, and incubate for another 45 min. In a typical assay using this protocol, reproducibility among triplicates should be >90%. Crude preparations of active rabbit anti-idiotypic antibody reduce the number of bound counts centrifuged through the column by >90%. It should be noted that the anti-idiotypic antibody competitively blocks [^{3}H]morphine binding to monoclonal antimorphine antibody, which is reflected as decreased radioactivity in the column eluate. Thus, any AB3 (anti-anti-idiotypic antibody) that may be present in the polyclonal preparations would lead to an apparent decrease of AB2 activity.

6. Close examination of our antimorphine antibodies shows that they all bind morphine with high affinity, but show no crossreactivity with a pharmacologically active enkephalin derivative, D-Ala^{5}D-Leu^{5}enkephalin (DADLE). Their crossreactivities with classical opioids show several interesting features that indicate that the immunoglobulins recognize structural features known from structure–activity studies to be important for pharmacological activity *(22)*. It is interesting that none of the workers who have raised either anti-Type I or anti-Type II antiopioid antibodies have found measurable cross-Type reactivities. Binding isotherms determined from data obtained using the column assay and analyzed via Scatchard plots show that the dissociation constants for morphine binding to our antibodies vary from 5–30 nM. Note that this K_d value does not correspond to that of the polyclonal antiserum of the spleen donor before cell fusion. The MAb display a much higher affinity than the antiserum. Thus, residing within a population of lymphocytes producing "homogeneous" polyclonal antiopioid serum of relatively low affinity, there may

be cells producing high-affinity antibodies that recognize widely divergent haptenic structural features. The animals' responses to conjugated opioids follow typical maturation behavior—the antiserum affinity for opioids rises steadily over time. We have had problems with maintaining lines of antimorphine MAb producing hybridomas. After several passages, the cell lines appear to dedifferentiate and cease secretion of the antibodies. This problem is also observed with antiopioid receptor antibodies (*see* Note 10).

7. Both polyclonal and monoclonal antiopioid receptor anti-idiotypic antibodies have been used as tools for studying opioid receptor properties. Although the method for production of polyclonal anti-Ids is simpler than that for the production of monoclonal anti-Ids, there are several advantages associated with the use of the latter. Monoclonal hybridoma cells provide a constant source of concentrated antibody. This eliminates the need for additional processing to concentrate and purify limited amounts of low-titer antisera. The advantage of preparing polyclonal anti-idiotypic antibodies, however, is that the amount of time involved in acquiring the immunoglobulins is reduced. Moreover, this procedure circumvents the potential problem of autocrine inhibition of hybridoma growth by the secreted antiopioid receptor antibodies. Growth-inhibitory effects of these antibodies on tumor cells and splenocytes via activation of opioid receptors have been documented *(23–25)*. The immune and hybridoma cells are known to express opioid receptors.

8. Immunization with monoclonal AB1 Fabs raised against a subclass-specific ligand should heighten the production of AB2 displaying subclass-specific binding characteristics *(26)*, but because immunizing with monoclonal AB1 limits the selection of monoclonal AB2s to the specificity of the original ligand, it may be desirable to immunize with polyclonal antiligand Abs raised against more than one ligand in order to obtain several monoclonal AB2 lines producing anti-Ids with different specificities for the receptor. Using more than one type of ligand coupled to the protein carrier has been shown to produce a polyclonal antiligand response in which different clones show no crossreaction to other antigens *(12)*.

9. Immunization with antimorphine Fab conjugated to keyhole limpet hemocyanin (KLH) yields no better response than Fab fragments alone.

10. Difficulties have been reported with regard to the growth of anti-Id-secreting hybridomas *(12,27)*. Cupo et al. *(12)* have suggested that the growth difficulties encountered with hybridomas secreting antiopioid receptor antibodies may be the result of the autocrine inhibition of hybridoma growth by the secreted antireceptor Abs. Although not reported in the literature, other workers have observed loss of anti-idiotypic antiopioid

receptor antibody-producing hybridoma cell lines (personal communications), presumably via dedifferentiation (*see* Note 6).

11. The elution protocol has been developed to avoid contamination of rabbit antibodies with either morphine or morphine-binding materials.

12. The anti-idiotypic activity of the purified antibodies is examined by testing the ability of the AB2 to compete reversibly with the initial ligand, morphine, for the AB1-binding site. This means that when the AB1 is incubated with morphine first, the latter is displaced by the AB2 and vice versa. The column assay described earlier has proven to be a useful tool for performing the displacement experiments, but because unknown components in the growth media used for hybridoma culture apparently interfere with the above assay, the solid-state assay is preferred for monoclonal anti-idiotypic antibody screening. The latter assay has the advantages that growth media from antimorphine hybridoma cultures may be used as samples rather than purified antibodies. Moreover, smaller amounts of radioactive ligand are required. On the other hand, the latter point reduced the assay sensitivity and increases worries concerning the effect of plastic surfaces on binding properties of molecules. Typical results with this assay are as follows: blank, background cpm; medium control, twice background cpm; negative control, 450 cpm.

13. The immunoglobulin/ligand competition assays performed on our MAb suggest a direct competition for the morphine-binding site, rather than a nonspecific blocking caused by binding of the anti-Id to sites on the idiotypic Ab remote from the morphine-binding region. The rank order of affinities of the original hapten, morphine, for the MAb is reflected in the relative abilities of the anti-Ids to compete with morphine at the MAb-binding site. It has also been demonstrated that the anti-Ids behave like morphine in that they displace analogs whose structures differ only slightly from that of the original hapten. This implies that the image of the morphine molecule is conserved in the binding region of the anti-idiotypic antibodies. However, all workers have found that, regardless of the specificity of their AB1s, the resultant anti-idiotypic antiopioid receptor antibodies crossreact with the μ and δ (but not κ) receptor subclasses.

14. Once anti-idiotypic antibodies have been purified and analyzed with respect to anti-idiotypic character, the strategy to ascertain the antireceptor subclass specificity of AB2 involves assay for binding to membrane-bound opioid receptors in the presence and absence of subclass-selective drugs. Opioid receptor subclass-selective drugs have been developed by pharmacologists to bind very selectively to individual members of the putative receptor classes. This enables one to determine the binding constants of a drug to a single, specific receptor subclass by blocking the other subclasses

with large amounts of their selective antagonists. As in all AB2-receptor competition experiments, it is necessary to show reversibility of the competition. The only experiments that can be legitimately interpreted to show molecular mimicry are those in which specific binding of ligand in the presence of AB2 is observed while nonspecific binding is unchanged.

15. At the present time, extensive work is available *(22,28)* on the receptor-binding properties of one population of AB2 (raised against our monoclonal line designated 10C3). Guanidine-hydrochloride fractions from the affinity-purified AB2 have the following properties. They bind specifically and reversibly to both μ and δ receptors present in mammalian brain membrane homogenates, but not to ethylketocyclazocine κ receptors found in the same homogenates. Specific binding of AB2 has also been observed to membrane homogenates of cultured NG108-15 neuroblastoma x glioma cells, which have been induced to express opioid receptors using nerve growth factor (NGF) *(29)*, and to cultured rat embryonic forebrain and hindbrain cells. AB2 also blocks binding of ^{125}I-labeled β-endorphin to guinea pig membranes *(30)*.

References

1. Simon, E. J., Hiller, J. M., and Edelman, I. (1973) Stereospecific binding of the potent narcotic analgesic [3-H] etorphine to rat-brain homogenate. *Proc. Natl. Acad. Sci. USA* **70**, 1947–1949.

2. Terenius, L. (1973) Characteristics of the "receptor" for narcotic analgesics in synaptic plasma membrane fraction from rat brains. *Acta Pharmacol. Toxicol.* **33**, 377.

3. Pert, C. B. and Snyder, S. H. (1973) Opiate receptor: demonstration in nervous tissue. *Science* **179**, 1011–1014.

4. Evans, C. J., Keith, D. E. J., Morrison, H., Magendzo, K., and Edwards, R. H. (1992) Cloning of a delta opioid receptor by functional expression. *Science* **258**, 1952–1955.

5. Kieffer, B., Befort, K., Gaveriaux, R. C., and Hirth, C. G. (1992) The delta-opioid receptor: isolation of a cDNA by expression cloning and pharmacological characterization. *Proc. Natl. Acad. Sci. USA* **89**, 12,048–12,052.

6. Chen, Y., Mestek, A., Liu, J., Hurley, J. A., and Yu, L. (1993) Molecular cloning and functional expression of a μ-opioid receptor from rat brain. *Mol. Pharmacol.* **44**, 8–12.

7. Fukuda, K., Kato, S., Mori, K., Nishi, M., Takeshima, H., Iwabe, N., Miyata, T., Houtani, T., and Sugimoto, T. (1994) cDNA cloning and regional distribution of a novel member of the opioid receptor family. *Febs Lett.* **343**(1), 42–46.

8. Meng, F., Xie, G.-X., Thompson, R. C., Mansour, A., Goldstein, A., Watson, S. J., and Akil, H. (1993) Cloning and pharmacological characterization of a rat κ opioid receptor. *Proc. Natl. Acad. Sci. USA* **90**, 9954–9958.

9. Nisonoff, A. and Lamoyi, E. (1981) Implications of the presence of an internal image of the antigen in anti-idiotypic antibodies: possible application to vaccine production. *Clin. Immunol. Immunopathol.* **21**, 397–406.

10. Glasel, J. A. (1988) Opiate receptors and molecular shapes, in *Anti-idiotypes, Receptors and Molecular Mimicry* (Linthicum, D. S. and Farid, N. R., eds.), Springer-Verlag, New York, pp. 135–153.
11. Glasel, J. A. and Pelosi, L. A. (1986) Morphine-mimetic anti-paratypic antibodies: cross-reactive properties. *Biochim. Biophys. Resch. Commun.* **136**, 1177–1184.
12. Cupo, A., Conrath, M., Eybalin, M., Fourrier, O., Zouaoui, D., Kaldy, P., and Herbrecht, F. (1992) Monoclonal antiidiotypic antibodies against delta receptors as an electron microscopy probe. *Eur. J. Cell Biol.* **57**, 273–284.
13. Gramsch, C., Schulz, R., Kosin, S., and Herz, A. (1988) Monoclonal anti-idiotypic antibodies to opioid receptors. *J. Biol. Chem.* **263**, 5853–5859.
14. Ornatowska, M. and Glasel, J. A. (1992) Two- and three-dimensional distributions of opioid receptors on NG108-15 cells visualized with the aid of fluorescence confocal microscopy and anti-idiotypic antibodies. *J. Chem. Neuroanatomy* **5**, 95–106.
15. Agarwal, D. and Glasel, J. A. (1993) Co-localization of μ and δ opioid receptors on SK-N-SH cells detected by fluorescence microscopy using labeled anti-idiotypic antibodies. *Life Sci.* **52(18)**, PL193-PL198.
16. Hughes, J. (1983) Opioid peptides. *Brit. Med. Bull.* **39**, 1–106.
17. Ornatowska, M. and Glasel, J. A. (1991) Direct production of Fv fragments from a family of monoclonal IgGs by papain digestion. *Mol. Immunol.* **28**, 383–391.
18. Tung, A. S., Ju, S. T., Sato, S., and Nisanoff, A. (1976) Production of large amounts of antibodies in individual mice. *J. Immunol.* **116**, 676–681.
19. Hebert, G. A. (1976) Improved salt fractionation of animal serums for immuno-fluorescence studies. *J. Dent. Res.* **55**, A33–A37.
20. Simon, E. J., Dole, W. P., and Hiller, J. M. (1972) Coupling of a new active morphine derivative to sepharose for affinity chromatography. *Proc. Natl. Acad. Sci. USA* **69**, 1835–1837.
21. Porter, R. R. (1959) The hydrolysis of rabbit γ-globulin and antibodies with crystalline papain. *Biochem. J.* **73**, 119–126.
22. Glasel, J. A., Bradbury, W. M., and Venn, R. F. (1983) Properties of murine anti-morphine antibodies. *Mol. Immunol.* **20**, 1419–1422.
23. Sibenga, N. and Goldstein, A. (1988) Opioid peptides and opioid receptors in cells of the immune system. *Annu. Rev. Immunol.* **6**, 219–249.
24. Zagon, I. S. and McLaughlin, P. J. (1989) Naloxone modulates body and organ growth of rats: dependency on the duration of opioid receptor blockade and stereo-specificity. *Pharmacol. Biochem. Behav.* **33**, 325–328.
25. Zagon, I. S. (1989) Endogenous opioids and neural cancer—an immunoelectron microscopic study. *Brain Res. Bull.* **22**, 1023–1029.
26. Myers, W. E. and Glasel, J. A. (1986) Subclass specificity of anti-idiotypic anti-opiate receptor antibodies in rat brain, guinea pig cerebellum and neuroblastoma x glioma (NG108-15). *Life Sci.* **38**, 1783–1788.
27. Coscia, C. J., Szücs, M., Barg, J., Belcheva, M. M., Bem, W. T., Khoobehi, K., Donnigan, T. A., Juszczak, R., McHale, R. J., Hanley, M. R., and Barnard, E. A. (1991) A monoclonal anti-idiotypic antibody to mu and delta opioid receptors. *Mol. Brain Res.* **9**, 299–306.

28. Glasel, J. A. and Myers, W. E. (1985) Rabbit anti-idiotypic antibodies raised against monoclonal anti-morphine IgG block μ- and δ-opiate receptor sites. *Life Sci.* **36,** 2523–2529.
29. Inoue, N. and Hatanaka, H. (1982) Nerve growth factor induces specific enkephalin binding sites in a nerve cell line. *J. Biol. Chem.* **257,** 9238–9241.
30. Glasel, J. A. (1989) Production and properties of anti-morphine anti-idiotypic antibodies and their anti-opiate receptor activity, in *Methods in Enzymology* (Langone, J. J., ed.), Academic, San Diego, pp. 222–243.

CHAPTER 13

Catalytic Antibodies

Structure and Possible Applications

Howard Amital, Ilan Tur-Kaspa, Zeev Tashma, Israel Hendler, and Yehuda Shoenfeld

1. Antibodies as Enzymes

Despite major progress in various fields of chemical and molecular biology, generation of a synthetic molecule that possesses the catalytic qualities of enzymes has not been achieved. In order to overcome this obstacle, numerous attempts have been carried out to synthesize antibodies that express catalytic activity.

Antibodies possess antigen-binding sites complementary to the conformation of antigenic epitopes, analogous to the conformational relationship between substrates and the active sites of enzymes. Hence, it is likely that antibodies synthesized in response to a substrate will share some of the binding properties of the active site of enzymes. Moreover, it is plausible that a few of these antibodies may even display catalytic activity similar to enzymes. This expectation is derived from likely similarities in intermolecular bonding in enzyme–substrate and antibody–antigen complexes constituted by the hydrophobic effect and electrostatic and van der Waals forces.

Catalytic antibodies can be induced by immunogens that resemble the transition state of the substrate bound to the active site of the enzyme. The transition state is really an enzyme–substrate complex in which the spatial interrelation between the components determines the direction of the chemical reaction and the resulting products. It is clear, therefore, that

From: *Methods in Molecular Biology, Vol. 51: Antibody Engineering Protocols*
Edited by: S. Paul Humana Press Inc., Totowa, NJ

the specific structure of a hapten molecule chosen to induce a catalytic antibody will determine the nature and rate of the reaction *(1–3)*. The substrate itself can also elicit catalysts *(4)*, and autoantibodies display catalytic activity (*see* Section 3.). It is likely, therefore, that the natural immune repertoire will serve as a good source of catalysts.

Catalytic antibodies can be expected to be highly specific for their antigens, usually beyond the level of specificity detected between enzymes and their corresponding substrates. However, enzymes accelerate chemical reactions efficiently, by factors reaching 10^6 times the rate of the uncatalyzed reaction and about 10^3 times the rate of antibody-catalyzed reactions. As reviewed recently by Tawfik et al. *(5)*, acyl transfer reactions serve as representative examples of antibody-catalyzed reactions. The catalytic antibody is induced by a tetrahedral hapten. Most catalytic antibodies described have been generated by immunization with phosphonate-containing haptens. The reactions catalyzed by these antibodies include hydrolysis of esters, amides, and carbonates. Tawfik et al. *(5)* proposed that difluoroketones or boronic acid immunogens comply with all the spatial and electrical requirements important in the genesis of catalytic antibodies, and may even elicit antibodies showing increased catalytic activity compared to those described until now.

Placement of functional groups known to facilitate catalysis at locations in the proximity of antigen-binding residues in antibodies represents yet another way to make catalytic antibodies. This can be achieved either by chemical modification of antibodies or by genetic engineering of antibody-active sites. In this manner, chemically reactive groups like —SH and —OH known to mediate enzymatic catalysis could be employed for this purpose *(6)*. Structurally complex and foreign molecules, such as oximes (C=N—OH) which are known to promote the catalysis of phospho-organic esters, may be used as well *(7)*.

Like enzymes, catalytic antibodies may require cofactors to complete biochemical reactions *(8,9)*. Multiple cofactors are known to facilitate enzyme-catalyzed reactions, e.g., nicotinamide, flavin, thiolic, and imidazole moieties, and metal ions like zinc. The cofactor plays an essential role in immobilizing the substrate properly within the antibody-active site.

In practice, catalytic antibodies are generated by development of monoclonal antibody (MAb)-secreting hybridoma cells directed to various haptens, as discussed above. At the end of the procedure, numerous antibodies are produced. A minority of the antibodies display catalytic properties. Rapid screening methods can be applied to test the different antibodies and assess whether they can mediate the chemical reaction of interest. Isolation of the most efficient and specific catalytic antibody may yield a biochemical tool that can be produced in large amounts with minimal cost and effort.

Catalytic antibodies will probably find important applications in the future, particularly when enzyme alternatives for the catalysis of the chemical reactions are not available or when industrial quantities of catalysts are required. One of the potential impending contributions of catalytic antibodies will be their application in neutralization of chemical warfare agents.

2. Catalytic Antibodies to Organophosphorus Compounds

Organophosphorus compounds are widely used insecticidal toxins. They cause acetylcholine (ACh) to accumulate at cholinergic receptor sites, and to produce excessive stimulation of cholinergic receptors throughout the central and peripheral nervous system. Prior to World War II, only "reversible" anticholine esterase (AChE) agents were available. However, during the war, extremely toxic organophosphates were developed in Germany that were bound irreversibly by AChE. Nowadays, these hazardous agents are components of military arsenals worldwide and, unfortunately, have even come close to being used, as in the Iran-Iraq war. Less potent organophosphate compounds are mainly used as insecticides. Organophosphate intoxication causes central and peripheral nervous system manifestations, and proceeds to lethal cardiac and respiratory symptoms. Even though antidotal treatments with atropine derivatives and oximes have existed for many years, their beneficial effect is limited. The therapeutic efficacy of these agents is low, and they must be given shortly after the exposure to the toxin owing to the "aging" process that AChE–inhibitor complexes undergo. During this process, an irreversible bond is generated between the AChE esterase site and the toxin. This stable new bond, once created, is unresponsive to further therapeutic interventions. The "aging" process is relatively brief with the chemical warfare agent soman (pinacolylmethylphosphonofluoridate) *(10,11)*.

Because of the complexity of combating organophosphorus compound intoxication, several trials to develop an effective vaccine had been carried out. The development of protective antibody responses that can neutralize the toxic effects of organophosphorus compounds must occur prior to exposure to these agents. This could be done by active immunization. Passive immunization with high-affinity antibodies can also be done prior to the expected exposure to the toxic compounds.

Several difficulties became apparent during these trials: Organophosphorus compounds have a low molecular weight. Therefore, these agents are not immunogenic. In order to solve this problem, these compounds must be conjugated to carriers and used as haptens. This procedure reduces the specificity of the resulting antibodies for the hapten.

Even minute amounts of organophosphates used as immunogens may exert severe toxic effects. To overcome this obstacle, synthetic analogs that resemble the target molecule must replace the toxins in the immunogen. Obviously, this substitution can reduce the selectivity of the antibodies for the original target.

Most studies conducted until now dealt with soman as the target molecule *(12–17)*. Cleavage of the fluoridate bond within the soman molecule results in irreversible binding of soman to the serine amino acid located in the active site of the AChE. The pinocolyl group imparts lipophilic properties to the molecule, enabling it to penetrate the central nervous system easily.

The American Medical Corps conducted several studies attempting to generate catalytic antibodies against the soman toxin. Brimfield et al. *(13)* assessed the effectiveness of antisoman MAb. In an in vitro assay, they succeeded in reversibly blocking the binding of the toxin to the AChE. Mice were immunized with a soman analog in which the fluorine atom was exchanged with a methoxy group (CH_3O). The elicited antibodies reacted well with various soman derivatives, sometimes even more avidly than with soman itself. However, any chemical alterations made in the pinocolyl group reduced the antigenicity of the molecule *(13,14)*.

Glickson et al. *(14)* demonstrated that only 20% of the antibodies induced by a chemical analog of soman in which its fluorine atom was substituted with other atoms will react with the toxin. If the fluorine is substituted by a hydrogen atom, no crossreactivity with soman is observed at all. Interestingly, a common denominator in the high-affinity antibodies to soman was an overusage of the VH J558 gene in the heavy chain and of the Vκ1 gene in the light chain *(18)*.

Administration of the antiorganophosphorus antibodies to mice and rats prior to exposure with soman *(19)*, peroxon *(20)*, and Vx *(21,22)* rendered the animals partially protected. In these studies, the animals survived four LD_{50} doses of the toxins.

The progress made with catalytic antibodies seems very attractive to researchers in the field of chemical warfare. It looks rather promising that antibodies will not only bind organophosphates, but neutralize them as well. Preliminary results were obtained by inducing catalytic antibodies to soman by immunization of mice with oxyphosphoranes and halogenated phosphines. These molecules resemble the transition-state analog of organophosphates during enzymatic hydrolysis (21,22).

Two other interesting attitudes involving catalytic antibodies were recently reported: Gentry et al. (23) described antibodies that affect the catalytic activity of the AChE enzyme. These antibodies react with an antigenic site near the active site of enzyme, thus inhibiting the binding of soman. Izadyar et al. (24) described an anti-idiotype antibody to the antibody that reacts with active site of AChE. This anti-idiotype binding site had a conformation similar to the AChE active site. Moreover, it hydrolyzed an AChE substrate (although to a lesser degree). These studies suggest that catalytic antibodies may not only bind and neutralize toxins, but they also may serve as a reservoir that can replace damaged enzymes.

3. Autoimmune Aspects of Catalytic Antibodies

It is becoming apparent in recent studies that catalytic antibodies play a role in autoimmune processes, and they even may be apart of normal physiological environment. Human autoantibodies were reported to hydrolyze the 28 amino neuropeptide VIP (25). Catalytic activity has also been demonstrated in anti thyroglobulin autoantibodies in patients with Hashimoto's thyroiditis (26). These autoantibodies display a high degree of specificity for their target antigens, binding, and disintegrating the VIP and thyroglobulin molecules into small polypeptides.

Patients with asthma display increased anti-VIP antibodies with catalytic activity (27). Likewise, potent anti-DNA autoantibodies with catalytic activity have been found in patients with systemic lupus erythematosus (28). The catalytic antibody was properly associated with antibodies of the IgG isotype, and was clearly different from enzymatic deoxyribonuclease activity.

Anti-idiotypic antibodies directed against antitopoisomerase I have been found in patients with scleroderma, systemic lupus erythematosus, and rheumatoid arthritis *(29)*. These antibodies can potentially catalyze the hydrolysis of DNA in a way analogous to hydrolysis of an AChE substrate by anti-anti-AChE antibody *(24)*. It is quite possible that autoimmune pathogenetic processes occur after catalytic antibodies are induced via the idiotypic network. In other words, sequential idiotypic stimulation may eventually create an idiotype that closely resembles the inciting antigen. In the case of catalytic antibody generation, the original inciting antigen may be an enzyme. Catalytic activity of antibodies in autoimmune disease may lead to shedding of tissue debris into the peripheral circulation. This process could eventually augment the generation of antibodies against "normal" tissue components.

4. Conclusion

The comprehension of both physiological and pathological processes is changing with the acknowledgment of the existence of catalytic antibodies. Not only do these antibodies raise numerous fundamental questions about the mechanism of their genesis and pathophysiological role, but they may also yield important applications. Catalytic antibodies, as discussed above, may confer immunity to various toxins. They may even act as a huge reservoir to replace enzymes that undergo damage by environmental toxins. In the future, catalytic antibodies will probably serve as a source for enzyme replacement in genetic diseases.

References

1. Pollack, S. J., Jacobs, W. J., and Schultz, P.G. (1986) Selective chemical catalysis by an antibody. *Science* **234,** 1570–1573.
2. Tramontano, A., Janda, K. D., and Lerner, R. A. (1986) Chemical reactivity of an antibody binding site elicited by mechanistic design of a synthetic antigen. *Proc. Natl. Acad. Sci. USA* **83,** 6736–6740.
3. Lerner, R. A., Benkovic, S. J., and Schultz, P. G. (1991) At the crossroad of chemistry and immunology: catalytic antibodies. *Science* **252,** 658–667.
4. Paul, S., Sun, M., Mody, R., Tewary, H. K., Stemmer, P., Massey, R. J., Gianferrara, T., Mehrotra, S., Dreyer, T., Meldal, M., and Tramontano, A. (1992) Peptidolytic monoclonal antibody elicited by a neuropeptide. *J. Biol. Chem.* **267,** 13,142–13,145.
5. Tawfik, D. S., Eshhar, Z., and Green, B. S. (1994) Catalytic antibodies: a critical assessment. *Mol. Biotechnol.* **1,** 87–103.
6. Pollack, S. J., Nakayama, G. R., and Schultz, P. G. (1988) Introduction of nucleophiles and spectrophotometric probes into antibody combining sites. *Science* **242,** 1038–1040.
7. Pollack, S. J., Nakayama, G. R., and Schultz, P. G. (1989) Design of catalytic antibodies. *Methods Enzymol.* **178,** 551–568.

8. Iverson, B. L. and Lerner, R. A. (1989) Sequence specific peptide cleavage catalyzed by an antibody. *Science* **243**, 1184–1188.
9. Lerner, R. A. and Tramontano, A. (1988) Catalytic antibodies. *Sci. Am.* **258**, 58–60.
10. Dunn, M. A. and Sidell, F. R. (1989) Progress in medical defence against nerve agents. *J. Am. Med. Assoc.* **262**, 649–663.
11. Koelle, G. B. (1981) Organophosphate poisoning: an overview. *Fund. Appl. Toxic* **1**, 129–134.
12. Lenz, D. E., Brimfield, A. A., Hunter, K. W., Benschop, H. P., de Jong, L. P., Van Dijk, C., and Cloro, T. R. (1984) Studies using monoclonal antibody against soman. *Fund. Appl. Toxicol.* **45**, 5156–5164.
13. Brimfield, A. A., Hunter, K. W., Lenz, D. E., Benschop, H. P., Van Dijk, C., and de Jong, L. P. (1985) Structural and stereochemical specificity of mouse monoclonal antibodies to the organophosphorus cholinesterase inhibitor soman. *Mol. Pharmacol.* **28**, 32–39.
14. Glikson, M., Arad-Yellin, R., Ghozi, M., Raveh L., Green, B. S., and Eshhar, Z. (1992) Characterization of soman-binding antibodies raised against soman analogs. *Mol. Immunol.* **29**, 903–910.
15. Lenz, D. E., Yourick, J. J., Dawson, J. S., and Scott, J. (1992) Monoclonal antibodies against soman: characterization of soman stereoisomers. *Immunol. Lett.* **31**, 131–136.
16. Buenafe, A. C. and Rittenberg, M. B. (1987) Combining site specific of monoclonal antibodies to the organophosphate hapten soman. *Mol. Immunol.* **24**, 401–407.
17. Buenafe, A. C., Makowski, F. F., and Rittenberg, M. B. (1989) Molecular analysis and fine specificity of antibodies against an organophosphorus hapten. *J. Immunol.* **143**, 539–545.
18. Dunn, M. A. and Sidell, F. R. (1989) Progress in medical defence against nerve agents. *J. Am. Med. Assoc.* **262**, 649–663.
19. Sternberg, L. A., Sim, V. M., and Kavanagh, W. G. (1972) A vaccine against organophosphorus poisoning. *Army Conference Proc.* **3**, 429.
20. Rong, K. T. and Zhang, L. J. (1990) Immunologic protection against VS intoxication in experimental animals. *Pharmacol. Toxicol.* **67**, 255–259.
21. Brimfield, A. A. and Lenz, D. E. (1991) Progress in the production of catalytic antibodies as biological scavengers for organophosphorus poisons, in *Proceedings of the 1991 Medical Defence Bioscience Review*, US Army Medical Research Institute of Chemical Defense, Aberdeen Proving Ground, MD, pp. 431–438.
22. Brimfield, A. A., Lenz, D. E., Maxwell, D. M., and Broomfield, C. A. (1993) Catalytic antibodies hydrolyzing organophosphorus esters. *Chem.-Biol. Interactions* **87**, 95–102.
23. Gentry, M. K., Saxena, A., Ashani, Y., and Doctor, B. P. (1993) Immunochemical characterization of anti-acetylcholinesterase inhibitory monoclonal antibodies. *Chem. Biol. Interactions* **87**, 227–231.
24. Izadyar, L., Friboulet, A., Remy, M. H., Roseto, A., and Thomas, D. (1993) Monoclonal anti-idiotypic antibodies as functional internal images of enzymes active sites: production of a catalytic antibody with a cholinesterase activity. *Proc. Natl. Acad. Sci. USA* **90**, 8876–8880.

25. Paul, S., Volle, D. J., Beach, C. M., Johnson, D. R., Powell, M. J., and Massey, R. J. (1989) Catalytic hydrolysis of vasoactive intestinal peptide by human autoantibody. *Science* **244**, 1158–1162.
26. Li, L., Kaveri, S., Tyutyulkova, S., Kazatchkine, M., and Paul, S. (1994) Catalytic activity of anti-thyroglobulin antibodies. *J. Immunol.* **154**, 3328–3332.
27. Paul, S. (1994) Catalytic activity of anti-ground state antibodies, antibody subunits and human autoantibodies. *Appl. Biochem. Biotechnol.* **47**, 241–255.
28. Shuster, A. M., Gololobov, G. V., Kvashuk, O. A., Bogomolova, A. E., Smirnov, I. V., and Gabibov, A. G. (1992) DNA hydrolyzing autoantibodies. *Science.* **256**, 665–669.
29. Shuster, A. M., Gololobov, G. V., Kvashuk, D. A., and Gabibov, A. G. (1991) Antiidiotypic and natural catalytically active antibodies. *Mol. Biol. (Mosk.)* **25**, 593–602.

CHAPTER 14

Preparation and Assay
of Acetylcholinesterase Antibody

Alain Friboulet and
Ladan Izadyar-Demichèle

1. Introduction

In 1974, Niels Jerne *(1)* proposed a theory that pictured the immune
system as a network of idiotypic–anti-idiotypic interactions regulating
the immune response to an antigen. The theoretical basis for the construction of idiotypic structures mimicking external antigen results
from the fact that the conformation of some of the anti-idiotypic antibodies may be complementary to the three-dimensional structure of
the binding site of the first antibody, and therefore, represents the internal image of the original epitope. The experimental validation of this
concept has been provided by numerous studies where anti-idiotypic
antibodies were not only found to mimic the structure of antigens, but
were also able to induce a functional activity that mimics the physiological activity of the original antigen. As an alternative to the transition-state approach for eliciting catalytic antibodies, our approach
consists of exploiting the internal image properties of anti-idiotypic
antibodies to produce catalytic antibodies. In the first step, an antibody
is raised that recognizes the active site of an enzyme. The binding site
of this first antibody (Ab1) has structural features complementary to
those of the enzyme. This monoclonal Ab1 is selected based on its
ability to inhibit the enzymatic reaction. In the second step, Ab1 is
used as antigen to produce anti-idiotypic antibodies. Among these
anti-idiotypic antibodies (Ab2), some may represent internal images of

From: *Methods in Molecular Biology, Vol. 51: Antibody Engineering Protocols*
Edited by: S. Paul Humana Press Inc., Totowa, NJ

the enzyme active site. Owing to the enormous variability in the antibody population, it is possible that among the anti-idiotypic antibodies, a few not only possess the binding function for the substrate, but also catalyze its transformation. If this is the case, the combining site of such "enzyme-like" antibodies may possess not only the general structural features common with the enzyme active site, but also the amino acid residues essential for catalytic activity.

The first model examined in this strategy is acetylcholinesterase (AChE; EC 3.1.1.7). A monoclonal antibody (MAb) that inhibits AChE activity, AE-2, was produced by Fambrough et al. *(2)* against human erythrocyte AChE. The cell line (HB-73) secreting this IgG1 is available at the American Type Culture Collection (Rockville, MD). Although the epitope recognized by AE-2 has not been completely characterized, several reports strongly suggest that it covers at least part of the anionic subsite of the AChE active site *(3–5)*. In preliminary experiments, when rabbits were immunized by F(ab')$_2$ fragments of AE-2, a cholinesterase-like activity was characterized in a purified polyclonal IgG preparation from the serum of immunized animals *(6)*. However, the results obtained with the polyclonal antibodies may be complicated by the unknown composition of the polyclonal preparation. An MAb was developed, therefore, to determine the kinetic properties of the anti-idiotypic catalytic antibodies. Methods employed to prepare 9A8, a monoclonal IgM with a cholinesterase activity *(7)*, using IgG AE-2 as the Ab1 are described in this chapter.

2. Materials

2.1. Ascitic Tumor Production of Ab1

1. HB-73 cells, available at the American Type Culture Collection.
2. BALB/c mice, 4 mo old.
3. Pristane, stored at room temperature.

2.2. Protein-A Affinity Chromatography

1. Affi-Gel Protein-A MAPS II kit (BioRad, Richmond, CA) containing protein-A agarose, the binding buffer (pH 9.0), the elution buffer (pH 3.0), and the regeneration buffer.
2. 1*M* Tris-HCl, pH 9.0.
3. Phosphate-buffered saline (PBS): 1.5 m*M* KH$_2$PO$_4$ (0.2 g/L), 8.1 m*M* Na$_2$HPO$_4$ (1.15 g/L), 2.7 m*M* KCl (0.2 g/L), 140 m*M* NaCl (8.0 g/L).

2.3. Production of F(ab')₂ Fragments of Ab1

1. 0.2M sodium acetate buffer, pH 4.5.
2. Pepsin solution, made up freshly, 2 mg/mL in acetate buffer.
3. 1M Tris-HCl, pH 9.0.
4. PBS (*see* Section 2.2.).

2.4. Inhibition of AChE Activity by F(ab')₂ Fragments of Ab1

1. 50 mM carbonate buffer, pH 9.3: Add 7.5 mL 0.1M sodium carbonate to 42.5 mL 0.1M sodium bicarbonate.
2. Acetylcholinesterase (AChE) from human erythrocyte, commercially available (Sigma): 50 µg/mL in carbonate buffer.
3. Wash buffer: 0.1% Tween-20 in PBS.
4. 1% (w/v) gelatine in distilled water.
5. 100 mM phosphate buffer, pH 7.4: Add 19 mL 0.2M $NaH_2PO_4 \cdot 12H_2O$ (7.16 g/100 mL), to 81 mL 0.2M $Na_2HPO_4 \cdot 2H_2O$ (3.12 g/100 mL) and dilute to 200 mL with distilled water.
6. DTNB medium: 1 mM 5,5'-dithiobis(2-nitrobenzoic acid) (DTNB): 39.6 mg DTNB in 100 mL phosphate buffer.
7. 25 mM acetylthiocholine iodide: 7.2 mg in 1 mL phosphate buffer.

2.5. Immunization

1. Biozzi mice from Institut Curie, Paris, France.
2. Complete and incomplete Freund's adjuvant.

2.6. Cell Fusion

1. Autoclaved polyethylene glycol 4000 (PEG) diluted in PBS (50% v/v).
2. HAT-sensitive myeloma cells that do not produce endogenous immunoglobulin: SP2/0 cells (commercially available).
3. Growth medium: DMEM or RPMI 1640 supplemented with antibiotics (100 U/mL penicillin, 100 µg/mL streptomycin), 2 mM L-glutamine, 1 mM pyruvate. The RPMI medium is also supplemented with 150 mM D-glucose. Store at 4°C preferably for not more than 1 mo.
4. Fetal bovine serum.
5. HA medium: dissolve hypoxanthine and azaserine to growth medium to give a final concentration of 3.4 and 0.25 µg/mL, respectively.

2.7. Screening for Anti-Ab1 Antibodies and Subclass Determination

1. 50 mM carbonate buffer, pH 9.3: Add 7.5 mL 0.1M sodium carbonate to 42.5 mL 0.1M sodium bicarbonate and dilute to 100 mL.

2. Washing buffer: 0.1% Tween-20 in PBS.
3. 1% (w/v) gelatine in distilled water.
4. Peroxidase conjugated antimouse IgM (μ-chain-specific) or IgG (γ-chain-specific).
5. Citrate buffer, pH 5.0: Dissolve 0.53 g citric acid monohydrate and 1.72 g Na_2HPO_4, $12H_2O$ in 100 mL distilled water.
6. Azinobisethylbenzothiazoline sulfonate (ABTS): 0.3 mg/mL in citrate buffer with 0.03% H_2O_2.

2.8. Cloning

1. Splenocytes from nonimmunized mouse spleen.
2. Growth medium as described in Section 2.6.
3. Fetal bovine serum.

2.9. Purification of IgM

1. 100 mM $CaCl_2$ in distilled water.
2. High-salt buffer: 0.1M Tris-HCl pH 8.0, 1M NaCl.
3. Sephacryl S-200 (Pharmacia, Uppsala, Sweden).
4. PBS.
5. Mono Q HR 5/5 column (Pharmacia).
6. Elution buffers: Buffer A, 15 mM Tris-HCl, pH 9.0; buffer B, 15 mM Tris-HCl, pH 9.0, 200 mM NaCl.

2.10. Catalytic Activity Measurement

1. DTNB medium (*see* Section 2.4.).
2. Acetylthiocholine iodide at different concentrations in DTNB medium.

2.11. Active Site Titration

1. Diisopropylfluorophosphate (DFP) at different concentrations in 100 mM phosphate buffer, pH 7.4.
2. DTNB medium.
3. Acetylthiocholine iodide: 1 mM in DTNB medium.

3. Methods
3.1. Ascitic Tumor Production of Ab1

High concentrations of MAb can be obtained by growing a hybridoma line as an ascitic tumor in an animal. The animals have been previously primed with pristane to diminish the possibility of solid tumor formation.

1. Inject pristane ip in Balb/c mouse (0.6 mL/mouse).
2. Four days later, inject 2–4 × 10^6 cells/animal ip.

3. When the tumor is clearly visible, collect the ascitic fluid with a heparinized glass micropipet.
4. Spin out the cells, and freeze the ascitic fluid at –20°C.
5. Continue to tap the tumor. If the animals are distressed, kill them and aspirate the ascitic fluid.

3.2. Protein-A Affinity Chromatography

Affi-Gel Protein-A MAPS II Kit (BioRad) provides an improvement in protein-A agarose methods for purification of mouse IgG1 from ascites fluid and for the separation of F(ab')$_2$ fragments in a mixture (*see* Note 1). Improved results were also obtained with IgG2$_a$ and IgG2$_b$.

1. Pack a 1-mL protein-A agarose column for every 6–8 mg mouse IgG.
2. Equilibrate the column with 5 bed volumes of binding buffer (supplied in the kit). After equilibration, the pH of the column effluent should be equal to the pH of the binding buffer (pH 9.0).
3. Apply the sample to the column.
4. Wash the column with 15 bed volumes of binding buffer.
5. Elute IgG with 5 bed volumes of elution buffer, and then wash the column with an additional 10 vol of elution buffer to ensure total removal of IgG.
6. Neutralize the eluate immediately with 1*M* Tris-HCl buffer, pH 9.0, or alternatively dialyze against PBS.
7. Wash the column with 5 bed volumes of regeneration buffer. The column can be kept in PBS containing 0.05% sodium azide until reused.

3.3. Production of F(ab')$_2$ Fragments of Ab1

1. Add 50 μL of pepsin solution to 10 mL of IgG solution (1 mg/mL in PBS).
2. Add an equal volume of acetate buffer to the preparation.
3. Incubate for 16 h at 37°C.
4. After incubation, neutralize the mixture with 1*M* Tris-HCl, pH 9.0, to inhibit further proteolysis.
5. Centrifuge for 10 min at 800*g* to remove pepsin.
6. Dialyze the supernatant overnight against PBS at 4°C.
7. The products of digestion are separated by protein-A affinity chromatography (*see* Section 3.2., steps 1–4). F(ab')$_2$ fragments are not retained on the column and are collected during washing. From this stage on, the homogeneity of the F(ab')$_2$ preparation can be checked by polyacrylamide gel electrophoresis in denaturing and nondenaturating conditions. The ability of F(ab')$_2$ fragments to inhibit acetylcholinesterase activity is determined using a solid-phase test (*see* Section 3.4.).

3.4. Inhibition of AChE Activity by F(ab')₂ Fragments of Ab1

1. Incubate 100 μL/well AChE in carbonate buffer (50 μg/mL) overnight at room temperature in a 96-well polystyrene plate.
2. Rinse the wells three times with wash buffer.
3. Fill the wells with 1% (w/v) gelatine in PBS, and incubate for 1 h at 37°C to block further binding of protein to the surfaces of the wells. Then wash three times more with wash buffer.
4. Dispense different concentrations of F(ab')₂ fragments (from 0 to 100 μg/mL) into the wells (100 μL/well) and incubate for 1 h at 37°C.
5. Wash two times again with washing buffer, and then with phosphate buffer.
6. Fill the wells with 240 μL DTNB medium and add 10 μL acetylthiocholine (1 mM final concentration). Read absorbance as a function of time at 410 nm.

3.5. Immunization

Biozzi mice (Institut Curie) are used because of their high immunological responsiveness when immunized with antibodies.

1. Emulsify F(ab')₂ fragments of Ab1 in Freund's complete adjuvant at 37°C. Use an equal volume of adjuvant to immunogen.
2. Inject 100–150 μg F(ab')₂ fragments/animal ip in about 0.5 mL vol.
3. Similar booster injections in incomplete Freund's adjuvant are administered three times at 2-wk intervals.
4. After a fourth boost, tail bleed the mice for an antibody test. A few hundred microliters of serum should be sufficient.
5. Test the sera at various dilutions compared with a normal mouse control (for the test, *see* Section 3.7.). A well-immunized mouse should display antibody-binding activity at a dilution of 1/1000 (*see* Section 3.7.).
6. A final injection in incomplete Freund's adjuvant is administered 3–4 d before fusion.

3.6. Fusion

1. Grow HAT-sensitive myeloma cells (SP2/O) in growth medium complemented with 20% fetal bovine serum to give enough cells for the fusion.
2. Kill the immunized mouse by cervical dislocation 3–4 d after the final immunization, and aseptically remove its spleen.
3. Dissociate the spleen in growth medium by homogenizing with a loose-fitting hand-held Potter-Elvejehm homogenizer.
4. Wash the splenocytes and the myeloma cells separately in about 50 mL growth medium by centrifugation for 10 min at 800g.

5. Resuspend myeloma cells in about 50 mL growth medium, and count them in a hemacytometer. The spleen from a hyperimmunized mouse yields about 10^8 lymphocytes.
6. Combine the cell preparations in a ratio of 1 myeloma cell to 2 spleen cells, and centrifuge the mixed cells for 5 min at 800*g*. Then aspirate the medium completely.
7. Gently disrupt the pellet by tapping the bottom of the tube, and add 1 mL of prewarmed (37°C) PEG$_{4000}$ to the pellet dropwise over the course of 90 s, while the tube is rotated continually to mix the cells and PEG gently.
8. Add about 50 mL prewarmed growth medium with continued swirling. Immediately collect cells by centrifugation at room temperature (10 min at 800*g*).
9. Resuspend the pellet in growth medium supplemented with 20% fetal bovine serum (a volume sufficient to plate out the cells at 1.5×10^5 cells/ well [120 µL/well] in 96-well microtiter plates).
10. Four to five days later, add 120 µL/well of HA medium. Feed cells with HA medium on days 4 and 10. Then replace the medium progressively with normal growth medium supplemented with 10% fetal bovine serum.
11. At about 2–3 wk, when the colonies are visible with the naked eye, screen tissue-culture supernatants for the presence of anti-Ab1 antibodies.

3.7. Screening for Anti-Ab1 Antibodies

The supernatant fluids can be easily screened for the presence of anti-Ab1 antibodies by an ELISA using 96-well microtiter plates coated with F(ab')$_2$ fragments of AE-2. Negative controls are done using irrelevant monoclonal IgG and IgM produced under the same conditions.

1. Incubate 100 µL F(ab')$_2$ fragments of AE-2 in carbonate buffer (2.5 µg/ mL)/well in a 96-well polystyrene plate overnight at room temperature.
2. Rinse the wells three times with wash buffer.
3. Fill the wells with 1% (w/v) gelatine in distilled water, and incubate for 1 h at 37°C to block further binding of protein. Then wash three times with wash buffer.
4. Dispense samples of hybridoma supernatants into the wells (100 µL/well), and incubate for 1 h at 37°C.
5. Wash three times again with wash buffer.
6. Incubate the wells with 1/1000 diluted peroxidase conjugated antimouse IgM (µ-chain-specific) or IgG (γ-chain-specific) (100 µL/well) for 1 h at 37°C. Wash three times.
7. Add working solution of fresh ABTS in citrate buffer (100 µL/well), and read absorbance at 405 nm after about 30 min of incubation.

3.8. Cloning

Hybridoma wells displaying binding activity are grown from a single cell to obtain MAb. This cloning process is most easily performed by growing up hybridomas at low cell densities. The presence of feeder cells (mouse splenocytes or peritoneal macrophages) is necessary to support growth of the hybrids at the limiting dilution cloning stages.

1. Prepare splenocytes from mouse spleen as described in the fusion protocol (*see* Section 3.6.). Plate out 4 × 96-well-plates/spleen in growth medium containing 10% fetal bovine serum (100 µL/well).
2. Two days later, count the number of cells in antibody-positive hybridoma wells. Dilute the cells to give final concentrations of 0.1 and 0.5 cells/well.
3. Distribute hybridoma cells at each density in a 96-well-plate (100 µL/well) containing feeder cells.
4. When visible colonies appear, screen for antibody activity (*see* Section 3.7.), and grow the positive wells.
5. Freeze positive cells (*see* Note 2), and repeat the cloning if necessary. When a cell line is truly cloned, all wells positive for growth are also positive by screening.

To obtain sufficient quantities of antibody for an enzymatic assay, each positive clone is used to generate ascitic tumors in animals (*see* Section 3.1.). The antibodies are then purified before catalytic activity is measured. Monoclonal IgG is purified as described in Section 3.2.

3.9. Purification of Murine IgM MAb

Various methods have been described for the purification of murine monoclonal IgM. To reach the highest purity with ascitic fluids as starting material, a three-step procedure is followed. The first step consists of euglobulin precipitation. The two following steps consist of gel-filtration and ion-exchange chromatography. These purifications can be performed using classical liquid chromatography or FPLC. Here we describe the use of a classical LC gel-filtration column and an FPLC anion-exchange column.

3.9.1. Euglobulin Precipitation

1. Add $CaCl_2$ (25 mM final concentration) to ascitic fluid to induce fibrin formation. Remove the fibrin by filtration on Whatman paper.
2. Following filtration, dialyze ascitic fluid for a few hours at 4°C against 100 vol of deionized water. Then centrifuge (30 min at 22,000g).
3. The resulting precipitate is dissolved in the high-salt buffer (0.1M Tris-HCl, pH 8.0, 1M NaCl).

4. A second cycle of dialysis and precipitation is recommended to increase IgM purity.
5. The immunoglobulin preparation is adjusted to a protein concentration of 5–10 mg/mL and stored at 4°C or –20°C.

3.9.2. Gel Filtration

Molecular sieving performed by gel permeation occurs by separation based on molecular size and conformation of the proteins mixture. IgM antibodies are large molecules (900 kDa) that can be separated by gel-exclusion chromatography using Sephacryl S-200.

1. Equilibrate a 2.6 × 70 cm column (Sephacryl S-200) with 2 bed volumes of PBS. The maximal flow rate is 2.5 mL/h.
2. Calibrate the column with protein standards to determine column performance. The volume of the sample should be 1–2% of the total gel bed volume.
3. Apply a sample of the immunoglobulin preparation at a maximum concentration of 10 mg/mL (1–2% of the total gel bed volume).
4. Collect the first peak of material absorbing at 280 nm in the void volume.

3.9.3. Ion-Exchange Chromatography

Immunoglobulins have long been purified by ion-exchange chromatography. IgM can be purified by a rapid method using FPLC anion-exchange chromatography on a Mono Q HR 5/5 column.

1. Equilibrate the column in buffer A at a flow rate of 1 mL/min until a stable baseline is reached on the absorbance monitor (280 nm).
2. Inject 1.5 mL of gel-filtration purified IgM into the system at a maximum concentration of 1 mg/mL.
3. Wash the column with 4 mL buffer A.
4. Increase progressively the ionic strength by running a linear gradient from 0 to 100% of buffer B (0–200 m*M* NaCl) over 20 min at a flow rate of 1 mL/min.
5. Collect 30-s fractions (500 μL) from the column. Monitor protein elution at 280 nm. Monoclonal IgM 9A8 elutes at 50–60 m*M* NaCl.
6. Dialyze against deionized water.
7. Assay each fraction for binding of Ab1 F(ab')₂ fragments by ELISA (*see* Section 3.7.).

3.10. Catalytic Activity Measurement
(see *Notes 3* and *4*)

The antibodies are tested for their catalytic activity by Ellman's method *(8)*.

1. In 1-mL spectrophometer cuvets (path length 1 cm), add 5–30 μg antibody in 950 μL of DTNB medium.
2. Add 50 μL of acetylthiocholine at different dilutions (up to 10 mM final concentration) in DTNB medium.
3. Gently mix and follow the increase in absorbance in a spectrophotometer at 412 nm against a blank without antibody or with an antibody that does not bind Ab_1 F(ab')$_2$ fragments.

3.11. Active Site Titration

To calculate precisely the catalytic constant, one needs to know the concentration of catalytic active sites in the preparation. This can be performed by titration using an irreversible inhibitor.

1. Mix 10 μL antibody preparation with DFP solutions at different concentrations (90 μL). The concentration of DFP is varied from 0.1- to 5-fold the estimated concentration of antibody-binding sites (IgM, 10; IgG, 2).
2. Incubate at room temperature for 2, 4, 6, and 12 h.
3. After incubation, add 0.9 mL DTNB medium containing 1 mM acetylthiocholine, and measure the residual catalytic activity at 412 nm. Completion of the reaction is confirmed when the measured residual activity is constant at each of the inhibitor concentrations.
4. The concentration of catalytic active sites is deduced by plotting the residual activity as a function of inhibitor concentration. The x-intercept of the curve obtained by a linear-regression fit to the data points represents the concentration of catalytic sites (Fig. 1). The value obtained must be close to the concentration of antibody-binding sites. This determination allows calculation of the rate constant of the reaction (k_{cat}; V_{max} in mol min^{-1}/catalytic site concentration in mol) with good accuracy. The rate constant of the uncatalyzed reaction (k_{uncat}) is determined under the same experimental conditions in the absence of antibody, permitting calculation of the acceleration factor (k_{cat}/k_{uncat}). Inhibition constants can be determined by measuring rates in the presence of reversible and irreversible inhibitors following classical enzymological protocols.

4. Notes

1. The Affi-Gel Protein-A MAPS II kit contains a sufficient quantity of reagents to purify approx 500 mg of mouse IgG1. For all sample sizes, short columns (10–15 cm or shorter) are recommended, since better linear flow rates obtained in short columns facilitate the washing and regeneration steps.

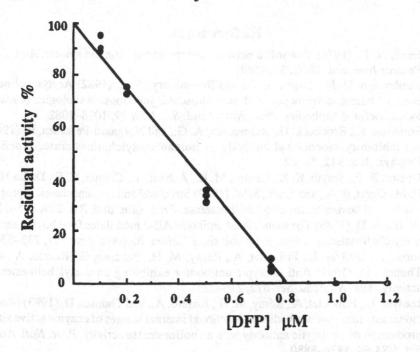

Fig. 1. Active site titration of acetylcholinesterase activity of MAb 9A8 preparation with DFP.

2. Cells can be stored for future use in frozen state. Cells in exponential growth are centrifuged and resuspended in 10% (v/v) dimethyl sulfoxide/ growth medium at a density of 0.5×10^6 cells/mL. Freeze the cells in vials by cooling at about 1°C/min by placing the cells in a polystyrene container in a −80°C freezer. When frozen, vials are placed in a liquid nitrogen container. When required, cells can be unfrozen by rapidly warming to 37°C in a water bath.

3. Among 600 MAb obtained, only 13 (IgG and IgM) were found positive for binding to F(ab')$_2$ fragments of MAb AE-2. Only one of the tested antibodies (IgM 9A8) was found positive for catalytic activity.

4. Several controls must be done to ensure that the measured catalytic activity is not the result of a contaminating enzyme. A single criterion may not be sufficient to rule out possible contamination of the preparation by an enzyme. Possible control experiments include: (a) Inhibition of the catalytic activity by Ab1. This can be determined by replacing AChE with Ab$_2$ in the procedure described in Section 3.4. (b) Demonstration of constant specific activity of the antibody preparation after repeated cycles of purification.

References

1. Jerne, N. K. (1974) Towards a network theory of the immune system. *Ann. Inst. Pasteur Immunol.* **125C**, 373–389.
2. Fambrough, D. M., Engel, A. G., and Rosenberry, T. L. (1982) Acetylcholinesterase of human erythrocytes and neuromuscular junctions: homologies revealed by monoclonal antibodies. *Proc. Natl. Acad. Sci. USA* **79**, 1078–1082.
3. Sorensen, K., Brodbeck, U., Rasmussen, A. G., and Norgaard-Pedersen, B. (1987) An inhibitory monoclonal antibody to human acetylcholinesterase. *Biochim. Biophys. Acta* **912**, 56–62.
4. Doctor, B. P., Smyth, K. K., Gentry, M. K., Ashani, Y., Cistner, C. E., De La Hoz, D. M., Ogert, R. A., and Smith, S. W. (1989) Structural and immunochemical properties of fetal bovine serum acetylcholinesterase. *Prog. Clin. Biol. Res.* **289**, 305–316.
5. Wolfe, A. D. (1989) The monoclonal antibody AE-2 modulates fetal bovine serum acetylcholinesterase substrate hydrolysis. *Biochim. Biophys. Acta* **997**, 232–235.
6. Joron, L., Izadyar, L., Friboulet, A., Rémy, M. H., Pancino, G., Roseto, A., and Thomas, D. (1992) Anti-idiotypic antibodies exhibiting an acetylcholinesterase activity. *Ann. NY Acad. Sci.* **672**, 216–223.
7. Izadyar, L., Friboulet, A., Rémy, M. H., Roseto, A., and Thomas, D. (1993) Monoclonal anti-idiotypic antibodies as functional internal images of enzyme active sites: production of a catalytic antibody with a cholinesterase activity. *Proc. Natl. Acad. Sci. USA* **90**, 8876–8880.
8. Ellman, G. L., Courtney, K. D., Andres, V., and Featherstone, R. M. (1961) A new and rapid colorimetric determination of acetylcholinesterase activity. *Biochem. Pharmacol.* **7**, 88–95.

CHAPTER 15

DNA Hydrolysis by Antibodies

Alexander G. Gabibov
and Oxana Makarevitch

1. Introduction

Catalysis of various chemical transformations by antibodies opens broad perspectives in the fundamental and applied branches of life science *(1)*. Antibodies are ideally suited for therapeutic applications owing to their capability of homing to a particular target. In addition, they happily withstand stringent conditions and, therefore, are easy to isolate and manipulate. These advantages have provoked considerable interest in the idea that new catalytic antibodies could substitute for enzymes in therapy.

The hypotheses that natural catalytic antibodies (abzymes) originate as anti-idiotypic antibodies *(2)* and unequivocal proof for autoantibody-mediated peptide *(3)* and DNA cleavage *(4)* suggest that catalysis is an additional function of antibody molecules in vivo. One can expect that the number of known substrates of natural catalytic autoantibodies will increase rapidly in the near future. The search for novel abzymes appears most promising in various pathological states. However, the physiological role of the catalytic activity of natural antibodies remains unknown. The data obtained to date allow the hope that measurement of the incidence and the level of activity of natural abzymes in blood will prove useful in the development of prognostic criteria and monitoring of disease.

In the initial stage of our studies, we attempted to find DNA-hydrolyzing antibodies (DNA-abzymes) in autoimmune diseases known to be associated with high levels of anti-DNA autoantibodies in blood. We

From: *Methods in Molecular Biology, Vol. 51: Antibody Engineering Protocols*
Edited by: S. Paul Humana Press Inc., Totowa, NJ

found DNA-hydrolyzing activity in autoantibodies isolated from the sera of patients with systemic lupus erythematosus (SLE), scleroderma (Scl), and rheumatoid arthritis (RA). Further studies led to discovery of DNA-abzymes in chronic lymphoid leukemia (HLL) and AIDS. The frequency of incidence of the DNA-abzymes differs in different diseases.

One concern in the investigation of abzyme activity is the problem of possible contamination by enzymes with properties similar to those attributed to antibodies. Even a negligible quantity of an enzyme with relatively high turnover number could lead to false-positive results. Thus, several control experiments are necessary to prove that the activity is the result of an antibody and not a contaminant. The following criteria can be considered as evidence for natural abzyme activity:

1. Electrophoretic homogeneity of catalytic antibody preparations checked by silver staining.
2. Retention of catalytic activity after antibodies are incubated at low pH ("acid shock" experiment; *see* Section 3.2., step 13).
3. Removal of the catalytic activity by immobilized protein-G or antihuman IgG (or an antibody directed against the particular isotype of the putative catalytic antibody).
4. Presence of the catalytic activity in the purified Fab fragments and its absence in the F_c fragment.
5. Differences in the substrate specificity of the antibody preparation and suspected enzyme contaminants.
6. Presence of catalytic activity in the expression product of cDNA encoding the antibodies.

1.1. Purification of DNA-Hydrolyzing Autoantibodies

The procedure for purification of DNA-hydrolyzing autoantibodies from human serum is based on two main properties of these newly described biocatalysts, namely their antibody nature and DNA-binding capacity. Here, ammonium sulfate precipitation, protein-G affinity chromatography, and HPLC ion-exchange steps were chosen from the arsenal of immunochemical purifications protocols. Affinity chromatography on a support-coupled DNA was employed to take into account the specificity of the antibodies for DNA.

Briefly, the complete abzyme-purification procedure is as follows (Scheme 1). After a two-step ammonium sulfate precipitation procedure, the crude antibody preparation is subjected to two rounds of pro-

Blood sera

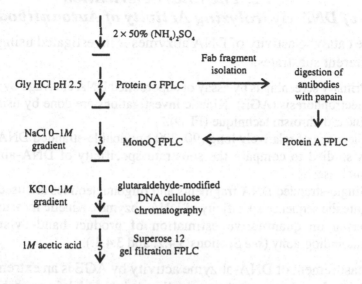

Scheme I. Preparation of DNA-hydrolyzing antibody.

tein-G affinity chromatography. A cation-exchange chromatography (Mono Q column) is used as the next purification step in order to remove any minor remaining impurities. The antibodies are further fractionated on DNA-cellulose to yield the DNA-binding antibody fraction. Gel filtration in acid is used as the last purification step to dissociate antibody–DNA complexes and possible protein contaminants bound to antibodies.

Primary screening for DNA-hydrolyzing activity in human serum involves examination of catalytic activity of a relatively large number of autoantibody samples. Because of its rapidity and efficiency, protein-G affinity chromatography is the purification method of choice for this purpose. The resulting antibody preparation is subjected to the supercoiled DNA-cleavage test. This very sensitive technique serves as our primary criterion for detection of DNA-abzymes (*see* Section 3.4.1.). Usually, two repeat cycles of the protein-G chromatography are sufficient to sift out samples without abzyme activity. Antibody preparations displaying positive response in the supercoiled DNA cleavage test are then subjected to additional purification to confirm catalytic activity.

1.2. The Characterization
of DNA-Hydrolyzing Activity of Autoantibodies

The catalytic activity of DNA abzymes is investigated using a number
of different substrates:

1. Primary screening is by assay of supercoiled DNA cleavage by agarose gel
   electrophoresis (AGE). Kinetic investigations are done by using the flow
   linear dichroism technique (FLD).
2. Cleavage of relatively long (90–300 bp) double-stranded DNA fragments
   is studied to compare the substrate specificity of DNA-abzymes and
   nucleases.
3. Single-stranded DNA fragments and oligonucleotides are used to investigate the sequence specificity of DNA abzymes. Kinetic measurements are
   based on quantitative estimation of product bands visualized by
   autoradiography (*see* Sections 3.4.2. and 3.4.3.).

Measurement of DNA-abzyme activity by AGE is an extremely sensitive procedure, because, theoretically, a single nick in supercoiled plasmid DNA is sufficient for unwinding of the supercoil, resulting in
decreased migration of the relaxed plasmid in the gel.

Kinetic measurements of DNA-abzyme activity can be performed also
in the presence of DNA polymerase I (holoenzyme). This approach is
based on the nicking capacity of DNA-abzymes when incubated with
plasmid DNA. The radiolabeled dNTPs provided in the reaction mixture
are then incorporated in the nicked DNA by DNA polymerase I *(4)* in
the well-known nick translation reaction. The incorporation rate of the
^{32}P-labeled nucleotides in this assay principally reflects the level of
DNA-abzyme nicking activity.

1.3. The FLD Technique: General Information

The FLD method is an alternative approach to measuring the rate of
nuclease-mediated supercoiled DNA unwinding. Nuclease activity is
monitored continuously, and the sensitivity of the method permits detection of abzyme-mediated supercoiled DNA cleavage.

The FLD method is based on the fact that oriented DNA molecules are
generally characterized by different absorption of light with different
planes of linear polarization, thus displaying linear dichroism (LD) (for
review, *see 5,6*). The magnitude of LD is defined as:

$$\Delta A = A_{\parallel} - A_{\perp} \qquad (1)$$

where A_1 and $A_\perp$ are the absorbances of polarized light parallel and perpendicular to the orientation axis, respectively. LD is usually expressed in a dimensionless parameter, the so-called reduced linear dichroism LD value, defined as $\Delta A/A_{ISO}$, where A_{ISO} is the isotropic absorption of an unoriented sample. Long polymers, such as DNA, can exist in a partially oriented state by shear flow. Changes in the length, conformation, or stiffness of the molecule influence the magnitude of the LD signal. This technique has previously been applied to study nuclease and DNA-abzymes reactions. The plasmid DNA molecules are oriented by the flow gradient provided by solution pumping through the flow cell. In order to estimate the FLD magnitudes for different forms of plasmid DNA, standard samples of relaxed circular and linear forms are also assayed (supercoiled plasmid DNA digested by DNase I and *Eco*RI,respectively). Kinetic constants can be determined by FLD curve fitting using the integral form of the Michealis-Menten rate equation at the initial stages of the reaction as:

$$D'_i - D_i = V_m \cdot \Delta - K_m(app) \ln (D_\infty - D_i/D_\infty - D'_i) \tag{2}$$

where: D_i and D_i' are the FLD signals at times t_i and t_i', respectively, D_∞ is the signal at time t_∞ (corresponding to achievement of maximal rate), and Δ is a time constant ($t_i' - t_i$).

2. Materials (*see* Note 1)
2.1. Isolation of DNA Autoantibodies
from Human Serum

1. Ammonium sulfate 50%.
2. Buffer A: 20 mM Tris-HCl, pH 7.5, 50 mM NaCl.
3. Buffer B: 100 mM glycine-HCl, pH 2.7, 50 mM NaCl.
4. HR 5/5 protein-G Superose FPLC column (Pharmacia) or similar column.

2.2. Purification
of DNA-Hydrolyzing Autoantibodies

1. Buffer C: 20 mM Tris-HCl, pH 9.0.
2. Buffer D: 20 mM MOPS, pH 7.0, 50 mM NaCl.
3. Buffer E: 1M acetic acid, 100 mM NaCl.
4. HR 5/5 Mono Q column (Pharmacia) or similar column.
5. HR 10/30 Superose-12 FPLC column (Pharmacia, Uppsala, Sweden) or similar column.
6. Centricon-10 concentrators (Amicon, Beverly, MA).

7. DNA-cellulose from Sigma (St. Louis, MO). This can also be synthesized according to ref. *(7)*.

2.3. Fab Fragment Preparation (8)

1. Papain.
2. 1*M* cysteine.
3. 20 m*M* EDTA.
4. 100 mm sodium acetate buffer.
5. Iodoacetamide.
6. Protein-A FPLC column (Pharmacia) or similar column.

2.4. Activity Assays

2.4.1. Reaction with Supercoiled DNA

1. Supercoiled plasmid DNA preparation. Any conventional plasmid cloning vector is suitable *(9)*.
2. Assay buffer, buffer F: 20 m*M* Tris-HCl, pH 8.0, 50 m*M* NaCl, 5 m*M* MgCl$_2$.
3. 10X agarose gel electrophoresis sample buffer, buffer G: 0.25% Bromphenol blue, 0.25 xylene cyanol, 30% glycerol in water.
4. 50X TAE buffer, buffer H: 2*M* Tris-HCl, pH 7.4, 0.1*M* EDTA.
5. 0.8% Agarose gels in 1X TAE.

2.4.2. Reaction with Double-Stranded (ds) DNA Fragment (see Note 4)

1. 150–200 bp ds DNA fragment with 3'-ends labeled with DNA polymerase I or its Klenow (Promega, Madison, WI) fragment and α-^{32}P-deoxynucleoside triphosphates according to ref. *(10)*.
2. Buffer F *(see* Section 2.4.1.).
3. 10 mg/mL tRNA.
4. 2% sodium perchlorate in acetone.
5. 75% ethanol in water.
6. 10% polyacrylamide gels in 7.5*M* urea. The aezylamide:bis-acrylamide ratio is 19:1.
7. 10X TBE, buffer I: 0.89*M* Tris-borate, 0.02*M* EDTA.
8. Polyacrylamide gel electrophoresis sample, buffer J: 5% AGE sample buffer *(see* Section 2.4.1.), 95% formamide.

2.4.3. Reaction with 5' ^{32}P-Labeled Deoxyribooligonucleotides

1. 5' ^{32}P-labeled deoxyribooligonucleotides.
2. Buffer F: *(see* Section 2.4.1.).
3. 10 mg/mL tRNA.
4. 2% sodium perchlorate in acetone.

5. 80% ethanol.
6. 20% polyacrylamide gels in 7.5*M* urea.

2.4.4. FLD

1. Supercoiled phage or plasmid DNA.
2. Buffer F: (*see* Section 2.4.1.) containing 10% glycerol.
3. Spectropolarimeter: JASCO J500 C or similar instrument equipped with 260-nm achromatic quarter wavelength prism.
4. 1.6-mL LD flow-cell with optical path length 2 mm.
5. Peristaltic pump.

3. Methods

3.1. Isolation of Autoantibody Fraction from Human Serum (see Scheme 1 and Notes 1 and 2)

1. Precipitate 5 mL of human serum with 50% saturated ammonium sulfate.
2. Dissolve the precipitate in 1 mL buffer A. Centrifuge 15 min at 10,000*g*. Save the supernatant.
3. Repeat steps 1 and 2 using 1 mL of 50% saturated ammonium sulfate for precipitation.
4. Apply the globulins dissolved in buffer A from step 3 to an HR 5/5 FPLC protein-G Sepharose column.
5. Wash the column with 20 column volumes of buffer A.
6. Elute the IgG fraction from the column with 5 mL of buffer B at flow rate 0.5 mL/min.
7. Immediately adjust pH of the antibody preparation to 8.0 by addition of 2*M* Tris-HCl, pH 9.0.
8. Repeat protein-G Sepharose chromatography (steps 4–7).
9. Check the DNA-hydrolyzing activity of the antibody preparation as described in Section 3.4.1. (*see* Note 2).

3.2. Purification of DNA-Hydrolyzing Autoantibodies

1. Dialyze the antibody preparation from step 8, Section 3.1., for 6 h at 4°C against buffer C (10 vol, two changes).
2. Apply the dialyzed preparation to an HR 5/5 MonoQ FPLC column equilibrated with buffer C.
3. Wash the column with 20 column volumes of buffer C.
4. Elute antibodies with 0–1*M* linear gradient of NaCl in buffer C over 30 min at flow rate 1 mL/min. Collect 1-mL fractions.

5. Assay DNA-hydrolyzing activity of effluent fractions (Section 3.4.1.).
6. Dialyze active fraction at 4°C for 6 h against buffer D (10 vol, three changes).
7. Apply the dialyzed preparation on the DNA-cellulose affinity column (0.5 × 2 cm) equilibrated with buffer D.
8. Wash the column with 10 column volumes of buffer D.
9. Elute the DNA-binding antibodies with the linear gradient of KCl (0–1M) in buffer D (flow rate 0.5 mL/min). Collect the eluate in 12 separate fractions (1.5 mL each).
10. Dialyze collected fractions separately for 6 h at 4°C against buffer D (10 vol, three changes).
11. Check the DNA-hydrolyzing activity of the antibodies from step 10 as in Section 3.4.1.
12. Pool active fractions, and concentrate to 10 mg protein/mL by ultrafiltration using Centricon-10 devices.
13. Apply 0.5 mL of the antibodies (5 mg) on the HR 10/30 Superose 12 gel-filtration column equilibrated with buffer E. Perform gel filtration at flow rate of 0.5 mL/min in buffer E.
14. Collect fractions corresponding to the molecular weight of IgG (150 kDa), and adjust pH to 8.0 by addition of 2M Tris-HCl, pH 9.0.
15. Dialyze against two changes of buffer D for 6 h at 4°C.
16. Determine the protein concentration using the Bradford technique (or similar procedure) and the purity of the preparation by SDS-polyacrylamide gel electrophoresis followed by silver staining (11).

3.3. Antibody Fab Fragment Preparation

1. Dialyze 2 mL of protein-G purified antibodies (5 mg/mL) against 100 mM sodium acetate, pH 5.5.
2. Add 100 μL of 1M cysteine and 100 μL of 20 mM EDTA to the antibody preparation. Final concentrations are 50 mM cysteine and 1 mM EDTA.
3. Add 10 μg of papain for each milligram of antibodies, mix well, and incubate at 37°C for 8–12 h.
4. Add iodoacetamide to a final concentration of 75 mM. Mix well, and incubate at room temperature for 30 min.
5. To separate Fab and F_c fractions, apply the mixture from step 4 on an HR 5/5 protein-A FPLC column.
6. Wash the column with buffer A. Collect fractions containing the Fab fragment.
7. Wash the column with buffer B. Collect fractions containing the F_c fragment.
8. Adjust pH of both preparations to 8.0 by addition of 2M Tris-HCl, pH 9.0.
9. Check the preparations for purity and DNA hydrolyzing activity of the fractions.

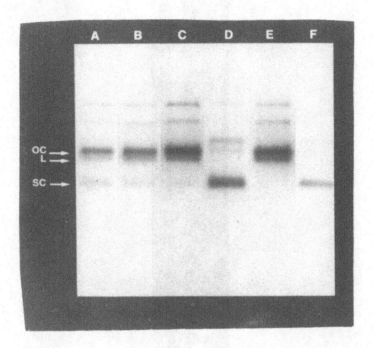

Fig. 1. Agarose gel electrophoresis of plasmid DNA treated with DNA-hydrolyzing antibodies. Plasmid DNA forms are indicated as: SC—supercoiled; L—linear, OC—open circle. A. Protein-A purified IgG fraction (*see* Scheme 1, step 2). B. DNA-cellulose-purified IgG fraction (*see* Scheme 1, step 4). C. IgG fraction subjected to "acid shock" (step 5). D. F_c fragment. E. Fab fragment. F. Background reaction.

3.4. Activity Assay (see Notes 3–5)

3.4.1. Reaction with Supercoiled DNA (see Fig. 1)

1. Mix 1 μg of supercoiled DNA with 2–10 μg of antibody in buffer F. Total reaction volume is 20 μL.
2. Incubate at 37°C overnight (*see* Note 5).
3. Add 2 μL of buffer G.
4. Electrophorese the sample in a 0.8% agarose gel in 1X TAE.
5. Stain the gel with ethidium bromide (2 μg/mL).

3.4.2. Reaction with 3' ^{32}P-Labeled ds DNA Fragment (see Fig. 2 and Note 4)

1. Mix 0.1–0.3 pmol of 3' ^{32}P-labeled ds DNA fragment (150-bp *EcoRI/BglI* fragment from pUC 19) with 2–10 μg of antibody in buffer F. Total reaction volume is 20 μL.

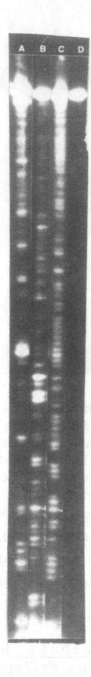

Fig. 2. Autoradiogram showing polyacrylamide gel electrophoresis of a 3' ^{32}P-labeled EcoRI/BglI fragment (150 bp) of pUC 19 treated with: (A) DNA hydrolyzing antibodies, and (B) DNase I. (C) Shows the pattern resulting from limited cleavage of the substrate at G and A (10), and (D), the background reaction.

2. Incubate at 37°C overnight.
3. Add 1 μL of tRNA and 200 μL of 2% sodium perchlorate in acetone.
4. Keep for 30 min at –20°C.
5. Centrifuge 10 min at 10,000*g*.
6. Remove the supernatant.
7. Add 200 mL of 75% ethanol, and vortex vigorously.
8. Spin for 10 min at 10,000*g*.
9. Remove the supernatant.
10. Repeat steps 7–9. Dry the pellet *in vacuo* for a few minutes.
11. Dissolve dried samples in 2–3 μL of buffer J, and run electrophoresis in a denaturing polyacrylamide gel.

3.4.3. Reaction with 5' ³²P-Labeled Deoxyribooligonucleotides

This reaction is studied essentially as in Section 3.4.2. Various single-stranded homopolymers and heteropolymers (6–30 bases) can be used as substrate (*see* ref. *4*).

3.4.4. FLD Assay of Supercoiled DNA Cleavage (see *Fig. 3* and *Note 5*)

1. Mix 1 μg of supercoiled plasmid DNA with 1–10 μg of the antibody preparation in 200 μL of buffer F.
2. Place the LD flow cell containing the reaction mixture into the spectropolarimeter.
3. Pump buffer F through the a flow cell at flow rate of 15 μL/s using a peristaltic pump. The average flow gradient in the cell is 6000/s (*see* refs. *5,6* for discussion of this method).
4. Monitor the LD signal over 30–60 min.

4. Notes

1. Glassware and reagents used in work with the antibody preparations must be sterilized. Buffers for chromatography are boiled and filtered through a nitrocellulose membrane (0.22 μm). Reaction buffers and plasticware are autoclaved (30 min, 121°C). Store the assay buffer (buffer F) used for the antibody-activity determination in small aliquots at –20°C.
2. Initial screening for catalytic activity in collections of human sample is carried out at this step. Samples exhibiting abzyme activity should be subjected to further purification and assayed for activity again.
3. Preparations of phage and plasmid DNAs used as substrates should contain no less than 80% supercoiled DNA. Stock plasmid solutions are conveniently kept at 0.5–1.0 mg DNA/mL, minimizing dilution of the assay buffer during activity measurement. EDTA in the plasmid storage buffer

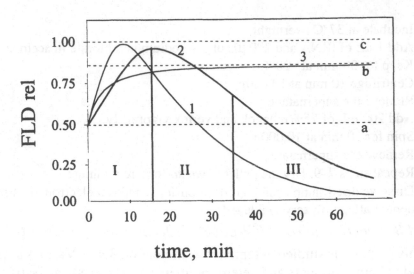

time, min

Fig. 3. Assay of supercoiled plasmid DNA cleavage by DNase I (curve 1), DNA-hydrolyzing antibodies (2), and *Eco*R1 (3) using FLD. Relative FLD signals corresponding to the supercoiled, linear, and relaxed CNA forms are shown by dotted lines (a, b, and c respectively). I, relaxation stage; II, linearization stage; III, degradation to small fragments.

    (10 mM Tris-HCl, pH 7.5, 1 mM EDTA) is diluted sufficiently that it does not interfere with the hydrolysis reaction.

4. Any ds DNA fragment with recessed 3'-ends labeled with ^{32}P according to ref. *(10)* can be used as substrate.

5. Decrease the reaction time if required to obtain partial conversion (as opposed to complete conversion) of the supercoiled form to the circular form as seen by agarose gel electrophoresis.

Acknowledgments

    The authors express their gratitude to Sudhir Paul for fruitful discussions. They are also grateful to A. M. Shuster, G. V. Gololobov, and D. V. Schouzov for their help in methods development and A. V. Kolesnikov for valuable help in the manuscript preparation and review. This work was supported in part by US Public Health Service grant R03 TW00287.

References

1. Suzuki, H. (1994) Recent advances in abzyme studies. *J. Biochem.* **115,** 623–628.
2. Bronstein, I. B., Shuster, A. M., Schevchenko, L. V., Gromova, I. I., Kvashuk, O. A., Geva, O. N., and Gabibov, A. G. (1989) Topoisomerase I from the human

placenta. Functional Activity of the cDNA expression Products. *Molekularnaya Biologiya* **23**, 1553–1557.

3. Paul, S., Volle, D. J., Beach, C. M., Jonson, D. R., Powell, M. J., and Massey, R. J. (1989) Catalytic hydrolysis of vasoactive intestinal peptide by human autoantibody. *Science* **244**, 1158–1162.

4. Shuster, A. M., Gololobov, G. V., Kvashuk, O. A., Bogomolova, A. E., Smirnov, I. V., and Gabibov, A. G. (1992) DNA hydrolyzing autoantibodies. *Science* **256**, 665–667.

5. Rodger, A. (1993) Linear dichroism. *Methods Enzymol.* **226**, 238–258.

6. Wilson, R. W. and Schellman, J. A. (1978) The flow linear dichroism of DNA: comparison with the bead-spring theory. *Biopolymers* **17**, 1235–1248.

7. Romanov, V. V. and Starostina, V. K. (1987) Immobilization of nucleic acids with glutaraldehyde. *Biotechologija (in Russian)* **3**, 618–623.

8. Harlow, E. and Lane, D. (1988) Digesting antibodies with papain to isolate Fab fragments, in *Antibodies. A Laboratory Manual,* Cold Spring Harbor Laboratory, Cold Spring Harbor, NY, pp. 628,629.

9. Zasloff, M., Ginder, D. G., and Fensenfeld, G. (1978) A new method for the purification and identification of covalently closed circular DNA molecules. *Nucleic Acids Res.* **5**, 1139–1151.

10. Maxam, A. and Gilbert, W. (1977) Sequencing end-labeled DNA with base-specific chemical cleavages. *Proc. Natl. Acad. Sci. USA.* **74**, 500–560.

11. Wray, W., Boulikas, P., Wray, W. P., and Hancock, R. (1981) Silver staining of proteins in polyacrylamide gels. *Anal. Biochem.* **118**, 197–201.

Screening Strategies for Catalytic Antitransition-State Analog Antibodies

Alfonso Tramontano

1. Introduction

Monoclonal antibodies (MAb) with prespecified enzyme-like catalytic activity are obtained from the immune response against transition-state analogs (TSA). The premise for generating antibody catalysts, as put forth by Jencks *(1)*, was validated through early examples of specific hydrolytic catalysts for ester and carbonate substrates *(2,3)*. The initial success with TSA of acyl transfer processes as haptens led to derivation of antibodies as catalysts for a variety of reactions *(4)*. This approach has been expanded to include haptenic molecules not directly related in structure to a deduced feature of the reaction's transition state, but that could deploy groups in the antibody that participate in a catalytic mechanism not otherwise available for the reaction in ordinary immunological recognition *(5)*. The unifying concept in these approaches is the insight to the reaction mechanism that allows the construction of a suitable mimic of the transition-state or other high-energy structures. Individual approaches explore the scope of the antibody's enzymatic qualities and the validity of the design strategy for generating the catalyst. The success of these endeavors typically requires several screening steps for the identification of a catalyst among a set of MAb obtainable from hybridoma cloning experiments.

From: *Methods in Molecular Biology, Vol. 51: Antibody Engineering Protocols*
Edited by: S. Paul Humana Press Inc., Totowa, NJ

The production and characterization of catalytic antibodies entails standardized immunochemical methodology, but may also require specific methods development predicated on the particular study or target reaction. In general, criteria for the experimental design should be considered in context with standard immunological methods. An appreciation of the requirements for catalysis of the reaction of interest as well as kinetic data for uncatalyzed rates of the specific substrates are useful before launching an effort to produce potential catalytic antibodies. It is also necessary to assess the practical limits of new assays that might be employed in screening and characterization of antibody catalysts. Several approaches have been devised for identifying catalytic antibodies as obtained from hybridoma culture supernatants. The conventional method relies on preliminary screening for hapten binding to reduce the number of clones for catalytic activity screening to a small manageable number. The application of immunoassay procedures for identification of high-affinity antibodies is integral to hybridoma development (6).

The design of new methodologies is driven by diverse concerns. Direct screening of antibodies in culture supernatants for catalytic activity has generally been impractical owing to the modest activities that have so far characterized these catalysts and the demand for relatively large quantities of antibody for detection. Nevertheless, direct screening remains desirable, since it would not only minimize the labor and expense of overproduction of antibodies, such as by ascites production, but also eliminate the assumption that catalytic antibodies are an exclusive subset of the high-affinity anti-TSA clones. As a result of these constraints, alternative procedures have been sought to approximate direct screening. Maintenance and simplification of a set of hybridomas in culture are critical features of a specific direct or indirect assay method. In any procedure, the selected hybridomas should be subcloned and preserved as soon as practical to guard against loss of the line or overgrowth by unwanted clones. Therefore, it is necessary that an assay have a convenient turnaround time to expedite processing and reduction of a hybridoma population. This chapter considers the technical aspects, capacities, merits, generality, advantages, and disadvantages of several available strategies (summarized in Table 1). Realization of the theoretical and practical limitations of antibody catalysis may ultimately derive from the greater use of these procedures.

1.1. Immunoassay for TSA Binding

Prescreening of antibodies in culture supernatants by immunoassay against the TSA is defensible on the grounds that catalysts should be found among the antibodies that bind tightly to molecules that accurately mimic the transition state for the catalytic process. Although this has been the traditional approach to discovery of catalytic antibodies, the process does not guarantee that selected cultures will yield catalysts. This poses a considerable obstacle, since a significant investment of time and labor is required to produce the MAb in sufficient quantity for a definitive enzymatic assay.

1.1.1. ELISA Against TSA

Antibodies that specifically bind the TSA hapten have been identified by ELISA against hapten conjugated to a protein different from the carrier used for immunization. This ensures against selection of anticarrier antibodies. Nevertheless, the antihapten group is composed of predominantly noncatalytic antibodies. This can be rationalized to some extent as the potential for diverse modes of recognition between antibody and hapten, with the recognition mode that is propitious to catalysis occurring in a fraction of all the possibilities. The degree of correspondence between hapten binding and catalytic activity is of practical concern, since the effort for maintenance, subcloning, propagation, ascites production, and purification of antibody for each candidate culture becomes progressively more onerous with increasing number of clones. A probability of less than one catalyst in 10 or 20 antihapten antibodies could discourage screening efforts, despite the merit of the experimental design.

The actual proportion of catalysts to noncatalysts within the set of anti-TSA antibodies could be taken as a measure of the ability of the hapten to mimic features of the transition state. Only limited experimental work has been reported to support this premise (7). A more general correlation has been suggested to describe the relationship between TSA affinity and catalytic efficiency (8). As a corollary to this argument, it could be suggested that the relative catalytic efficiencies of a set of antibodies against a common TSA will follow the order of their affinities. Though specific examples appear to fit the theoretical relationship, more systematic analysis gives less evidence for its support (for example, *see* ref. 9).

Table 1

Comparison of Techniques for Screening Catalytic Antibodies in Hybridoma Culture Supernatant

	ELISA, anti-TSA	CIEIA, short TSA	Direct enzyme assay	Capture/immobilized antibody	catElisa
Format	96-well plate	96-well plate	Microtiter plate	Microtiter plate or tubes	96-well plate
Throughput capacity	10^3–10^4 (typical for manual or automated plate manipulation)	10^3–10^4 (typical for manual or automated plate manipulation)	10^3–10^4 (small number of plates)	<10^3 samples	10^3–10^4 (small number of plates)
Independent steps	No	No	No	Yes (adsorb/separate)	No
Time for completion	3–6 h	3–6 h	Depends on catalyst efficiencies; prolonged for low activity catalysts	8–16 h	3–6 h
Sample requirement	100 µL	100 µL	Unknown	3–50 mL (depends on Ig concentration)	100 µL

Sensitivity	High (for binding)	High (for binding)	Variable	Variable	High
Special requirements	None	Ligands smaller than the hapten that specifically define the transition-state structure	Sensitive radiometric or spectrometric method; compatible media or buffer	General anti-Ig affinity adsorbent	Highly specific antiserum against products with little crossreaction with substrates
Advantages	Rapid and sensitive for high-affinity clones	Rapid and sensitive for high-affinity clones; restricts number anti-TSA clones based on affinity	Potentially provides direct access to most active catalysts	Adaptable to any substrate and analytical method; reduces interference from contaminants and media	Provides direct access to high-activity clones
Disadvantages	Uncertain correlation with catalytic activity	Uncertain correlation with catalytic activity; not amenable to all types of reactions	Restricted substrates; interference from contaminants and background rates; few successful examples	Uses large quantities of supernatants; time-consuming and tedious to manipulate samples	Restricted substrates (immobilized); difficulty of obtaining anti-product antiserum

1.1.2. Competitive Binding to Small TSA (CIEIA)

Although a hapten may be designed to present features of the transition state, antibody recognition of ground-state features in the hapten is inevitable. This can explain the high proportion of noncatalytic antihapten antibodies, as well as the poor correlation between affinity and activity in a set of catalytic antibodies to a particular TSA. Competitive binding for smaller molecules that retain only the groups necessary for mimicking the bond changes in the transition state has been suggested as a strategy for further delimiting anti-TSA antibodies *(10)*. The method can be developed as a straightforward extension of the immunoassay procedure, provided that appropriately trimmed or shortened TSA are available. Affinity for the trimmed molecule is expected to be attenuated relative to the original hapten. Therefore, the concentration needed for effective competition with preadsorbed hapten is likely to be high. An upper limit to its concentration should be empirically determined at which the compound does not nonspecifically compete with hapten using an unrelated antibody–antigen pair.

1.2. Direct Kinetic Screening

Immunoassays for TSA binding eliminate many hybridoma clones that potentially produce antibodies with catalytic activities comparable to or greater than those found in the set of TSA binders. This assertion remains moot, since activities of confirmed catalytic antibodies are difficult to detect as provided in hybridoma culture supernatants. It is impractical to overproduce and purify more than a few candidates for rigorous activity assays. Therefore, techniques to screen antibody from hybridoma cultures for catalytic activity and circumvent traditional affinity-based prescreening are of considerable interest. Methodology for such direct assays has been based on design of chromogenic or fluorogenic substrates, allowing the detection of small levels of product formation in the presence of dilute antibody solutions (for example, *see* ref. *11*). In practice, such methods are compromised by spontaneous breakdown of the substrate, interference from enzyme contaminants or other components of the culture supernatants, and other nonspecific processes leading to high background. Limited substrate turnover or inhibition of the antibody by other culture components can also attenuate the signal-to-noise ratio. These latter problems are difficult to anticipate and therefore not amenable to technical solution. Therefore, in principle, direct screening of antibodies in cell culture is feasible for specific reactions of stable substrates, provided that the catalysts can attain specific activities that are several orders of magnitude greater that those thus far observed for anti-TSA antibodies.

1.3. Indirect Kinetic Screening

Novel immunoenzymatic assays appear to offer a practical compromise to the problems and demands associated with catalytic antibody screening. Several formats have been described that combine the multistep operations of microtiter plate immunoassays with reaction-specific analysis of enzymatic assay. Though adaptable to other reactions than those for which they were developed, these assays are not universal. Hydrolytic reactions have characteristics that are particularly suitable to these formats, and this accounts in part for the emphasis on esterase and amidase activity of antibodies. The throughput capacities are similar to conventional immunoassays, although the convenience and sensitivity of the assays may be compromised by excessive manipulations, slow reaction rates, or turnaround times. Alternative methods utilize specific immunoadsorbents to capture antibody from dilute solution, which permits separation from the media and subsequent kinetic assay as appropriate to the reaction. These procedures often require more supernatant than is available from the well of a microtiter plate, as well as the stepwise manipulation of individual samples. Thus, the application may be limited to small hybridoma culture collections.

1.3.1. Pooled Antibody Capture

Catalytic assays that are based on spectrophotometric changes are potentially very sensitive. Interference from agents in the crude cultures can be alleviated by affinity separation and transfer of the antibodies into the appropriate assay buffer. The problem of sample manipulation, which can discourage screening of large hybridoma collections, can be made manageable by devising pooling strategies (6). Batch or column affinity purification of several hundred pooled samples is handled with ordinary laboratory equipment and plasticware. The choice of affinity matrix is critical for efficient capture of all potential catalytic antibodies. Protein-A and protein-G Sepharose are the most convenient and cheapest materials for employment in multiple small-column purifications. However, these supports are isotype-specific. Protein-A binds efficiently to murine IgG2 and IgG3, but not to IgG1 subclass. Protein-G has broader specificity and many desirable characteristics for capture of all IgG subtypes. Immobilized anti-IgG is another acceptable matrix, but is generally more expensive and has variable binding efficiency and capacity. Since only small volumes of supernatant are used, the amount of the affinity matrix can be minimized. A bed volume of 0.2–0.1 mL gel/sample is adequate for these applications.

After sequential loading, washing, and elution steps, antibodies are contained in a small volume of buffer solution that is sufficient for assay by spectrophotometric or radiometric techniques. Reasonable estimates for detection limits may be based on antibody concentrations in hybridoma supernatants. Assuming typical antibody concentrations of 2–50 μg/mL, a 0.2-mL vol of each supernatant provides approximately 3–60 pmol of each antibody in the assay. A 2–3-mL vol of supernatant is more practical for adequate amounts of antibody from low-density cultures. Successful detection of antibody activity depends on the catalytic efficiencies and assay sensitivity. At 10–100 turnovers of substrate in a 1-mL vol, low nanomolar to submicromolar concentrations of product should be released, which is near the detection limit of fluorimetric analysis. Incubation times can be varied to achieve this limit of detection, provided that nonspecific signal or background reactions do not interfere.

1.3.2. Immobilized Antibody

A variation of the antibody capture assay that requires fewer manipulations has been examined in early detection of antibodies with amidase activity *(12)*. Antibody is captured from the supernatants on an anti-IgG affinity matrix, and the immobilized antibodies are incubated directly in enzyme assay buffer. The technique assumes that immobilization of the antibody on the gel does not significantly affect its catalytic activity. The final step can employ any analytical procedure for detection of the reaction product. This typically requires filtration or washing to separate the assay mixture from the matrix and spectrophotometry or other method of analysis. Limitations of the method include the requirement for filtration microtiter plates and other equipment for accurately dispensing and washing gel in a 96-well plate format. Although the method could in principle be applied for primary screening of the hybridomas obtained soon after the fusion, the number of plates involved and the limited volume of supernatants prohibit this. As with the antibody-capture technique, the method is more suited to secondary screening of a restricted set of clones selected by immunoassay.

1.3.3. catELISA

A unique immunoassay variant that was devised specifically for catalytic antibody screening is dubbed catELISA *(13)*. The method, which is an adaptation of ELISA, allows direct screening of primary cultures from hybridoma fusion. The assay utilizes a substrate–carrier conjugate as the immunosorbent and requires a product-specific antiserum that does not crossreact with the substrate. Preincubation of the adsorbed substrate with culture supernatants generates an immobilized product when a catalyst is present. Subsequent washing, incubation with the antiproduct reagent, and development then identify cultures that contain specific catalytic antibodies. The antiproduct reagent should be developed from a species different from that used for hybridoma development to avoid detecting monoclonals that simply bind to the products or the substrate.

The application of a catELISA strategy to esterase antibodies has provided a practical demonstration of the screening dilemma and the advantanges of bypassing affinity-based assays for prescreening. Conventional immunoassay identified nearly 1000 hapten-binding clones, whereas the catELISA method distinguished only nine clones as positive for esterase activity. These results also illustrate the variable selectivity of antihapten ELISA. In some hybridoma screening experiments, relatively few antihapten antibodies are distinguished, whereas in others, hundreds of clones may be found. The widely used ELISA techniques encompass a variety of procedures and diverse reagents. The difficulty of standardizing assay procedures further complicates the correlation of results among different laboratories.

Clearly the catELISA technology requires strategic development of materials and methods for the specific assay. In addition, the catalytic process should lend itself to the design of substrates and products that remain immobilized to carriers or supports while being acted on by the catalyst. Nevertheless, this methodology has placed proper focus on the screening technology as a critical bottleneck in the production of catalytic antibodies.

New techniques are expected to arise in response to the challenge of catalytic antibody development in recombinant systems where expression levels and activities are similarly restricted. A schematic illustration of the routes available for screening and the processing steps to identify catalytic antibodies from cloned hybridomas (or other cells expressing antibody) is shown in Fig. 1.

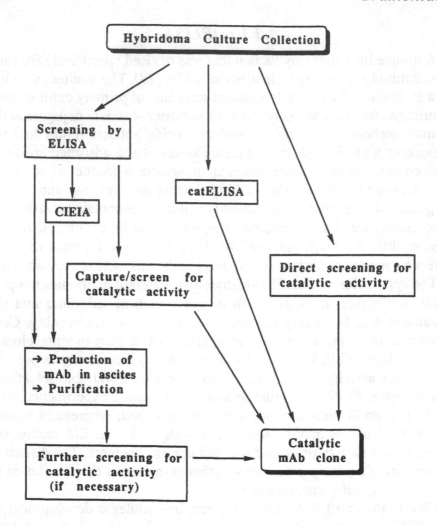

Fig. 1. Schematic representation of routes for catalytic antibody screening indicating the stages of assay and sequence for evaluating samples derived from hybridomas.

2. Materials
2.1. ELISA (see Note 1)

1. Buffer A (phosphate-buffered saline [PBS]): 10 mM Na$_2$HPO$_4$, and 2 mM KH$_2$PO$_4$, pH 7.2, 140 mM NaCl, 2 mM KCl, and 0.05 % NaN$_3$.
2. Buffer B: 10 mM Tris-HCl, pH 8.0, 0.1% Tween 20, and 0.05% NaN$_3$.
3. 1% Bovine serum albumin (BSA) (fraction V): 1% w/v in buffer A.

4. Rabbit antimouse-alkaline phosphatase conjugate: Commercial preparations typically supplied as a 1 mg/mL solution (*see* Note 2).
5. Buffer C: Diethanolamine 10% v/v aqueous solution, pH 9.8, 10 mM MgCl$_2$, and 1 mM ZnCl$_2$.
6. *p*-Nitrophenylphosphate, sodium salt (PNPP): Supplied as a powder (store desiccated).

2.2. CIEIA (see Note 3)

10X Solution of competitive ligands: 10 mM in distilled water or as otherwise appropriate to the standard ELISA procedure.

2.3. Antibody Capture

1. Reusable columns can be prepared from a 1-mL syringe barrel by plugging the tip with cotton. A reservoir constructed from a 30-mL syringe barrel is attached to the column with a luer lock or a simple gasket.
2. 10X buffer A: 0.5M Tris-HCl, pH 7.8, and 0.1% NaN$_3$.
3. Buffer B: 100 mM glycine-HCl, pH 2.8, and 0.05% NaN$_3$.
4. Antibody affinity gel: Immobilized protein-A, protein-G, or antimouse IgG-coupled to Sepharose or agarose (*see* Note 4).

2.4. Immobilized Antibody

1. Antibody affinity gel: *see* Section 2.3., item 4.
2. 96-well filter plates.
3. Phosphate-buffered saline, PBS: see Section 2.1., buffer A.

3. Methods

3.1. Antihapten ELISA (see Note 1)

1. Coat a set of 96-well microtiter plates with 50–200 μL/well of a solution of hapten–BSA conjugate (10 μg/mL in buffer A). Incubate at 37°C for 30 min to 1 h.
2. Wash plates with 3 × 200 μL of buffer B. An automatic or manual plate washing device is convenient.
3. Coat all wells with 200 μL of 1% BSA solution, and incubate for 15 min at 37°C.
4. Repeat wash step 2.
5. Transfer 100 μL/well of supernatants from hybridomas to the assay plates with a multichannel pipeter, and incubate for 30 min at 37°C.
6. Repeat wash step 2 and tap the inverted plate on a paper towel to dry the wells.
7. Prepare a 1:1000 dilution of the enzyme conjugate in 1% BSA solution, add 100 μL/well, and incubate for 30 min at 37°C.

8. Repeat wash step 2.
9. Add to each well 100 µL of a fresh solution of 1 mg/mL PNPP in buffer C. Incubate for 15–30 min, and read absorbance visually or with ELISA plate reader at 400 nm.

3.2. CIEIA: TSA Competitive Inhibition (see Note 3)

1. Follow the standard ELISA procedure as described above through step 4.
2. In alternate wells on the microtiter plate, mix 100 µL of hybridoma supernatants (*see* Note 5) that have previously tested positive and 10 µL of a stock solution of the competitive ligand. Fill the adjacent wells with 100 µL of the corresponding supernatants and 10 µL buffer A containing no competitor. Incubate the plate at 37°C for 1–3 h.
3. Complete the standard ELISA procedure above from steps 6–9.

3.3. Antibody Capture

1. Pool 3–10 mL of each hybridoma supernatant into groups of five or more (*see* Note 6).
2. For each pooled supernatant, load a column with about 0.2 mL of affinity gel.
3. Pass each supernatant through a column by gravity filtration. Volumes smaller than 20 mL can be reloaded for a second pass to increase antibody capture.
4. Wash the columns with 3 mL of buffer A.
5. Elute the bound protein with buffer B, collecting 1-mL aliquots in sterile Eppendorf tubes containing 50 µL of 10X buffer A.
6. Pool fractions containing protein as judged by 280-nm absorbance (*see* Note 7).
7. Aliquots may be employed in the appropriate catalysis assay (*see* Note 8).

3.4. Immobilized Antibody

1. Transfer individual hybridoma supernatants or pools into 15-mL conical tubes.
2. Add 140 µL of a 50% slurry of affinity gel to each tube, and mix by inverting slowly end over end for 18 h (*see* Note 9).
3. Allow the gel to settle to the bottom by standing the tubes upright or by brief centrifugation. Remove most of the supernatant by decanting, and transfer the gel samples in a small volume of slurry to individual wells of a 96-well filter plate.
4. Wash the gel samples by filtration with 3 × 200 µL PBS containing 0.05% Tween-20 and 2 × 200 µL PBS.
5. Add the assay buffer containing substrate to the wells, and incubate as appropriate.

6. Collect samples at convenient time intervals by filtration or pipeting, and analyze accordingly (*see* Note 8).

3.5. catELISA (see Note 3)

1. Adsorb the substrate–BSA conjugate (1–10 µg/mL) onto 96-well microtiter plates as described for the ELISA Section 3.1.
2. Follow the standard ELISA procedure through step 6, increasing the time of incubation of the supernatants (step 5) on the plate to 3 h.
3. Prepare a solution of the antiproduct antiserum in PBS containing 0.04% Tween-20 at the predetermined dilution that gives minimal ELISA reactivity with the substrate conjugate (reported example used 1:5000), and coat the plate with 100 µL/well. Incubate at 37°C for 30–60 min.
4. Complete the standard ELISA procedure above from steps 6–9 (*see* Note 10).

4. Notes

1. The described ELISA protocol uses an alkaline phosphatase conjugate and is representative of the method. However, enzymes, reagents, and incubation times vary in other commonly used assays.
2. Commercial antibody–enzyme conjugates are prepared by diverse methods that determine their stability and preferred method of use. The method described employs a conjugate prepared by glutaraldehyde coupling. For methods of preparation, *see* ref. 6.
3. Materials and methods used for catELISA and CIEIA should be based on the corresponding ELISA protocol.
4. Commercial gels are supplied as slurries in neutral buffer containing a preservative. The gel should be washed either before or after loading onto the column with buffer B, followed by equilibration with buffer A.
5. Supernatants should be titered as necessary to establish conditions where the ELISA signal (optical density) is responsive to 1:1 dilution of the sample. Competitive binding can be confirmed by using the free hapten in competition with the conjugated hapten on the plate.
6. Proteins contributed from the media constitute the principal source of contaminant to antibodies in hybridoma supernatants. Hybridomas may be cultured in serum-free media or with low fetal bovine serum, when tolerated, to reduce the unwanted proteins, such as bovine γ-globulin, that copurify with the MAb.
7. Antibody is typically found in the first 1-mL fraction eluted with low-pH buffer from a small protein-G Sepharose affinity column.
8. Typical enzymatic assay employing UV/vis or fluorescence spectrophotometric measurement can be set up in appropriate cuvets or 96-well plate

formats. Sufficient sample should be available to allow use of the antibody without further dilution in the analytical device, which can read volumes of 1 mL or less.

9. The slow rate of antibody capture in batch immunoadsorption may affect the efficiency of the assay. Concentrating the samples by ultrafiltration or adjusting the buffer conditions for optimal binding may improve efficiency by increasing the rate of capture (*see* ref. *6*).

10. The enzyme–antibody conjugate used in catELISA should be an appropriate reagent for detection of antibody from the species used to produce the antiproduct antiserum.

References

1. Jencks, W. P. (1969) *Catalysis in Chemistry and Enzymology*, McGraw-Hill, New York.
2. Tramontano, A., Janda, K. D., and Lerner, R. A. (1986) Catalytic antibodies. *Science* **234,** 1566–1570.
3. Pollack, S. J., Jacobs, J. R., and Schultz, P. G. (1986) Selective chemical catalysis by an antibody. *Science* **234,** 1570–1573.
4. Lerner, R. A., Benkovic, S. J., and Schultz, P. G. (1991) At the crossroads of chemistry and immunology: catalytic antibodies. *Science* **252,** 659–667.
5. Shokat, K. M., Leumann, C. J., Sugasawara, R., and Schultz, P. G. (1989) A new strategy for the generation of catalytic antibodies. *Nature* **338,** 269–271.
6. Harlow, E. and Lane, D. (1988) *Antibodies: A Laboratory Manual*, Cold Spring Harbor Laboratory, Cold Spring Harbor, NY.
7. Janda, K. D., Weinhouse, M. I., Danon, T., Pacelli, K. A., and Schloeder, D. M. (1991) Antibody bait and switch catalysis: a survey of antigens capable of inducing abzymes with acyl-transfer properties. *J. Am Chem. Soc.* **113,** 5427–5434.
8. Benkovic, S. J., Napper, A. D., and Lerner, R. A. (1988) Catalysis of a stereospecific bimolecular amide synthesis by an antibody. *Proc. Natl. Acad. Sci. USA* **85,** 5355–5358.
9. Miyashita, H., Hara, T., Tanimura, R., Tanaka, F., Kikuchi, M., and Fujii, I. (1994) A common ancestry for multiple catalytic antibodies generated against a single transition-state analog. *Proc. Natl. Acad. Sci. USA* **91,** 6045–6049.
10. Tawfik, D. S., Zemel, R. R., Arad-Yellin, R., Green, B. S., and Eshhar, Z. (1990) Simple method for selecting catalytic monoclonal antibodies that exhibit turnover and specificity. *Biochemistry* **29,** 9916–9921.
11. Gong, B., Lesley, S. A., and Schultz, P. G. (1992) A chromogenic assay for screening large antibody libraries. *J. Am. Chem. Soc.* **114,** 1486,1487.
12. Martin, M. T., Angeles, T. S., Sugasawara, R., Aman, N. I., Napper, A. D., Darsley, M. J., Sanchez, R. I., Booth, P., and Titmas, R. C. (1994) Antibody-catalyzed hydrolysis of an unsubstituted amide. *J. Am. Chem. Soc.* **116,** 6508–6512.
13. Tawfik, D. S., Green, B. S., Chap, R., Sela, M., and Eshhar, Z. (1993) catELISA: a facile general route to catalytic antibodies. *Proc. Natl. Acad. Sci. USA* **90,** 373–377.

CHAPTER 17

Expression of Chimeric Immunoglobulin Genes in Mammalian Cells

Sergey M. Deyev and Oleg L. Polanovsky

1. Introduction

The ability to make monoclonal rodent antibodies has revolutionized immunology. To reduce the immunogenicity of these antibodies for human in vivo use, methods have been developed to create artificial recombinant antibodies *(1)*. Chimeric recombinant antibodies containing mouse variable domains and human constant domains are characterized by essentially the same antigen-binding properties as the mouse antibodies from hybridomas. The immunogenicity of the chimeric antibodies is lower owing to replacement of mouse constant domains for human ones. Various humanized, reshaped, and other antibody constructs have been created in different laboratories *(1)*.

For expression of antibody constructs, appropriate gene constructs can be inserted into mammalian cells using transfection methods. Expression of both the heavy and light immunoglobulin chain genes is under the control of regulatory elements, promoters, and enhancers. These elements are housed upstream and downstream of the transcription start site, respectively. DNA-binding transcription factors recognize these genetic elements and participate in the initiation of transcription. The development of recombinant DNA techniques has allowed us to construct a heterologous transcription machinery with a high level of expression. These systems may be used for immunoglobulin gene expression in different cell types. It is not the purpose here to review all available expression

From: *Methods in Molecular Biology, Vol. 51: Antibody Engineering Protocols*
Edited by: S. Paul Humana Press Inc., Totowa, NJ

constructs and procedures. Instead, as an example, we shall describe below the strategy for construction of chimeric immunoglobulin genes and expression of these genes under the control of the cytomegalovirus promoter, as well as expression of an immunoglobulin gene tandem under the control of the T7 RNA polymerase promoter *(2)*.

1.1. Strategy to Identify Expressible Immunoglobulin Genes

Hybridoma cells have karyotypes different from ordinary diploid cells. There is varying chromosomal ploidy in hybridoma cells. J_H-C_H and J_κ-C_κ rearranged loci may be represented by several alleles. Only one allele in each case is responsible for the synthesis of the antibody heavy (H) and light (L) chain. We used a DNA region containing the third and fourth J_H exons as the probe to detect H-chain RNA. This probe was used because the distal J_H4 segment and its 3'-flank are preserved and can be detected using hybridization analysis when the V_H gene is translocated to any J_H segment.

In the hybridoma PTF-02, the J_H-C_H locus is represented by three alleles, each of which is different from embryonic genes. The strategy chosen for cloning of the antibody genes from this hybridoma cell line was based on the hybridization analysis data. Incomplete *Eco*RI and *Bgl*II hydrolysates of PTF-02 DNA were used to compile a genomic library. Three clones containing the J_H-C_H locus were identified. Only one of them (clone HII) contained both V_H and $C_{\gamma l}$ regions. Two other clones contained incomplete portions of these regions. The presence of the gene responsible for H-chain synthesis in clone HII was confirmed by comparison of the DNA sequence of this clone with the sequence of the heavy polypeptide chain synthesized by hybridoma cell line PTF-02.

Hybridization analysis of the original PTF-02 hybridoma line revealed three κ genes. One of them corresponds to a fetal gene that is lost after continuous cultivation of the hybridoma. *Eco*RI, *Bam*HI, and *Hin*dIII digests were used to analyze the two remaining alleles (κ-1 and κ-2). A 2.7-kb J_κ-probe was used for the hybridization analysis and screening of gene libraries. One of the genes (κ-1) originates from the myeloma used for fusion. The second gene (κ-2) originates from the antitransferrin producing lymphocyte partner used in cell fusion. This gene was analyzed in detail. For this purpose, a 7.5-kb *Bam*HI fragment containing both V_κ and C_κ exons was digested with *Eco*RI, *Hin*dIII, and *Pst*I restriction endonucleases and subcloned in plasmid pUC19. The nucleotide sequences of the leader exon, the V_κ exon joined with J_5 segment, and adjacent 5'-region accommodating regulatory transcription sequences were determined. Both H- and L-chain genes encoding the antibody polypeptide chains were cloned and sequenced in this way.

1.2. Expression of an Immunoglobulin Gene Tandem Under the Control of T7 RNA Polymerase

The entire gene tandem composed of H- and L-chain genes and appropriate introns and spacer between the genes is placed under the control of the T7 bacteriophage RNA polymerase promoter (Fig. 1). The transfected cells contain in their genome a modified semisynthetic gene for T7 RNA polymerase *(3)*. The modification of the polymerase consists of replacement of the N-terminal segment with amino acids 124–133 of the SV40 viral large T-antigen, coded for by a synthetic nucleotide sequence. This sequence is the signal for nuclear localization of the protein, allowing the modified polymerase to penetrate effectively from the cytoplasm into the nucleus and providing for nuclear translation under T7 promoter control.

The V_H-gene from mouse hybridoma and the human C_ε-gene are inserted into pGEM1 plasmid under the control of bacteriophage T7 RNA polymerase promoter. The sticky ends of the *Hind*III fragment of the V_H-gene and *Bam*HI fragment of C_ε-gene are blunted with Klenow fragment of DNA polymerase, and the intermediate is ligated by its blunt ends, yielding plasmid pIG.1e. *Escherichia coli* (strain *DH5α*) cells are transformed with a vector pIG.1e. The clones containing inserts are screened and analyzed using restriction endonucleases. The *Pst*I site is replaced with a *Hind*III site, yielding plasmid pIG.2e.

The mouse V_κ-gene (from the same hybridoma) and the human C_κ gene are inserted into pUC19, yielding plasmid pIG.3k. *E. coli DH5α* cells are transformed with the plasmid pIG.3k, and clones containing the ligation product are treated with *Hind*III. The sticky ends are blunted and then religated, yielding plasmid pIG.4k.

Plasmid pIG.4k is cloned in *E. coli JM103*. *Eco*RI sites at both ends of V_κ-C_κ genes tandem are then replaced with *Hind*III sites, yielding plasmid pIG.5k. The final construct consists of the V_κ-C_κ gene fused to the 3'-end of the $V_H C_\varepsilon$ gene. Both genes are in the sense orientation. The structure of the final plasmid (pIG.6ek) is shown in Fig 1.

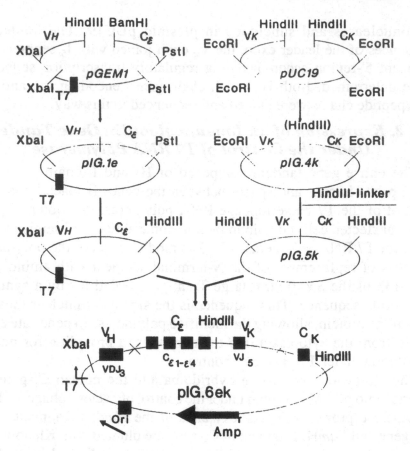

Fig. 1. Design of plasmid pIG.6ek containing the mouse/human immunoglobulin gene tandem. Location of H- and L-chain genes of immunoglobulins is
shown with black boxes; T7—T7 bacteriophage RNA polymerase promoter;
ori—origin of replication.

1.3. Expression of H- and L-Chain Genes Under the Control of Cytomegalovirus (CMV) Promoter

E. coli cells (strain *JM103*) were used for cloning the plasmids, as
described below. Restriction digestion was carried out according to ref.
(4). Three buffers (*see* Section 2.) may be used: high, low, and medium
ionic strength (*see* Note 1).

Plasmid pCMV was cut using *Eco*RI and *Sac*I restriction endonucleases. The fragments were separated by polyacrylamide gel electro-

phoresis. The 293-bp *Eco*RI-*Sac*I fragment containing the CMV promoter was eluted and cloned into pUC.19. After transformation, colonies with the insert were selected on the plates containing X-gal and isopropylthio-β-galactoside (IPTG). This plasmid (pUC.CMV.293) was analyzed by double cleavage with *Eco*RI + *Sac*I.

The V_HC_ϵ fragment from plasmid pIG.1e (Fig. 1) was then cloned into plasmid pUC.19.CMV.293. To do this, plasmid pIG.1e was cut with restriction endonucleases *Xba*I and *Pst*I. DNA fragments were separated in a 1% low-melting agarose gel. The V_HC_ϵ fragment was eluted from the gel, blunted with Klenow's fragment, and cloned into plasmid pUC.19.CMV.293 that had previously digested with *Sma*I. Colonies with inserts were selected, and the orientations of inserts were determined by restriction analysis of plasmid DNA.

Plasmid pUC.pur.CMV.$V_\kappa C_\kappa$ was obtained in the following way (Fig. 2). Fragment $V_\kappa C_\kappa$ was cut out from plasmid pIG.5k using restriction endonuclease *Hind*III. The fragment was isolated by electrophoresis in 1% low-melting agarose, eluted from the agarose, and cloned into plasmid pUC.CMV.293 that had previously been digested at the *Hind*III site. Colonies with the inserts were selected. $V_\kappa C_\kappa$ cloning and orientation were confirmed by restriction analysis. Plasmid pUC.CMV.$V_\kappa C_\kappa$ was cut with *Eco*RI and then subjected to limited hydrolysis with restriction endonuclease *Hind*III. The obtained fragments were separated in an agarose gel. Fragment *Eco*RI-CMV.$V_\kappa C_\kappa$-*Hind*III was eluted and cloned into plasmid pUC.pur, cleaved in advance with *Eco*RI. Sticky *Eco*RI ends of the plasmid and the insert were ligated, insert *Hind*III end and the plasmid *Eco*RI end were blunted with Klenow's fragment, and blunt ends of both fragments were ligated.

Plasmid pUC.pur was obtained from plasmid pPAC1. It carries the N-acetyl transferase gene from *Streptomyces alboniger*, conferring puromycin resistance to mammalian cells on transfection. The correctness of cloning was checked by sequencing the obtained plasmids from the CMV promoter side.

2. Materials

1. 2*M* CaCl$_2$ stock solution sterilized in autoclave or by filtration through nitrocellulose filter.
2. Geneticin G-418 selection medium: RPMI-1640 medium supplemented with 10% fetal calf serum and Geneticin G-418 (Gibco; 400 μg/mL for CHO cells; 1.5 μg/mL for SP2/0 cells).

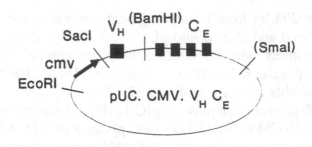

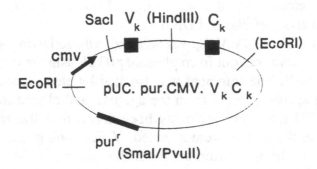

Fig. 2. Structure of plasmids containing H- and L-chain chimeric immunoglobulin genes placed under the control of cytomegalovirus (CMV) promoter; pur—puromycin resistance gene.

3. Chinese hamster ovary (CHO) cells are maintained in a 5% CO_2 incubator using RPMI medium supplemented with 10% fetal calf serum.

4. SP2/0 myeloma cells are maintained in a 5% CO_2 incubator using RPMI-1640 medium supplemented with 10% fetal calf serum.

5. CHO and SP2/0 cell lines containing in their genome a semisynthetic T7 RNA polymerase gene and steadily expressing this enzyme (obtained from A. Lieber, ref. 3).

6. Recombinant DNA constructs: Various vectors with inserted gene fragments were created by recombinant DNA methods (see Section 1.). These constructs are dissolved in sterile distilled water at a final concentration of 1 µg/mL and stored at –20°C.

7. Antibodies for radioimmunoassay: Rabbit antihuman whole IgE and anti-ε-chain antibodies (ISN Flow, UK) dissolved in the PBS buffer to a

final concentration 10 µg/mL. These antibodies do not crossreact with other isotypes of immunoglobulins.

8. DNA probes: As J_H probe, an *Eco*RI-*Bam*HI fragment (1.9 kb) from fetal mouse locus was used. This fragment contained J_H3 and J_H4 segments. A *Hind*III-*Hind*III fragment of fetal mouse $J_κ$ locus was used as the $J_κ$ probe. This probe contained $J_κ1$-$J_κ5$ segments.

9. Plasmids: pGEM1 (Promega) containing T7 RNA polymerase promoter; pSV2-neo containing the neomycin resistance gene.

10. Antibiotics: Puromycin and geneticin (G418).

11. Buffers for restriction endonuclease digestion:

    High salt: 50 m*M* Tris-HCl, 100 m*M* NaCl, 10 m*M* MgCl$_2$, 1 m*M* dithio-threitol, pH 7.5.

    Medium salt: 10 m*M* Tris-HCl, 50 m*M* NaCl, 10 m*M* MgCl$_2$, 1 m*M* dithio-threitol, pH 7.5.

    Low salt: 10 m*M* Tris-HCl, 10 m*M* MgCl$_2$, 1 m*M* dithiothreitol, pH 7.5.

    *Sma*I buffer: 15 m*M* Tris-HCl, 15 m*M* KCl, 6 m*M* dithiothreitol MgCl$_2$, 6 m*M* 2-mercaptoethanol, pH 8.5.

12. 10X MOPS buffer: 0.2*M* 3-[*N*-Morpholino]propanesulfonic acid, 0.05*M* Na acetate, pH 7.0, 0.01*M* disodium EDTA.

13. 2X HBSP buffer: 1.5 m*M* Na$_2$HPO$_4$, 10 m*M* KCl, 280 m*M* NaCl, 12 m*M* glucose, 50 m*M* HEPES, pH 6.95.

14. 10X PBS buffer: 80.06 g NaCl, 2.01 g KCl, 29 g Na$_2$HPO$_4$·12 H$_2$O (or 11 g Na$_2$HPO$_4$), and 2.04 g KH$_2$PO$_4$ in 1 L water. The pH of this buffer is 7.2.

15. 20X SSC buffer: Dissolve 175.3 g NaCl and 88.2 g Na$_3$ citrate·2H$_2$O in 1 L water. Adjust pH to 7.0.

16. 10X nick-translation buffer: 0.5*M* Tris-HCl, pH 7.6, 0.1*M* MgSO$_4$, 10 m*M* dithiothreitol, 500 mg/mL bovine serum albumin. Filter, sterilize, and store in 0.5-mL aliquots at –20°C.

17. Separate solutions in sterile distilled water of dATP, dCTP, dGTP, and dTTP, each at 0.2 m*M*. Adjust pH to 7.0–7.5 and store at –20°C.

18. α-^{32}P-dCTP (Amersham).

19. DNA polymerase I: 5 U/mL (Amersham or Boehringer Mannheim). Store at –20°C.

20. DNase I: 5 mL (Fermentas, Riga, or Boehringer Mannheim). Store at –20°C. Each aliquot is used only once.

21. Yeast tRNA stock solution: 10 mg/mL.

22. Hybond N filter membrane (Amersham).

23. Prehybridization buffer: 50% deionized formamide, 5X SSC, 5X Denhardt's solution, denatured salmon sperm DNA concentration (250 µg/mL final, diluted from stock solution in 50 m*M* sodium phosphate buffer, pH 6.5).

24. Hybridization buffer: 50% deionized formamide, 5X SSC, 1X Denhardt's solution, 100 µg/mL denatured salmon sperm DNA.
25. ELISA substrate buffer: 27 g/L citric acid, 35.6 g/L Na$_2$HPO$_4$·12 H$_2$O.
26. ELISA plate reader: Multiscan MCC-340, "Lab Systems," Finland.
27. IgE.
28. Monoclonal biotin-conjugated antihuman IgE.
29. Streptavidin–horseradish peroxidase conjugate.
30. o-Phenylenediamine and H$_2$O$_2$.
31. Bio-Rad (Richmond, CA) electrotransfer cells.
32. Electrotransfer buffer: 25 mM Tris-HCl, pH 8.3, 192 mM glycine, 0.02% SDS, 20% methanol.
33. Amido black 10B.
34. ^{125}I-protein A (Amersham).
35. XAR-5 X-ray film (Kodak).

3. Methods

3.1. Transfection of Mammalian Cells (see Notes 2 and 3)

3.1.1. Transfection of CHO Cells by Calcium Phosphate Method

1. Prepare cells at the stationary growth stage in a volume of 5 mL.
2. At least 3 h in advance, renew the culture medium (DMEM with 10% FCS) *(4)*.
3. Prepare calcium-phosphate precipitates as follows: To 213.5 µL of autoclaved water in a glass tube, add 4.5 µL of the DNA to be transfected (6–12 µg), 1.0 µL DNA of plasmid pSV2neo (0.25 µg/mL). The ratio of DNA to be transfected and plasmid DNA should be 50:1. While mixing on a vortex mixer, add 30 µL of 2.0M CaCl$_2$. Immediately thereafter, add dropwise 250 µL of 2X HBSP buffer. Fine precipitates should be formed. The suspension may be kept for 10 min and then poured into the flask containing the cells. In cotransfection experiments, plasmids puc.CMV.V$_H$C$_\epsilon$ and pUC.pur.CMV.VκCκ are mixed in equimolar concentration: 213 µL H$_2$O, 30.0 µL of 2M CaCl$_2$, 250.0 µL of 2X HBSP, and 3.5 µL (3.5 µg) of each plasmid.
4. Place the flasks in a CO$_2$ incubator at 37°C.
5. Change the medium after 4–18 h incubation.
6. Add 50.0 µL of Geneticin solution (40 mg/mL) each third day for 2 wk (final concentration of geneticin is 400 µg/mL for CHO cells).

3.1.2. Electroporation of SP2/0 Cells (see Notes 4 and 5)

1. Cells from one 260-mL culture flask are used per 96-well plate (*see* step 6, this section).

2. Collect the cells, count them under a microscope, and pellet for 5 min at 1000 rpm.
3. Suspend the pellet in 50% conditioned medium to a concentration of 5×10^6–1×10^7 cells/mL.
4. Add DNA to 50 µg/mL. Pour the suspension into electroporation cuvets. Apply electrical pulse. Pulse parameters: 400–450 V, 50 ms, space between electrodes, 2 mm (rectangular pulse).
5. Transfer cells from cuvets into sterile tubes with 50% conditioned medium containing the antibiotic. Selection in geneticin (1–1.5 µg/mL) is done at 5×10^4 cells/mL and in puromycin (5 µg/mL) at 2.5×10^4 cells/mL.
6. Dispense the cells into 96-well plates at 200 µL/each well.
7. Change the medium containing antibiotic geneticin in 8–24 h, and the medium that contains puromycin, in 24–48 h.
8. Five days later, change half of the medium. Fresh medium should contain the antibiotic at the same concentration as the original culture. Fifty percent conditioned medium should be used for cell growth until colonies are formed. The selection for antibiotic should be stopped at the time when viable cells disappear in a control culture subjected to the transfection and selection procedure without DNA (usually about 10 d) (*see* Note 4).

3.2. Northern Hybridization

3.2.1. RNA Electrophoresis in 1% Agarose Gel in the Presence of Formaldehyde

1. Dissolve 1 g of agarose in 85 mL of boiling water, and add 10 mL of 10X MOPS buffer stock solution.
2. Cool to 50°C. Working in a fume hood, add 5.4 mL of 37% formaldehyde solution. Mix by swirling.
3. Pour the mixture into the gel base plate. Use 1X MOPS buffer as electrode buffer.
4. Prepare RNA sample as follows: Add 2.5 µL of 10X MOPS buffer and 4.0 µL of 37% formaldehyde to 12.5 µL of deionized formamide. Add 5–10 µg of RNA (6 µL). Incubate the mixture for 5 min at 65°C, then cool on ice, and add 2.5 µL of 50% (v/v) glycerol containing 0.1 mg/mL of Bromphenol blue.

3.2.2. RNA Transfer to the Filter

1. Fill a cuvet with the transfer buffer (20X SSC or 20X SSPE), place a transfer plate into the cuvet, and cover with the three sheets of Whatman 3MM filter paper moistened with buffer so that the edges of the paper are hanging out from the plate edges and touching the transfer buffer.

2. Place the gel on the plate with Whatman 3MM with the holes downward (*see* Note 6).
3. Cut out a Hybond N filter sheet corresponding to the size of the gel. Moisten it in distilled water and then in transfer buffer. Place the filter on the gel (*see* Note 6). Drape three sheets of Whatman filter paper wetted with the transfer buffer over the Hybond filter membrane.
4. Place paper towels (5–10 cm) over the gel sandwich.
5. Place a glass plate and an appropriate object weighing 0.5–1.0 kg on the paper towels, and keep for 8–16 h.
6. When the transfer is over, carefully disassemble the gel sandwich. Wash the membrane in 2X SSC or 2X SSPE to remove adherent agarose.
7. Dry the membrane for 30 min.
8. Wrap the filter in Saran Wrap, and place RNA-side down on a transilluminator for 2–5 min (recommended wavelength, 312 nm).

3.2.3. RNA Hybridization with a Labeled DNA Probe

1. Place the Hybond filter in a double-walled plastic bag and pour prehybridization buffer into the bag. Heat-seal the bag. Carry out prehybridization for 3–5 h at 42°C.
2. Open the bag, remove the prehybridization buffer, and pour the hybridization buffer into the bag. Add hybridization buffer (50–100 µL/1 cm^2 of filter surface). Add denatured DNA probe (5–10 ng/mL) labeled in vitro with ^{32}P by nick-translation (*see* Section 3.3.). Incubate the filter with the labeled probe for 12–15 h.
3. Wash the filter in 0.5% SDS in 2X SSC twice for 15 min each at room temperature, once in 0.5% SDS in 2X SSC at 60°C for 30 min, and once in 0.5% SDS in 0.1X SSC at 60°C for 30 min.
4. Dry the filter and carry out autoradiography.

3.3. Nick Translation

Nick translation is used for the preparation of labeled DNA probes. Nicks are generated at random locations by limited digestion of the DNA with DNase I. The nicks are then repaired with DNA polymerase I.

1. Add the following reactants in 1.5-mL sterile microfuge tube: 2.5 mL of 10X nick-translation buffer, 2.5 mL of each dNTP (0.2 mM), 5 mL of α-^{32}P-dCTP, 5 U of DNA polymerase I, 0.5 mL of DNase I, 0.1–0.5 mg of substrate DNA, and sterile distilled water to a total volume of 25 mL.
2. Incubate at 15°C for 20 min (*see* Note 7), and place the tube on ice.
3. Add 2.5 mL of tRNA stock solution.
4. Separate the labeled DNA from free nucleotides by passage through a G-50 Sephadex column. Collect effluent fractions.

5. Pool the fractions containing the peak of radioactivity.
6. Calculate the specific activity of the labeled DNA as total radioactivity in the excluded peak (corrected for counting efficiency) divided by the weight of DNA added to the reaction mixture.

3.4. ELISA

1. Coat 96-well microtiter plates (Nunc) with monoclonal antibodies (MAb) against human IgE (concentration 10 μg/mL) in 0.05M sodium carbonate buffer, pH 9.6, for 18 h at 4°C (100 μL/well).
2. Block nonspecific binding sites with 1% BSA in PBS for 1 h (100 μL).
3. Dispense samples and IgE standards into the wells in triplicate, and incubate for 2 h (100 μL/well) (*see* Note 8).
4. Add 100 μL biotin-conjugated MAb to human IgE (diluted 1:500 in PBS containing 0.2% BSA and 0.05% Tween-20). Incubate for 1 h. This antibody is directed against an antigenic determinant different from that recognized by the immobilized anti-IgE antibody.
5. Wash wells three times with 200 μL PBS containing 0.05% Tween-20.
6. Add streptavidin–horseradish peroxidase (100 μL/well) (diluted 1:500 in 0.1% PBS containing BSA and 0.05% Tween-20). Incubate for 1 h at room temperature.
7. Wash wells five times with PBS containing 0.05% Tween-20 (200 μL each).
8. Develop color reaction with 0.4 mg/mL *o*-phenylenediamine and 0.03% H_2O_2 in ELISA substrate buffer (100 μL) for 20 min at room temperature in dark.
9. Stop the reaction by addition of 100 μL of 5% H_2SO_4. Measure optical density at 492 nm using an ELISA plate reader.

3.5. Immunoblotting

This is done to confirm expression of correct-sized antibody H (~60 kDa) and L chains (~30 kDa).

1. Apply marker proteins and samples (cell lysates prepared by detergent extraction or sonication) to the polyacrylamide gel for electrophoresis. Three identical sample series are applied to the same gel. One-third of the gel corresponding to one of the replicate sample series is cut out with a razor blade and stained with Coomassie blue.
2. Perform electrotransfer on nitrocellulose filters using the remaining two-thirds portion of the gel. This can be done using special transfer cells like those sold by Bio-Rad. The transfer buffer is 25 mM Tris-HCl, pH 8.3, 192 mM glycine, 0.02% SDS, and 20% methanol. The following transfer conditions are used: voltage 80 V, current strength 0.2 ρ, transfer time 2 h.

3. Stain one-half of the filter with 0.1% amido black 10B in 7% acetic acid for 30 min, and wash in 7% acetic acid to check the quality of electrotransfer. Wash the second half of the filter twice in PBS with 0.05% Tween-20, each time for 15 min.
4. Incubate the filter in PBS containing 1% BSA without Tween-20 for 1 h at room temperature. Then wash.
5. Incubate the filter with polyclonal rabbit antibodies against human immunoglobulin E (10–20 µg/mL) in PBS containing 0.2% BSA and 0.05% Tween-20 for 1 h at room temperature. Wash the filter three times for 5 min each in PBS containing 0.05% Tween-20.
6. Incubate the filter with the solution of ^{125}I-protein A (50 µCi) in PBS containing 0.2% BSA and 0.05% Tween-20 for 1 h at room temperature. Wash the filter five times for 15 min each with PBS containing 0.05% Tween-20. Dry the filter and expose it to X-ray-film in light-tight cassets at –70°C.

4. Notes

1. All restriction endonucleases used in this chapter were active in the buffer "medium salt" (*see* Section 2.).
2. Usage of transfection technique depends on cell type. Adherent cells (CHO) should be transfected by calcium phosphate gel precipitation. Electroporation is preferable for transfection of suspension (nonadherent) cell culture (Sp2/0).
3. The pH of 2X HBSP buffer is 6.95. It is adjusted with 1.0*N* NaOH. The buffer is then filtered through a nitrocellulose filter (0.22 µm). The pH of this buffer is extremely important for obtaining fine precipitates.
4. The cells should be at the logarithmic stage of growth at the time of electroporation. To this end, change half of the medium in a culture that has almost reached the monolayer stage 1 d prior to the electroporation.
5. Conditioned medium is defined here as the supernatant collected from a cell monolayer after 1 d of culture. Although the nutrients in this medium are partly exhausted, the medium contains growth factors. These factors allow the antibiotic resistant single cells to survive even when the bulk of the cells are dying.
6. Be careful to prevent trapping of air bubbles between the gel and filter.
7. To optimize the nick translation system, it is desirable to calibrate the time needed for 30–40% incorporation of free label into DNA. Typically, optimal incorporation is achieved within 20–40 min.
8. To block nonspecific binding, dilute samples with PBS containing 0.1% Tween-20.

References

1. Morrison, S. L. (1992) In vitro antibodies: strategy for production and application. *Annu. Rev. Immunol.* **10,** 239–265.
2. Deyev, S. M., Lieber, A., Radko, B. V., and Polanovsky, O. L. (1993) Production of recombinant antibodies in lymphoid and nonlymphoid cells. *FEBS Lett.* **330,** 111–113.
3. Lieber, A., Sandig, V., Sommer, W., Bahring, S., and Strauss, M. (1993) Stable high-level gene expression in mammalian cells by T7 RNA phage polymerase. *Methods Enzymol.* **217,** 47–66.
4. Sambrook, J., Fritsch, E., and Maniatis, T. (1989) *Molecular Cloning: A Laboratory Manual*, vol. 2. Cold Spring Harbor Laboratory, Cold Spring Harbor, NY.

CHAPTER 18

Single-Chain Anti-DNA F$_v$

Michael Polymenis and B. David Stollar

1. Introduction

Antibodies to native B-DNA are common in systemic lupus erythematosus (SLE), and their measurement serves as a diagnostic and prognostic marker of the disease (1). Autoreactive antibodies are also found in the sera of normal individuals (2). Natural autoantibodies crossreact with a variety of conserved, and seemingly unrelated, autoantigens. Most of these antibodies are of low affinity, although rare exceptions of high affinity natural anti-DNA antibodies have been reported (3). The role of cells that make natural autoantibodies and whether they are progenitors of cells that make disease-associated autoantibodies remains unclear (4).

Nucleic acids by themselves are not significantly immunogenic, but can be high mol-wt haptens. That is, when they are presented in a complex with carrier polypeptides, antibodies specific to the nucleic acid can be obtained. In this way, antibodies against nucleic acids of varying structure, composition, and conformation have been prepared and characterized (5). An important question is the relationship between experimentally induced antinucleic acid antibodies and autoantibodies from autoimmune subjects. Both groups are usually IgG, mutated, and have high affinity for the antigen. It has been suggested that the genetic origin of the two groups of antibodies can be the same, since the genes of two experimentally induced anti-Z-DNA antibodies were most homologous with genes of anti-DNA autoantibodies from autoimmune mice (6). Furthermore, from sequence comparisons and structural studies, immunization-induced and autoimmune antinucleic acid antibodies are indistinguishable (7,8).

From: Methods in Molecular Biology, Vol. 51: Antibody Engineering Protocols
Edited by: S. Paul Humana Press Inc., Totowa, NJ

The very high specificity of the induced antibodies for their antigen makes them ideal for studying the structural elements required for antigen recognition *(9)*. Therefore, the characterization of induced anitnucleic acid antibodies helps our understanding of antibody-nucleic acid interactions that are important in mediating autoimmunity. Furthermore, a more detailed characterization of anti-DNA antibodies will improve their many uses as selective reagents against various forms of nucleic acids. These goals can be achieved with the use of recombinant DNA technology to produce anitnucleic acid antibodies and manipulate them at will.

1.1. pIg20: A Vector for Expression of Soluble Single-Chain-Variable Fragment (scF$_v$) in E. Coli

In addition to being economical and very fast, expression of antibody fragments in *Escherichia coli* exploits the well-established bacterial gene technology for manipulations that can be made directly on the expression vector. The pIg20 vector uses the very specific and powerful T7 RNA polymerase promoter to drive scF$_v$ expression *(10)*. The *E. coli* strain used for expression, BL21(DE3)-pLysE, carries a chromosomal copy of the T7 RNA polymerase gene under the inducible *lac*UV5 promoter *(11)*.

In the scF$_v$ construct, the V$_H$ is upstream of the V$_L$ domain. The two domains are connected with a (GGGGS)$_3$ flexible peptide *(12)*. At the 5'-end of the scF$_v$, a leader peptide from bacterial alkaline phosphatase (*Pho*A) targets the expressed protein for secretion out of the cytoplasm (*see* Note 1). At the 3'-end of the scF$_v$, five His residues allow for the application of metal-chelating chromatography for product purification. However, detection and purification of the scF$_v$ are more efficient with a 3'-end fusion of one B domain (58 amino acids) of *Staphylococcus aureus* protein-A, exploiting the well-characterized interaction of this domain with the Fc portion of IgG (*see* Note 2). This domain can be removed proteolytically with thrombin digestion after the scF$_v$ is purified, using a unique thrombin-site engineered between the His$_5$ segment and the protein-A domain. A schematic map of the pIg20 expression vector is shown in Fig. 1.

Individual (or libraries of) antibody V$_H$ and V$_L$ domains can be inserted into the pIg20 vector at unique sites *(Xma*I and *Xba*I for V$_H$, *Bgl*II and *Nco*I for V$_L$), after they are polymerase chain reaction (PCR)-amplified with oligonucleotides that encode for these restriction sites.

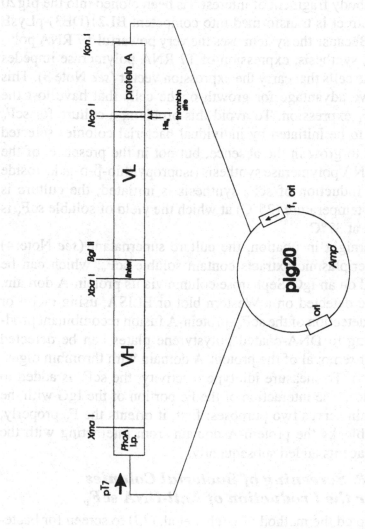

Fig. 1. A schematic map of the pIg20 scF$_v$ expression vector is shown. For a detailed description, *see* Section 1.1.

1.2. Production, Purification, and Detection of Anti-DNA scF$_v$

Once the antibody fragment of interest has been cloned into the pIg20 vector, the construct is transformed into competent BL21(DE3)-pLysE bacterial cells. Because the system uses the very powerful T7 RNA polymerase for scF$_v$ synthesis, expression of T7 RNA polymerase impedes the growth of the cells that carry the expression vector (*see* Note 3). This offers a selective advantage for growth of the cells that have lost the plasmid for scF$_v$ expression. To avoid this problem, a culture for scF$_v$ production has to be initiated by individual bacterial colonies selected for their ability to grow in the absence, but not in the presence, of the inducer of T7 RNA polymerase synthesis (isopropylthio-β-D-galactoside [IPTG]). After induction of scF$_v$ synthesis is initiated, the culture is placed at lower temperature (25°C) at which the yield of soluble scF$_v$ is higher than it is at 37°C.

After an overnight incubation, the culture supernatant (*see* Note 4) and bacterial periplasmic extracts contain soluble scF$_v$, which can be directly purified on an IgG-Sepharose column via its protein-A domain. The scF$_v$ can be detected on a Western blot or ELISA, using rabbit or human IgG for detection of the scF$_v$–protein-A fusion recombinant product *(10)*. Binding to DNA-coated polystyrene plates can be detected directly, or after removal of the protein-A domain with thrombin digestion (*see* Note 5). To measure idiotype reactivity, the scF$_v$ is added to IgG-coated plates. The interaction of the Fc portion of the IgG with the protein-A domain serves two purposes: first, it orients the F$_v$ properly, and second, it blocks the protein-A domain from interacting with the anti-idiotype reagents added subsequently.

1.3. Screening of Bacterial Colonies for the Production of Anti-DNA scF$_v$

We have adapted the method of Dreher et al. *(13)* to screen for bacterial colonies that produce anti-DNA scF$_v$. In this very sensitive technique, bacterial colonies are grown on a low-protein-binding filter (Durapore) on top of a nitrocellulose filter that is coated with rabbit IgG. The two-filter sandwich is then cultured at room temperature on top of a fresh agar plate for scF$_v$ synthesis. This arrangement allows the bacterial cells to produce and secrete soluble scF$_v$ (fused to the protein-A domain), which, after it passes through the low-protein-binding filter, is captured

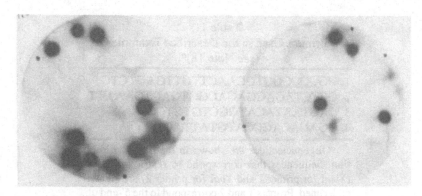

Fig. 2. Autoradiogram showing the screening of bacterial colonies that were able to bind to brominated d(G-C)$_n$, which was [^{32}P]-labeled *(10)*. Brominated d(G-C)$_n$ adopts the Z-DNA left-handed conformation in physiological conditions.

on the IgG-coated nitrocellulose filter. To detect anti-DNA scF$_v$, the nitrocellulose filter is removed and incubated with the radiolabeled nucleic acid of interest in the presence of a large excess of irrelevant nucleic acid. Autoradiography identifies the positive bacterial clones. We have applied this sensitive technique to detect bacterial colonies that produce anti-Z-DNA scF$_v$ (Fig. 2).

1.4. Mutagenesis and Segment Swapping

Once an anti-DNA scF$_v$ of interest has been cloned in the pIg20 vector, its primary sequence can be modified to study structure–function relationships. For site-directed mutagenesis and segment swapping we have used the PCR-based overlap extension method *(14)*. For each mutation (or set of mutations), two complementary mutagenic oligonucleotides (sense and antisense) are made that encode the designed replacements. In addition, one needs the two primers that were used for the insertion of the V domain in the pIg20 vector.

Initially, two different PCRs are done. In both reactions, the V domain serves as template. The antisense mutagenic oligonucleotide serves as a downstream primer in a PCR with the upstream primer corresponding to the 5'-end of the V domain. In a separate PCR, the sense mutagenic oligonucleotide is the upstream primer, whereas the downstream primer is complementary to the 3'-end of the V domain. The products of the two reactions have overlapping ends, which correspond to the sequence of the mutagenic oligonucleotides. After the products are purified by elu-

Table 1
Primers Used in the Described Example
(*see* Note 18)[a]

1. GG<u>CCCGGG</u>TGCAACTTGTTGAGTCTG
2. GC<u>TCTAGA</u>GGAGACGGTGACTGAAATT
3. CAGTAATACATGGCTGTGTCC
4. GGACACAGCCATGTATTACTG

[a]Oligonucleotides are shown in the 5' to 3' direction. Sequences that correspond to restriction sites
(*Xma*I for primer 1 and *Xba*I for primer 2) are shown
underlined. Primers 1 and 2 correspond to the 5'-end of
Z22 V_H and 3'-end of Z22 J_H, respectively. Primers 3
and 4 are complementary to each other, and correspond
to an FR3 sequence common to Z22 and Z3-3 V_H.

tion from an agarose electrophoresis gel, they are mixed, heated, and
allowed to anneal at their complementary region. This annealed product
serves as a template in a final PCR, where it is amplified using the primers complementary to the ends of the V domain, and can then be cloned
directly in the pIg20 vector. If two different V domains are used to
generate the products of the first two PCRs, then the annealed product,
which will be amplified in the final PCR, will be a chimera. In this
way, segment swapping and complementarity determining region
(CDR) grafting can be performed easily. The method is fast, efficient,
and does not require the presence of any restriction sites in the sequence
to be mutated.

2. Materials

2.1. PCR Amplification of H- and L-Chain V Domains

1. *Taq* polymerase (5 U/μL).
2. DNA, plasmid, or cDNA, with the template of interest.
3. Primer oligonucleotide solutions (as an example, *see* primers 1 and
   2, Table 1, for the V_H amplification of the mouse anti-Z-DNA MAb Z22):
   6 μ*M*.
4. 10X *Taq* polymerase buffer: 0.5*M* KCl, 100 m*M* Tris-HCl, pH 9.0, 15 m*M*
   MgCl$_2$, 1% Triton X-100.
5. dNTP's solution: 1.25 m*M* of dATP, dGTP, dTTP, and dCTP.
6. Mineral oil.
7. Sterile distilled water.
8. Thermo-cycling instrument.

2.2. Cloning into the pIg20 Vector

1. pIg20 plasmid DNA.
2. Restriction enzymes (5–10 U/μL): *Xma*I and *Xba*I for cloning the V$_H$ domain, *Bgl*II and *Nco*I for the V$_L$ domain.
3. 10X Restriction enzyme buffer: 20 m*M* Tris-acetate, 10 m*M* magnesium-acetate, 50 m*M* potassium-acetate, 1 m*M* DTT, pH 7.9.
4. Phenol/chloroform/isoamyl alcohol (25:24:1). Phenol is saturated with 100 m*M* Tris-HCl, pH 8.0.
5. Chloroform/isoamyl alcohol (24:1).
6. Absolute ethanol at –20°C.
7. 10*M* ammonium acetate.
8. 70% ethanol at –20°C.
9. 1% Agarose gel TAE buffer (40 m*M* Tris-acetate, 1 m*M* EDTA).
10. GeneClean DNA purification kit (Bio101, La Jolla, CA).
11. TE Buffer: 10 m*M* Tris-HCl, pH 8.0, and 1 m*M* EDTA.
12. T4 DNA ligase (5 U/μL).
13. 5X T4 DNA ligase buffer: 250 m*M* Tris-HCl, pH 7.6, 50 m*M* MgCl$_2$, 5 m*M* ATP, 5 m*M* DTT, 25% (w/v) polyethylene glycol-8000.
14. *E. coli* competent cells (*see* Note 6).
15. LB media: 10 g/L bacto-peptone, 5 g/L bacto-yeast extract, 10 g/L NaCl, pH 7.0.
16. Ampicillin: 50 mg/mL.
17. LB agar plates supplied with 100 μg/mL ampicillin.
18. Plasmid DNA purification kit (Promega, Madison, WI).
19. DNA sequencing kit with Sequenase® (US Biochemicals, Cleveland, OH).
20. Microcentrifuge.
21. Incubator or water bath.
22. Sterile distilled water.

2.3. Expression and Purification of Anti-DNA scF$_v$

1. Competent *E. coli* BL21(DE3)-pLysE cells.
2. LB media: 10 g/L bacto-peptone, 5 g/L bacto-yeast extract, 10 g/L NaCl, pH 7.0.
3. Ampicillin: 50 mg/mL.
4. Chloramphenicol: 20 mg/mL in ethanol.
5. LB agar plates supplied with 200 μg/mL ampicillin and 20 μg/mL chloramphenicol.
6. Isopropyl-β-D-thiogalactopyranoside (IPTG): 1*M*.
7. TES buffer: 0.2*M* Tris-HCl, pH 8.0, 0.5 m*M* EDTA, 0.5*M* sucrose.
8. IgG-Sepharose beads (Pharmacia, Piscataway, NJ).

9. TBST buffer: 50 m*M* Tris-HCl, pH 7.6, 150 m*M* NaCl, 0.05% Tween-20.
10. HAc buffer: 0.5*M* acetic acid adjusted to pH 5.0 with ammonium acetate.
11. 5 m*M* Ammonium acetate, pH 5.0.
12. Elution buffer: 0.1*M* acetic acid adjusted to pH 3.4 with ammonium acetate.
13. Ammonium carbonate solution: 1.5*M*.
14. Centrifuge.
15. Sterile distilled water.

2.4. Screening Bacterial Colonies for Anti-DNA scF$_v$ Expression

1. Durapore filters (Millipore, Bedford, MA).
2. Nitrocellulose filters (Schleicher and Schuell, Keene, NH).
3. LB media: 10 g/L bacto-peptone, 5 g/L bacto-yeast extract, 10 g/L NaCl, pH 7.0.
4. Ampicillin: 50 mg/mL.
5. Chloramphenicol: 20 mg/mL in ethanol.
6. LB agar plates supplied with 200 μg/mL ampicillin and 20 μg/mL chloramphenicol.
7. IPTG: 1*M*.
8. PBS buffer: 8 g/L NaCl, 0.2 g/L KCl, 1.44 g/L Na_2HPO_4, 0.24 g/L KH_2PO_4, pH 7.4.
9. Rabbit γ-globulin solution: 0.1 mg/mL in PBS.
10. Binding buffer: 25 m*M* HEPES, pH 7.9, 3 m*M* $MgCl_2$, 4 m*M* KCl, 0.25% nonfat milk.
11. Tween-20.
12. Salmon sperm DNA.
13. Blocking buffer: 5% nonfat milk and 0.1% Tween-20 in PBS.
14. Target DNA radiolabeled with [^{32}P] by any of the commonly used methods *(15)*.
15. Exposure cassette and film for autoradiography.

3. Methods
3.1. PCR Amplification of Antibody V Domains

1. To prepare a 100-μL PCR reaction, add the following components to a sterile 0.5-mL polypropylene tube in the described order: 53 μL of sterile distilled water, 10 μL of the 10X *Taq* polymerase buffer, 16 μL of dNTP's solution, 10 μL of each primer solution, 0.5 μL of DNA template solution (*see* Note 7), 0.5 μL of *Taq* polymerase.
2. Overlay on top of the solution 50 μL of mineral oil.
3. Place the reaction tube(s) in the thermo-cycling instrument.

4. Program the instrument for 25 cycles with the following segments per cycle: 1 min at 94°C, 2 min at 52°C (*see* Note 8), 1 min at 72°C.

3.2. Cloning Antibody V Domains into the pIg20 Expression Vector

1. To determine whether the PCR was successful, a small sample (5 μL) of each reaction can be analyzed using standard agarose gel electrophoresis techniques *(15)*.
2. Transfer the remainder of the PCR reaction (avoiding the mineral oil on the surface) to a clean polypropylene tube, and add to it 200 μL of sterile distilled water.
3. Add an equal volume of chloroform/isoamyl alcohol solution, vortex for 1 min, and spin it in a microcentrifuge for 2 min.
4. Transfer the aqueous phase to a clean tube, and add an equal volume of phenol/chloroform/isoamyl alcohol. Vortex the sample for 1 min, and spin it in a microcentrifuge for 2 min.
5. Transfer the aqueous phase to a clean tube, and repeat step 3.
6. Transfer the aqueous phase to a clean tube, add 2 vol of absolute ethanol, and 0.2 vol of 10*M* ammonium acetate. Vortex the sample and spin it in a microcentrifuge at 4°C for 30 min. Discard the supernatant, wash the precipitate with 70% ethanol, and let the pellet dry.
7. Resuspend the pellet in 16 μL of sterile distilled water, add 2 μL of 10X restriction enzyme buffer, and 1 μL of each of the two restriction enzymes (*Xma*I and *Xba*I for cloning the V$_H$ domain, *Bgl*II and *Nco*I for the V$_L$ domain). Incubate at 37°C overnight.
8. In a separate tube, under identical conditions, digest the pIg20 plasmid DNA (2–3 μg) with the same enzymes that were used to digest the V-domain PCR product.
9. Separate the digestion products by electrophoresis on an agarose gel (1% agarose in TAE buffer) under standard conditions *(15)*.
10. Gel-purify separately the bands of the vector and PCR insert using the GeneClean kit, according to the manufacturer's instructions. At the final step, elute the DNA in 15 μL total volume of TE buffer.
11. Set up ligation reactions. In a polypropylene tube, add 6 μL insert DNA, 1 μL vector DNA, 2 μL 5X T4 DNA ligase buffer, and 1 μL T4 DNA ligase. As a negative control set up a ligation reaction in the same way as above, except that sterile distilled water is substituted for insert DNA (*see* Note 9). Incubate overnight at 10°C.
12. Transform competent *E. coli* with the ligation reactions (*see* Note 10). Aliquot 50 μL of competent cells for each transformation to a 15-mL polypropylene tube, and immediately add 1 μL of the ligation reaction.

Mix by pipeting several times, and leave on ice for 25 min. Heat-shock at 42°C for 45 s, and store on ice for 2 min. Add 0.3 mL of LB media and incubate at 37°C on a shaker for 45 min. Plate 100 μL on an LB agar plate that contains 100 μg/mL ampicillin (*see* Note 11). Incubate overnight at 37°C.

13. Pick individual colonies for growth in 3 mL of LB media (supplied with 100 μg/mL ampicillin). Culture on a shaker overnight at 37°C.
14. Extract plasmid DNA, using the plasmid DNA purification kit according to the manufacturer's instructions.
15. Sequence the individual clones to verify the presence and integrity of the V domain in the pIg20 expression vector, using the DNA sequencing kit according to the manufacturer's instructions.

3.3. Expression and Purification of Anti-DNA scF$_v$

1. Transform competent BL21(DE3)-pLysE cells with the pIg20 vector, which contains the anti-DNA scF$_v$ of interest (*see* Note 12).
2. Transfer the bacterial colonies with sterile toothpicks on two replica LB agar plates (supplied with 200 μg/mL ampicillin and 20 μg/mL chloramphenicol). One of the two replica plates includes 0.5 m*M* IPTG. Incubate at 37°C overnight.
3. Identify colonies that grew in the absence, but not in the presence, of IPTG (*see* Note 13).
4. Transfer a few IPTG-sensitive colonies in a 3-L flask that contains 0.5 L of LB media supplied with 20 μg/mL ampicillin and 20 μg/mL chloramphenicol (*see* Note 14). Incubate at 37°C, with shaking, until a density with A_{550} of 0.6 has been reached.
5. Add IPTG to 0.5 m*M* final concentration. Incubate overnight at 25°C, with shaking (*see* Note 15).
6. Transfer the culture to 250-mL bottles, and centrifuge at 5,000*g* for 20 min.
7. Collect the supernatant. Resuspend the bacterial pellet in 10 mL ice-cold TES buffer/1 L of culture. In a separate tube, which can withstand high centrifugal forces, add 12 mL of ice-cold sterile distilled water, 4 mL ice-cold TES buffer, and the resuspended bacterial pellet. Mix and leave on ice for 30 min.
8. Spin the suspension for 10 min at 15,000*g* and collect the supernatant, which contains the soluble periplasmic bacterial extract (*see* Note 16).
9. Mix the culture media and soluble periplasmic extracts, and filter through a 0.2-μm low-protein-binding filter to remove any debris that may be present.
10. Transfer 2 mL of IgG-Sepharose into a 1.5 × 10 cm column. Pack the resin by washing it extensively with TBST buffer.

11. Equilibrate the column with 2 bed volumes each of: HAc, TBST, HAc, TBST.
12. Prior to applying the sample for purification, the pH of the eluate should be neutral. Apply directly the media-periplasmic extract sample. The purification should be done at 4°C, and the flow rate should not exceed 0.5 mL/min.
13. Wash with 10 bed volumes of TBST. Then add 2 bed volumes of NH_4Ac buffer. Elute with elution buffer. Collect 1.5-mL fractions and neutralize with 200 µL ammonium carbonate solution.
14. Measure the A_{280} of the fractions, and identify the ones that contain protein. The eluted material can be analyzed by SDS-PAGE and tested for DNA binding with common techniques, such as ELISA. Western blotting can be performed using IgG to detect the scF_v–protein-A recombinant protein *(10)*.

3.4. Screening Bacterial Colonies for Anti-DNA scF_v Expression

1. Transform BL21(DE3)-pLysE cells with a library of anti-DNA scF_vs cloned in the pIg20 vector, as in Section 3.3., step 1.
2. With sterile toothpicks, transfer individual colonies on replica LB agar plates (supplied with 200 µg/mL ampicillin and 20 µg/mL chloramphenicol), and incubate at 37°C overnight.
3. Incubate a nitrocellulose filter (the size of the agar plate) with the rabbit γ-globulin solution at room temperature for 2 h. Then incubate with IPTG (0.5 m*M* in PBS) at room temperature for 2 h.
4. Place the nitrocellulose filter on top of an LB agar plate (supplied with 200 µg/mL ampicillin, 20 µg/mL chloramphenicol, and 0.5 m*M* IPTG). Air bubbles between the filter and the plate should be avoided.
5. Place the Durapore filter on top of one of the replica plates with the bacterial colonies. After 20 min, lift the Durapore filter and place it on top of the nitrocellulose filter (which in turn is on top of the agar plate), with the bacterial colonies facing up. Invert the plate and incubate at room temperature overnight.
6. Remove the nitrocellulose filter and incubate it with the blocking solution for 2 h at room temperature.
7. Transfer the nitrocellulose filter in binding buffer, which also contains 0.1% Tween-20, 10 µg/mL irrelevant nucleic acid, and 50 ng/mL of the ^{32}P-labeled nucleic acid of interest. Incubate on a shaker overnight at 4°C.
8. Wash the nitrocellulose filter several times in binding buffer. Place it on a filter paper and cover with a plastic sheet. Perform autoradiography under standard conditions *(15)*. Positive colonies can be picked and grown from the additional replica plate prepared in step 2 *(see also* Note 17).

3.5. Mutagenesis and/or Segment Swapping

1. Perform the first PCRs as in Section 3.1. (*see* Table 1, and Note 18 for primers and templates used).
2. Load 25 µL of the PCR reactions on an agarose gel (1% agarose in TAE). Perform gel electrophoresis and ethidium bromide staining under standard conditions (*15*).
3. Using a micropipetor, remove 3 µL of agarose gel containing the PCR products of correct size. These agarose pieces are placed directly in a 0.5-mL polypropylene tube that contains the following: 47.5 µL sterile distilled water, 10 µL 10X *Taq* polymerase buffer, 16 µL of dNTP's solution, 10 µL of each primer solution (primers 1 and 2, Table 1), and 0.5 µL of *Taq* polymerase (*see* Note 19).
4. Perform the PCR amplification and cloning of the product as in Sections 3.1. and 3.2., respectively.

4. Notes

1. Use of the secretion signal increases the likelihood of obtaining soluble product, since most of the scF$_v$ that remains in the cytoplasm usually forms insoluble aggregates.
2. The protein-A domain may also increase the total yield of soluble scF$_v$ by increasing its solubility and/or stability.
3. The growth of the cells is inhibited because T7 RNA polymerase depletes the nucleotide pool. Even a very low amount of T7 RNA polymerase, produced by the basal activity of the *lac*UV5 promoter, is enough to provide a growth disadvantage. This problem is solved to some extent by the presence of an additional plasmid in the cells, pLysE. This plasmid drives the expression of T7 lysozyme, which binds and inactivates the constitutively expressed T7 RNA polymerase. This inhibition is overcome once the inducer is added and scF$_v$ synthesis begins. For additional information, *see* Studier et al. (*11*).
4. The secretion leader peptide targets the scF$_v$ to the periplasm and not to the medium. However, most of the secreted recombinant protein is found in the medium, possibly because of cell lysis. Continuous shaking of BL21 cultures in rich medium can result in cell lysis.
5. An effective thrombin can be purchased from Hematologic Technologies Inc. (Essex Junction, VT). Digestion is performed according to the manufacturer's instructions.
6. *E. coli* cells can be made competent by any of the commonly used methods (*15*).
7. If the V domain of interest is already cloned in a plasmid, then the amount of DNA template in 0.5 µL of plasmid miniprep is more than enough for

the PCR reaction. However, if for any reason it is thought that the amount of template is not enough, one can add more template and adjust accordingly the amount of distilled water. One should also prepare a separate reaction in the same way, but without any template DNA present. This negative control will ensure that the obtained product is not the result of contamination.

8. We routinely use 5–10°C below the melting point of the primer–template duplex as the annealing temperature.

9. This is a control for the restriction enzyme digestion. The vector DNA should not re-ligate to itself, since it was digested with two different restriction enzymes, resulting in no bacterial colonies on transformation. However, if the digestion with the two enzymes was not complete, then single-cut vector DNA will be present. If the separation of single-cut and double-cut vector DNA molecules on the agarose gel is not sufficient, they will be copurified. Then the single-cut DNA will re-ligate to itself, resulting in background colonies on transformation. The background will be very high, since the efficiency of the re-ligation of single-cut vector DNA is much higher than the ligation of double-cut vector DNA with insert (unimolecular vs bimolecular reaction).

10. To avoid problems that may arise from loss of the plasmid in *E. coli* BL21(DE3)-pLysE (*see* Section 1.2.), all the plasmid manipulations should take place in a different strain, such as the commonly used DH5α, JM109, or HB101. Once the cloning into the pIg20 vector has been completed, then the new construct can be transferred in *E. coli* BL21(DE3)-pLysE for scF$_v$ expression. In addition to transforming bacteria with the ligation reactions, supercoiled plasmid DNA should also be used in a separate transformation, as a control for the transformation efficiency.

11. The pIg20 vector carries ampicillin resistance.

12. Perform the transformation as in Section 3.2., step 12. The pLysE plasmid (already present in the cells) carries chloramphenicol resistance. Therefore, transformants are selected on LB agar plates supplied with 200 μg/mL ampicillin (for pIg20 selection) and 20 μg/mL chloramphenicol (for pLysE selection).

13. Growth should be completely inhibited on the plate that contains IPTG. If only partially IPTG-sensitive colonies are obtained, then these colonies should be streaked on a fresh LB agar plate (supplied with 200 μg/mL ampicillin and 20 μg/mL chloramphenicol). From these partially IPTG-sensitive colonies, the IPTG-sensitivity test should be repeated until completely sensitive clones are isolated.

14. Growth of BL21(DE3)-pLysE cells, carrying the pIg20 vector, in liquid media can be performed in the presence of 20 μg/mL ampicillin, instead of

the 200 µg/mL that are used for growth on agar plates. An increase to 200 µg/mL does not offer any significant advantage in inhibiting cells that do not carry the plasmid to overgrow the culture. Even a relatively small amount of pIg20-carrying cells secrete enough β-lactamase into the medium, which in turn overcomes the effect of high amounts of ampicillin to cells that do not carry the plasmid. Therefore, it is essential that the culture is started with completely IPTG-sensitive colonies.

15. During this incubation period, when anti-DNA scF$_v$ synthesis is induced, there is only minimal growth of the culture, since only IPTG-sensitive cells should be present.

16. Samples from total cell lysates, culture media, and periplasmic extracts can be analyzed by standard techniques, such as SDS-PAGE, for scF$_v$ production *(15)*.

17. Plasmid DNA from the colonies of interest should be prepared immediately to avoid loss of the plasmid owing to the reasons explained in Section 1.2.

18. As an example, we describe the graft of the CDR3/framework region (FR)4 region of the V$_H$ of Z22 MAb onto the V$_H$ segment of Z3-3, another V$_H$10-encoded V$_H$ cDNA *(16)*. In the first reaction, primers 1 and 3 were used with Z3-3 V$_H$ cDNA as a template, whereas in the second reaction, primers 4 and 2 were used with Z22 V$_H$ cDNA as a template (Table 1).

19. The agarose pieces contain the PCR products that will form the template for this PCR reaction. The primers in this PCR correspond to the 5'- and 3'-ends of the V$_H$ domain, and they will amplify only the annealed product of the first two PCRs.

Acknowledgment

This research was supported by grant GM32375 from the National Institute of General Medical Sciences, NIH.

References

1. Weinstein, A., Bordwell, B., Stone, B., Tibbetts, C., and Rothfield, N. F. (1983) Antibodies to native DNA and serum complement (C3) levels. *Am. J. Med.* **74,** 206–216.

2. Stollar, B. D. (1991) Autoantibodies and autoantigens: a conserved system that may shape a primary immunoglobulin gene pool. *Mol. Immunol.* **28,** 1399–1412.

3. Shefner, R., Kleiner, G., Turken, A., Papazian, L., and Diamond, B. (1991) A novel class of anti-DNA antibodies identified in BALB/c mice. *J. Exp. Med.* **173,** 287–296.

4. Schwartz, R. S. and Stollar, B. D. (1994) Heavy-chain directed B-cell maturation: continuous clonal selection beginning at the pre-B cell stage. *Immunol. Today* **15,** 27–32.

5. Stollar, B. D. (1989) Immunochemistry of DNA. *Intern. Rev. Immunol.* **5,** 1–22.

6. Brigido, M. M. and Stollar, B. D. (1991) Two induced anti-Z-DNA monoclonal antibodies use V$_H$ gene segments related to those of anti-DNA autoantibodies. *J. Immunol.* **146,** 2005–2009.

7. Krishnan, M. R. and Marion, T. N. (1993) Structural similarity of antibody variable regions from immune and autoimmune anti-DNA antibodies. *J. Immunol.* **150,** 4948–4957.

8. Barry, M. M., Mol, C. D., Anderson, W. F., and Lee, J. S. (1994) Sequencing and modeling of anti-DNA immunoglobulin F$_v$ domains. Comparison with crystal structures. *J. Biol. Chem.* **269,** 3623–3632.

9. Stollar, B. D. (1994) Molecular analysis of anti-DNA antibodies. *FASEB J.* **8,** 337–342.

10. Brigido, M. M., Polymenis, M., and Stollar, B. D. (1993) Role of mouse V$_H$10 and V$_L$ gene segments in the specific binding of antibody to Z-DNA, analyzed with recombinant single chain F$_v$ molecules. *J. Immunol.* **150,** 469–479.

11. Studier, F. W., Rosenberg, A. H., Dunn, J. J., and Dubendorff, J. W. (1990) Use of T7 RNA polymerase to direct expression of cloned genes. *Methods Enzymol.* **185,** 60–89.

12. Huston, J. S., Levinson, D., Mudgett-Hunter, M., Tai, M.-S., Novotny, J., Margolies, M. N., Ridge, R. J., Bruccoleri, R. E., Haber, E., Crea, R., and Oppermann, H. (1988) Protein engineering of antibody binding sites: recovery of specific activity in an anti-digoxin single-chain F$_v$ analogue produced in *Escherichia coli. Proc. Natl. Acad. Sci. USA* **85,** 5879–5883.

13. Dreher, M. L., Gherardi, E., Skerra, A., and Milstein, C. (1991) Colony assays for antibody fragments expressed in bacteria. *J. Immunol. Methods* **139,** 197.

14. Ho, S. N., Hunt, H. D., Horton, R. M., Pullen, J. K., and Pease, L. R. (1989) Site-directed mutagenesis by overlap extension using the polymerase chain reaction. *Gene* **77,** 51–59.

15. Sambrook, J., Fritsch, E. F., and Maniatis, T. (1989) *Molecular Cloning: A Laboratory Manual,* Cold Spring Harbor Laboratory, Cold Spring Harbor, NY.

16. Polymenis, M. and Stollar, B. D. (1994) Critical binding site amino acids of anti-Z-DNA single chain F$_v$ molecules. Role of heavy and light chain CDR3 and relationship to autoantibody activity. *J. Immunol.* **152,** 5318–5329.

CHAPTER 19

Molecular Cloning of Antiground-State Proteolytic Antibody Fragments

Qing-Sheng Gao and Sudhir Paul

1. Introduction

The variable regions of antibody subunits are the "business ends" of these molecules responsible for interactions with antigens and activation of the biological functions of the constant regions. Rearrangement of variable-, diversity-, and joining-region genes and the hypermutability of the complementarity determining regions (CDRs) permit development of new antigen-binding specificities. With the discovery of natural catalytic activity in autoantibodies (1–3) and the confirmation of this phenomenon (4,5), it has become clear that hypervariability in antibody genes may permit a natural evolution of enzyme-like sites in antibodies. Additional evidence for this hypothesis consists of observations that monoclonal antibodies (MAb) to a natural antigen, vasoactive intestinal polypeptide (VIP), display proteolytic activity (6,7). As the first step toward establishing the physicochemical basis of the catalytic activity, we have cloned and expressed the light (L)-chain subunit and single-chain F_v (scF_v) fragment of one such antibody. The recombinant L chain and the scF_v display interactions with VIP typical of an antibody-combining site. Both molecules are efficient catalysts (8). The distinctive feature of catalytic hydrolysis of VIP by these recombinant proteins is high-affinity substrate binding (low K_m), a property not shared by conventional enzymes. The L chain also catalyzes the hydrolysis of a protease substrate unrelated in sequence to VIP, but this activity appears to be the result of low affinity recognition of basic residues (8). By primary structure analyses, molecular modeling, and kinetic examination of the

From: *Methods in Molecular Biology, Vol. 51: Antibody Engineering Protocols*
Edited by: S. Paul Humana Press Inc., Totowa, NJ

catalytic activities, it appears that the residues in the antibody active site providing important contributions in the binding and hydrolysis steps may be different. Site-directed mutagenesis of the recombinant protein active sites is ongoing to validate this hypothesis.

The L chain and scF$_v$ were cloned in a phagemid vector pCANTAB5*his$_6$* described by McCafferty et al. *(9)*. The vector contains a gene3/*pel*B signal peptide sequence facilitating transport of recombinant proteins into the periplasm (Fig. 1). The recombinant proteins are expressed at reasonably high levels (0.5–10 mg/L). A 10-residue c-*myc* tag permits detection of the proteins by immunoblotting and a hexahistidine tag at the C-terminus permits rapid metal-affinity chromatography. The proteins can be expressed in soluble form in *E. coli* HB2151 or on the surface of phage particles as a fusion protein in *E. coli* TG1 cells. Expression of the recombinant proteins is under control of the *lacZ* promoter and is induced by IPTG. The insert cDNA is introduced into the vector using *Sfi*I and *Not*I restriction sites.

2. Materials (*see* Note 1)

2.1. RNA and cDNA Preparation

Buffers are prepared in "Milli-Q" water. RNA preparation should be done with buffers made from diethylpyrocarbonate (DEPC)-treated water. Gloves should be worn to prevent RNase contamination.

1. RNA extraction buffer: 4M guanidine thiocyanate, 25 mM sodium citrate, pH 7.0, 0.5% N-lauroylsarcosine. This solution is stable and can be stored indefinitely at room temperature. Just before use, add 0.1M β-mercaptoethanol.
2. DEPC-treated water: Add 0.1 mL of DEPC to 100 mL water. Shake vigorously to dissolve DEPC. Incubate the solution at 37°C for at least 12 h and then autoclave for 15 min at 15 lb/in^2 to inactivate remaining DEPC.
3. TE buffer: 10 mM Tris-HCl, pH 8.0, 1 mM EDTA.
4. Phenol saturated with TE buffer.
5. Chloroform/isoamyl alcohol: 24:1 (v/v) mixture.
6. 3M sodium acetate, pH 5.2: Dissolve 408 g sodium acetate 3H$_2$O and adjust pH to 5.2 with acetic acid. Make up to 1 L.
7. Absolute ethanol stored at –20°C.
8. 75% ethanol prepared in DEPC-treated water.
9. Isopropanol.
10. Oligonucleotide primers: 50 µM in TE buffer (*see* Table 1).
11. 25 U/µL Moloney murine leukemia virus (M-MuLV) reverse transcriptase and 10X reverse transcriptase buffer (500 mM Tris-HCl, pH

```
pUC119 - GTG AAA AAA TTA TTA TTC GCA ATT CCT TTA GTT GTT CCT TTC TAT GCG GCC CAG CtCG GCC ATG GCC CAG GTC CAA
                   signal peptide                                       SfiI      NcoI

CTG CAG GAG CTC GAG ATC AAA CGG GCtG GCC GCA cat cat cat cac cat cac ggg gcc gca gaa caa aaa ctc atc tca
 PstI       XhoI                 Not I             poly his                                         c-myc

gaa gag gat ctg aat ggg gcc gca tag - gene3
                                Amber
```

Fig. 1. Cloning region of phagemid vector pCANTAB5*his*$_6$.

Table 1
Oligonucleotide Primers for Anti-VIP (Clone c23.5) L-Chain and scF$_v$ cDNA
Amplification and Sequencing

V$_L$-Back

1	2	3	4	5	6	7

5' gtcctcgcaactgc<u>GGCCCAGC CGGCC</u>atggccGAY GTN GTN ATG ACN CAG AC
                 *Sfi*I

L-For

213	212	211	210	209	208	207	206

5' gagtcattct<u>GCGGCC GC</u> CTC ATT CCT GTT GAA GCT CTT GAC
            *Not*I

V$_H$-For

123	122	121	120	119	118	117	116

5' gagtcattct<u>GCGGCC GC</u> HGG ATA GAC LGA TGG GGQ TGT YGT
            *Not*I

Link-V$_L$-For

113	112	111	110	109	108	107

5' tcctttaccttcagacgatttcccagagccggaggtagaacc TGG TGC AGC ATC AGC CCG TTT
                    Linker

Link-V$_H$-Back

1	2	3	4	5	6	7	8

5' ggttctacctccggctctgggaaatcgtctgaaggtaaagga GAG GTG AAG CTG GTG GAR TCT GG
                    Linker

SEQBACK
5' CAGGAAACAGCTATGAC

fdSEQ1
5' GAATTTTCTGTATGAGG

Y: C/T, N: A/T/G/C, H: G/T, L: A/C/T, Q: G/C, R: A/G. Restriction recognition sequences are underlined with cleavage sites shown by gaps. Clamp sequences on the 5'-side of restriction sites facilitate digestion by enzymes. Nucleotides 28–33 in *V$_L$-Back* encode Met and Ala, which are required for signal peptidase cleavage of the recombinant proteins. Nucleotides shown in upper case at the 3'-termini of *Back* and *For* primers correspond to amino acid residues in L and H chains, indicated by position numbers above the codons (from the N-terminus). Linker sense and antisense sequences in *Link-V$_L$-Back* and *Link-V$_L$-For*, respectively, are in italics and correspond to a 14-residue flexible linker (Gly-Ser-Thr-Ser-Gly-Ser-Gly-Lys-Ser-Ser-Glu-Gly-Lys-Gly). SEQBACK and fdSEQ1 primers anneal to nucleotides 2206–2222 and 2404–2420, respectively, in pCANTAB5*his$_6$*.

8.3, 80 m*M* MgCl$_2$, 300 m*M* KCl, and 100 m*M* dithiothreitol; New England BioLabs).

12. 20–40 U/µL RNasin (Promega, Madison, WI).

13. GeneAmp PCR reagent kit (Perkin Elmer Cetus, Norwalk, CT) containing 5 U/µL Ampli*Taq* DNA polymerase, 10X PCR buffer (100 m*M* Tris-HCl, pH 8.3, 500 m*M* potassium chloride, 15 m*M* magnesium chloride, 0.01% gelatin), and 10 m*M* solutions of dATP, dGTP, dCTP, and dTTP.

14. TAE buffer: 40 mM Tris-acetate, pH 8.0, 1 mM EDTA. A 50X TAE stock solution can be prepared by mixing 242 g Tris base, 57.1 mL acetic acid, 100 mL 0.5M EDTA, and water to 1 L.
15. 1% agarose gel in TAE buffer containing 50 ng/mL ethidium bromide.
16. 6X agarose gel electrophoresis sample buffer: 40% (w/v) sucrose, 0.1% bromophenol blue and 0.1% xylene cyanol FF in water.
17. 100-bp DNA ladder (BRL, Gaithersburg, MD).
18. DNA Thermal Cycler (Perkin Elmer Cetus, 480).
19. GeneClean II DNA purification kit (Bio 101, La Jolla, CA).
20. UV transilluminator.
21. Spectrophotometer.
22. Heating blocks.
23. SpeedVac system (Savant, SC200, Farmingdale, NY).

2.2. cDNA Cloning and Insert Identification

1. Wizard Miniprep or Midiprep plasmid DNA purification kits (Promega).
2. 0.5 µg/µL pCANTAB5his_6 phagemid DNA in TE buffer (Cambridge Antibody Technology, Cambridgeshire, UK).
3. *E. coli* HB2151 K12Δ (lac-pro), ara. thi/F' proAB, *lac*I^q, *lac*Z ΔM15 (Cambridge Antibody Technology).
4. Restriction enzymes (10 U/µL): *Sfi*I with 10X NE buffer-2, *Not*I with 10X NE buffer-*Not*I (New England BioLabs, Beverly, MA).
5. GeneClean II DNA purification kit (Bio 101).
6. T4 DNA ligase (400 U/µL) and 10X reaction buffer (500 mM Tris-HCl, pH 7.8, 100 mM MgCl$_2$, 200 mM dithiothreitol 10 mM ATP, 500 µg/mL bovine serum albumin [BSA]; New England BioLabs, Beverly, MA).
7. Competent *E. coli* HB2151 cells for electroporation: Harvest 500 mL of the bacteria in midlog phase growth (OD$_{600}$ = 0.4–0.6; 1 OD$_{600}$ = 5 × 10^8 cells/mL) by centrifugation at 4000g for 15 min at 4°C. Wash the cells three times with 500 mL ice-cold 10% glycerol. Resuspend cells gently in 10% glycerol at a density of 3 × 10^{10} cells/mL. Freeze 100-µL aliquots on dry ice, and store at –80°C.
8. Gene pulser electroporator apparatus (Bio-Rad, Hercules, CA).
9. 100 mg/mL ampicillin in water: Filter-sterilize and store at –20°C.
10. SOC medium: 2% bacto-tryptone (Difco, Detroit, MI), 0.5% bacto-yeast extract (Difco), 10 mM sodium chloride, 2.5 mM potassium chloride, 10 mM magnesium chloride, 10 mM magnesium sulfate, and 10 mM glucose. Make up 20 g tryptone, 5 g yeast extract, and 0.5 g NaCl to 1 L with water, and autoclave. Add filter-sterilized 1M MgCl$_2$ (1 mL), 1M MgSO$_4$ (1 mL) and 20% glucose (5 mL) per 100 mL medium (after cooling).

11. 2YT medium: Mix 16 g bacto-tryptone (Difco), 10 g bacto-yeast extract (Difco), 5 g NaCl, and water to 1 L, and autoclave. When the medium cools, add ampicillin to 100 µg/mL and glucose to 2% w/v (glucose stock solution, 20% w/v) (*see* Note 1).

12. 2YT-induction medium: This is identical to the medium in step 11, with the exception that the glucose concentration is 0.1% w/v (*see* Note 1).

13. 2YT-ampicillin plates: Prepare and autoclave 1.5% bacto-agar (Difco) in 2 YT medium as in step 11. Cool to about 45°C, add ampicillin to 100 µg/mL and glucose to 2% w/v, and pour into Petri dishes.

14. Ampli*Taq* DNA polymerase and 10X PCR buffer.

15. Mineral oil.

16. Oligonucleotide primers: 50 µ*M* in TE buffer (*see* Table 1).

17. 1% agarose gel in TAE buffer.

18. Sequenase 2.0 DNA sequencing kit (US Biochemical, Cleveland, OH).

2.3. Recombinant Protein Expression, Identification, and Purification

1. 2YT medium and 2YT induction medium (*see* Section 2.2.).

2. 1*M* isopropylthio-β-D-galactoside (IPTG).

3. Lysis buffer: 1*M* sodium chloride, 10 m*M* sodium phosphate buffer, pH 7.2, 1 m*M* EDTA.

4. 96-well dot-blot apparatus (Bio-Rad).

5. Nitrocellulose membrane (0.2-µm Trans-Blot sheets, Bio-Rad).

6. Phosphate-buffered saline (PBS) pH, 7.4: 137 m*M* sodium chloride, 2.7 m*M* potassium chloride, 4.3 m*M* disodium hydrogen phosphate, 1.4 m*M* potassium dihydrogen phosphate.

7. 100 ng/mL human c-*myc* peptide 1 in PBS (Oncogene Science, Uniondale, NY).

8. Anti-c-*myc*: Ascites from murine 9E10 hybridoma (ATCC) diluted 1:500 in PBS containing 1% BSA.

9. Goat antimouse IgG (F$_c$-specific) conjugated to peroxidase (Sigma, St. Louis, MO) diluted 1:1000 in PBS 1% BSA.

10. Dot-blot blocking and wash solutions: PBS-5% BSA and PBS-1% BSA, respectively.

11. Substrate solution: Dissolve 3 mg 3,3'-diaminobenzidine (DAB) and 3 µL 30% hydrogen peroxide in 10 mL PBS. Prepare fresh.

12. UMAX Data Scanning System (UC630) equipped with Image 1.43a processing and analysis software (courtesy W Rasband, NIH Research Services Branch; e-mail, wayne@helix.nih.gov) and Adobe Photoshop.

13. Chelating-Sepharose Fast Flow gel and columns (Pharmacia, C 16/20 and C 10/20, Piscataway, NJ).

14. Ni^{2+} ion-charging solution: 0.2M nickel sulfate in water.
15. FPLC system (Pharmacia).
16. Buffer A: 50 mM Tris-HCl, pH 7.2, 0.025% Tween-20, 0.02% sodium azide.
17. Buffer B: 2M ammonium chloride in buffer A.
18. Buffer C: 50 mM sodium formate, 0.025% Tween-20, adjusted to pH 3.8 with formic acid.
19. Buffer E: 50 mM EDTA in buffer A.
20. Phast electrophoresis system (Pharmacia).
21. Phast SDS-polyacrymide gels (8–25%) and Phast isoelectric focusing gels (pH 3–9) (Pharmacia).

3. Methods

3.1. Total RNA Preparation from Hybridoma Cells (see Note 2)

1. Centrifuge about 1×10^7 cultured hybridoma cells for 10 min at 400g. Wash cells twice with PBS.
2. Lyse the cells in 1 mL of ice-cold RNA extraction buffer by pipeting up and down several times in a sterile microfuge tube on ice. Leave on ice for 10 min. Centrifuge at 16,000g at 4°C for 5 min.
3. To the supernatant from step 2, add 0.1 mL 3M sodium acetate, 1 mL TE-buffer saturated phenol, and 0.2 mL chloroform-isoamyl alcohol (24:1). Mix thoroughly by vortexing after addition of each reagent.
4. Incubate on ice for 5 min, and spin at 16,000g for 10 min at 4°C. Transfer the upper aqueous phase to a fresh tube. Avoid carryover material from the interphase (this contains proteins).
5. Extract the aqueous phase again as in steps 3 and 4, but without addition of sodium acetate in step 3.
6. Extract the aqueous phase with an equal volume of chloroform-isoamyl alcohol (24:1), and spin at 16,000g for 2 min at 4°C. Repeat this step if necessary until white interphase material between the aqueous and organic phases disappears.
7. Mix the aqueous phase from step 6 with an equal volume of isopropanol. Keep at –20°C for at least 1 h to precipitate total RNA.
8. Spin at 16,000g for 15 min at 4°C. Wash the resulting RNA pellets with 1 mL ice-cold 75% ethanol. Store the RNA at –80°C in 75% ethanol.
9. Just before use, spin down the RNA pellet at 16,000g for 10 min. Dry the pellet *in vacuo* (SpeedVac) for 5 min at room temperature. Dissolve RNA in 50 µL of DEPC-treated water.
10. Dilute 5 µL total RNA solution with 500 µL DEPC-treated water, and measure absorbance at 260 and 280 nm. The A_{260}/A_{280} ratio should be between 1.5 and 2. Calculate the total RNA concentration from the rela-

tionship: 1 A_{260} = 40 μg/mL RNA (1-cm path length). Typical yields are 50–150 μg of RNA/10^7 cells.

11. Electrophorese 5 μL of RNA preparation on a 1.4% agarose gel containing 50 ng/mL ethidium bromide. Good-quality RNA preparations are characterized by two sharp bands at 2.2 and 4.9 kb, corresponding to the 18S and 28S ribosomal RNA bands (*see* Note 2).

3.2. L-Chain cDNA Preparation (see Notes 3 and 4)

1. Mix 20–50 μg total RNA, 1 μg V_L-*For* primer, and DEPC-treated water to 20 μL in a 500-μL microfuge tube.
2. Incubate the tube at 70°C for 10 min, and place on ice.
3. Add 5 μL 10X reverse transcriptase buffer, 2.5 μL 10 m*M* dNTP mixture, 2 μL RNAsin, 25 U M-MuLV reverse transcriptase, and DEPC-treated water to 50 μL.
4. Incubate at 42°C for 1 h to permit synthesis of cDNA. Then heat at 95°C for 2 min. Store at –80°C if necessary.
5. Mix 5 μL RNA–cDNA mixture (from step 4), 5 μL 10X PCR buffer, 1 μL 10 m*M* dNTPs, 0.5 μg V_L-*For* primer, 0.5 μg V_L-*Back* primer, and add water to 50 μL in a 500-μL microfuge tube. Overlay the reaction mixture with 50 μL mineral oil.
6. Heat at 95°C for 5 min to melt duplexes.
7. Add 5 U Ampli*Taq* DNA polymerase. This "hot start" reduces mispriming.
8. Amplify cDNA by 25 PCR cycles. Each cycle consists of denaturation of DNA at 95°C 1 min, annealing at 62°C for 1 min, and extension at 72°C for 1 min (*see* Note 4).
9. Keep the reaction tube at 72°C for 10 min. Add 10 μL 6X agarose gel electrophoresis sample. Mix and spin briefly in a microfuge.
10. Electrophorese an aliquot of the colored liquid below the mineral oil on 1% agarose gel containing 50 ng/mL ethidium bromide. Use 100-bp DNA ladder for size comparison.
11. Using a UV transilluminator light, identify and cut the correct size band from the agarose gel. The size of the L-chain cDNA is 0.7 kb.
12. Use GeneClean DNA kit to purify the cDNA according to the protocol supplied by the manufacturer (Bio 101).

3.3. Preparation of Single-Chain F_v cDNA

3.3.1. Preparation of V_L and V_H cDNA (see Notes 3 and 4)

1. In two separate 500-μL microfuge tubes, mix 20–50 μg total RNA from step 11, Section 3.1. with 1 μg V_L-*For* primer or 1 μg V_H-*For* primer. Add DEPC-treated water to 20 μL.
2. Prepare reverse-transcribed V_L and V_H cDNA as in steps 2–4, Section 3.2.

3. Mix 5 µL RNA–cDNA mixture from step 2, 5 µL 10X PCR buffer, and 1 µL 10 mM dNTPs with 0.5 µg *Link-V_L-For* and 0.5 µg *L-Back* primers to prepare V_L cDNA or 0.5 µg *V_H-For* and 0.5 µg *Link-V_H-Back* primers to prepare V_H cDNA. Add water to 50 µL. Overlay with 50 µL mineral oil.
4. Heat at 95°C for 5 min to melt the RNA–cDNA duplex.
5. Add 5 U Ampli*Taq* DNA polymerase. Amplify cDNA by PCR 25 cycles (denaturation at 95°C for 1 min, annealing at 62°C for 1 min, extension at 72°C for 1 min; *see* Note 4).
6. Electrophorese and cut out PCR products on a 1% agarose gel as in steps 9–11, Section 3.2. The size of V_L-*Link* and *Link-V_H* fragments is about 0.4 kb each.
7. Use the GeneClean DNA purification kit to purify the cDNA according to the protocol supplied by the manufacturer (Bio 101).

3.3.2. Linkage by Overlap Extension and Amplification of scF_v cDNA (see Note 5)

1. Mix 50 ng each of V_L-*Link* and *Link-V_H* cDNA fragments (from step 7, Section 3.3.1.), 5 µL 10X PCR buffer, 1 µL 10 mM dNTPs, 0.5 µg V_L-*Back* primer, and 0.5 µg V_H-*For* primers. Add water to 50 µL. Overlay with 50 µL mineral oil.
2. Incubate the reaction mixture at 95°C for 5 min, and gradually change the temperature to 45°C over 15 min using the PCR thermocycler. Antisense and sense linker sequences in *Link-V_H* cDNA and V_L-*Link* cDNA will anneal in this step.
3. Add 5 U Ampli*Taq* DNA polymerase. Perform 25 PCR cycles (denaturation at 95°C for 1 min, annealing at 55°C for 1 min, extension at 72°C for 1 min). The product of this reaction is V_L-*Link-V_H* cDNA.
4. Incubate at 72°C for 10 min. Electrophorese to confirm production of scF_v cDNA, and purify the cDNA (~0.8 kb) as in steps 9–12, Section 3.2.

3.4. cDNA Cloning (see Notes 6 and 7)

1. Digest pCANTAB5*his_6* DNA, L-chain cDNA, and scF_v cDNA in separate reaction tubes with *Sfi*I (*see* Notes 6 and 7). In each case, mix 10 µL 10X NE buffer 2, 1–5 µg DNA, 100 U *Sfi*I, and add water to 100 µL in a 500-µL microfuge tube. Overlay with mineral oil, and incubate at 50°C overnight. Remove *Sfi*I using the GeneClean kit.
2. Mix *Sfi*I-digested DNA from step 1 with 10 µL 10X *Not*I-NE buffer and 50 U *Not*I. Add water to 100 µL. Incubate at 37°C for 5 h. Remove *Not*I using the GeneClean kit.
3. Ligate L-chain or scF_v cDNA into pCANTAB5*his_6* via *Sfi*I and *Not*I sites. Mix 4 µL 5X T4 ligase buffer, 50 ng *Sfi*I-*Not*I digested pCANTAB5*his_6*, 50 ng *Sfi*I-*Not*I digested cDNA fragments, 20 U T4 DNA ligase, and add

water to 20 µL. In a control reaction, mix all of the above solutions, except the *Sfi*I-*Not*I digested antibody cDNA (vector self-ligation control). Incubate at 15°C overnight. Purify the DNA using the Gene-Clean Kit, and add water to a final volume of 50 µL.

4. Infect *E. coli* HB2151 cells with the ligated DNA by electroporation. Mix 5 µL ligated DNA and 50 µL competent HB2151 cells (1.5×10^9 cells) in an ice-cold GenePulser cuvet (0.2 cm) on ice. Apply an electrical pulse (25 µF, 2.5 kV; pulse controller set to 200 Ω; this should yield a pulse with a time constant of 4.5–5 ms). Add 1 mL SOC medium immediately to the pulsed cells, and incubate at 37°C for 45 min.

5. Spread 200 µL transformed cell culture onto a 2YT-100 µg/mL ampicillin-2% glucose agar plate, and incubate at 30°C overnight. Single uncrowded colonies should be seen. Antibody cDNA reaction mixtures generally yield ten times more colonies than the vector self-ligation control reaction mixture.

3.5. cDNA Insert Identification by PCR (see Note 8)

1. Make 1 mL of a PCR-mix solution composed of 100 µL 10X PCR buffer containing 15 m*M* MgCl$_2$, 10 µL 10 m*M* dNTPs, 5 µg SEQBACK primer, and 5 µg fdSEQ primer. Add water to 1 ml. This mixture can be stored at –20°C for several months.

2. Add 5 U of *Taq* DNA polymerase to 100 µL PCR mix just before carrying out PCR. Transfer 15 µL of this mixture to each PCR tube.

3. Pick individual colonies from the plate in step 5, Section 3.4. with sterile tooth picks. Insert the toothpick end briefly into the PCR reaction mixture of step 2.

4. To grow the colonies in larger scale in liquid medium, insert each toothpick briefly into 0.5 mL 2YT-100 µg/mL ampicillin–2% glucose medium in 1.5-mL sterile microfuge tube. Cap tubes, and incubate at 37°C for 4 h. Store at 4°C until PCR screening is completed.

5. Layer PCR tubes from step 3 with 50 µL mineral oil, and carry out 25 PCR cycles each cycle: 95°C for 1 min, 40°C for 1 min, 72°C for 1 min.

6. Electrophorese in 1% agarose to identify amplified DNA. The L-chain cDNA insert yields a band at 0.9 kb, and the scF$_v$ cDNA insert, a band at 1 kb (*see* Note 8).

7. Grow up clones containing desired cDNA from the cultures in step 4 in 2YT-100 µg/mL ampicillin–2% glucose at 37°C overnight. Prepare stocks by mixing with an equal volume of 50% sterile glycerol and freeze at –80°C.

8. Purify phagemid DNA from selected clones using Wizard plasmid DNA miniprep kit.

9. Perform DNA sequencing of inserts according to the DNA sequenase kit manual (*see* Note 9). Primers used for insert identification (fdSEQ, and SEQBACK; *see* Table 1) can also be used for sequencing.

3.6. Periplasmic Extract Preparation (see Note 10)

1. Inoculate 5 mL of an overnight culture into 500 mL 2YT-100 µg/mL ampicillin–0.1% glucose in a 2-L flask, and grow at 37°C with rocking until OD_{600} reaches 0.8–0.9.
2. Add IPTG to a final concentration of 1 mM (from a 1M stock solution). Incubate at 30°C for 3 h with rocking.
3. Centrifuge at 4000g for 15 min.
4. Suspend the cell pellet in 15 mL of ice-cold lysate buffer. Mix well and incubate on ice for 15 min.
5. Centrifuge at 6000g for 15 min at 4°C to collect the supernatant (periplasmic extract). Filter the supernatant through a 0.45-µM nitrocellulose filter.
6. Dialyze periplasmic extract against buffer A (*see* Section 2.3.) at 4°C overnight, and store at –20°C.

3.7. Dot-Blots for c-myc Expression (see Note 11)

1. Soak a 0.22-µM nitrocellulose sheet in water, and then sandwich it securely in the 96-well dot-blot apparatus while still wet.
2. Transfer the samples into wells. Sample volumes from 10 to 500 µL can be used. It is advisable to keep sample and standard volumes identical in individual assays. Human c-*myc* peptide 1 is used as standard. The linear response range for the standard is 1–20 ng/well.
3. Apply vacuum to remove unadsorbed proteins. Then soak the nitrocellulose sheet in blocking buffer (5% BSA in PBS) for 1 h at room temperature with slow shaking.
4. Wash the sheet in wash buffer for 5 min, and then soak it in anti-c-*myc* antibody solution for 1 h at room temperature with shaking.
5. Wash the membrane three times in wash buffer (10 min each), and then soak it in peroxidase-conjugated goat antimouse IgG for 1 h at room temperature with shaking.
6. Wash twice in wash buffer (10 min each) and once in PBS. Develop color by soaking in DAB/hydrogen peroxide solution for 10 min.
7. Wrap the wet membrane with Saran Wrap, and estimate color intensities in individual wells using an image analyzer. Construct a standard curve using the data obtained with c-*myc* peptide standard (*x*-axis, log peptide concentration; *y*-axis, color intensity). Read unknown sample concentrations off the standard curve (*see* Note 11).

3.8. Immobilized Metal Chelating
Affinity Chromatography (see Notes 12 and 13)

Solutions used for chromatography are filtered on a 0.2-µm filter and degassed prior to use.

1. Pack 30 mL Chelating Sepharose Fast-Flow gel in C16/20 column, and charge with 60 mL of 0.2*M* nickel sulfate. Wash the column with 100 mL of water followed by 60 mL of buffer A (flow rate, 2 mL/min).
2. Remove any fine precipitates from the dialyzed periplasmic extract by filtration through a 0.22-μm filter.
3. Apply the sample (100 mL of periplasmic extract) to the column at 2 mL/min.
4. Wash the column with 60 mL of buffer B, 60 mL of buffer A, 60 mL of buffer C, and 120 mL of buffer A to remove weakly bound proteins.
5. Elute bound proteins with 60 mL of buffer E. The recombinant proteins elute in the later portion of the protein peak in buffer E identified by c-*myc* dot-blotting as in Section 3.7. (*see* Note 13).
6. Perform SDS-PAGE and silver staining to assess purity of the recombinant protein fractions (~28 kDa band). Western blotting of the gels can be done using anti-c-*myc* antibody or antimouse L-chain antibody to confirm the identity of the proteins.
7. Pool fractions containing the recombinant protein, and dialyze against excess buffer A at 4°C. Change buffer at least four times (every 6–12 h) to remove as much EDTA as possible.
8. Apply 50 mL of the dialyzed protein pool (total protein ~2.5 mg) to 8 mL chelating Sepharose packed in a C10/20 column at 1 mL/min flow rate (*see* Note 13).
9. Wash off weakly bound proteins with 25 mL buffer A, 25 mL of buffer B, 25 mL of buffer A, 25 mL of buffer C, and 50 mL of buffer A.
10. Elute recombinant protein with buffer E. Collect fractions and dialyze extensively against buffer A to remove EDTA.
11. Perform SDS-PAGE and IEF-PAGE to confirm purity. Both types of gels can be subjected to Western blotting as in step 6 to confirm protein identity (*see* Note 13).

3.9. Structure–Function Analysis

Molecular modeling can be done using AbM™ as described by Webster and Rees (Chapter 2) and solvent-accessible (and, thus, antigen-accessible) residues can be deduced for mutagenesis experiments (*see* Note 14). Binding and catalysis analyses can be studied using radioactive, fluorescent, or other probes. For demonstration of antibody catalysis, it is advisable to demonstrate constant specific activity following chromatography on columns that separate proteins based on different structural characteristics (e.g., charge, binding to tags like *his*$_6$, or molecular mass; *see* Note 15).

4. Notes

1. Glucose is used at 2% to inhibit *lac* promotor activity and minimize recombinant protein expression during cell growth. The *lac* promotor is induced efficiently in cultures containing 0.1% glucose after the sugar is consumed by proliferating bacteria.
2. Total RNA works well as template for cDNA synthesis in our hands. Well-defined ribosomal RNA bands indicate absence of extensive RNA degradation.
3. V_L-*Back* and V_H-*Back* primers contain sequences corresponding to sense codons for residues 1–7 and 1–8 of anti-VIP (clone c23.5) L and heavy (H) chains, respectively, determined by N-terminal amino acid sequencing of the purified proteins *(10)*.
4. Annealing temperature is an important variable in PCR amplification. Ideally, the melting temperatures (T_m) for the two primers should be similar. We perform PCRs using annealing temperatures about 10°C below the T_m. If the T_m is very high, annealing temperatures as high as 72°C can be used, and primer annealing and extension of the cDNA occur at the same temperature. Increased magnesium concentrations are permissive for heteroduplex formation, and nonspecific amplification can occur. For best results, it is useful to test several annealing temperatures and magnesium concentration in preliminary PCR trials.
5. Several methods are available to construct single-chain Fv (e.g., ref. *11*). In the present example, complementarity between linker antisense and sense sequences placed in the primers (Table 1) is utilized to achieve covalent linkage between V_L and V_H domains. Following linkage by overlap extension, scF$_v$ DNA is amplified by using PCR primers that anneal the 5'- and 3'-termini.
6. *Sfi*I and *Not*I sites are rare in antibody-variable genes. These enzymes can be used, therefore, for cloning of most V_L and V_H sequences.
7. Restriction digestion of the phagemid cDNA with both enzymes must be as complete as possible to prevent sticky-end vector self-ligation. Incomplete digestion is reflected by the presence of a large number of clones without cDNA inserts in Section 3.5.
8. The anti-VIP L-chain and scF$_v$ cDNAs are composed of 654 and 750 base pairs (bp), respectively. PCR using SEQBACK and fdSEQ primers and pCANTAB5*his$_6$* template without inserts yields a 224-bp product. The products using pCANTAB5*his$_6$* templates with L-chain and scF$_v$ inserts are 878 and 974 bp in size, respectively.
9. Polymerase errors can introduce mutations (about 1/1000 bases for *Taq*). There are many examples of altered binding affinity resulting from single

amino acid substitutions in CDRs *(12,13)*. Even recombinant protein expression levels can change on mutations in CDR and framework regions *(14)*. Unequivocal identification of catalytic residues in antibodies remains to be accomplished. As in enzymes, catalytic activity in antibodies is likely to be encoded by a few chemically activated amino acids. Chance mutations at these residues could lead to loss of activity. It is essential, therefore, to sequence the clones prior to detailed structure–function study of the recombinant proteins.

10. cDNA cloned in pCANTAB5 *his*$_6$ can be expressed in two ways. There is an amber stop codon between the cloned cDNA and the gene3 structural protein sequence. *E. coli* TG1 cells recognize the amber codon as Glu, and the recombinant protein is expressed as a protein3 fusion protein. *E. coli* HB2151 lack the amber suppressor mutation, and insert cDNA is expressed as a soluble molecule. A *pel*B/gene3 hybrid leader peptide directs secretion of the recombinant proteins to the periplasm. After 3–4 h of culture in 1 mM of IPTG at 30°C, most of the recombinant protein is found in the periplasm. Longer incubations in the inducing medium result in accumulation of antibody fragments in the culture medium.

11. A c-*myc* peptide sequence (10 residues) close to the C-terminus of the recombinant proteins permits rapid detection using anti-c-*myc* antibody. The dot-blot procedure described here is considerably more sensitive than the ELISA method reported in Chapter 26 (this vol.), although quantitation of the dot-blot signal is cumbersome. In most cases, signal quantitation is unnecessary (e.g., in identification of the protein at various chromatography steps). The signal is stronger in wet blots than in dry blots.

12. The antibody fragments contain a six-residue histidine tag located at the carboxy-terminus that binds immobilized nickel. The first round of chelating chromatography removes >85% of irrelevant periplasmic proteins. The metal binding strengths of different L-chain and scF$_v$ clones appear to be different, and the purity levels of the different proteins after the first round of chelating chromatography are not identical. The variations probably derive from conformational factors imposed by recombinant protein aggregation and noncovalent interactions with irrelevant proteins present in the periplasm.

13. The recombinant proteins do not elute immediately on passage of EDTA through the immobilized metal affinity column owing to the gel-filtration effect in the column. β-lactamase, a protein with approximately the same mass as the recombinant L chain and scF$_v$ (30 kDa), can be a coeluting contaminant. IEF-PAGE resolves the recombinant proteins from β-lactamase (pI between 4.5 and 5.2). Our initial attempts to purify recombinant L chain yielded pure β-lactamase, identified by N-terminal amino acid sequencing.

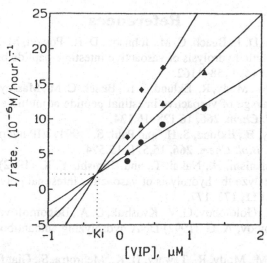

Fig 2. Inhibition of recombinant L chain-catalyzed hydrolysis of Pro-Phe-Arg-methylcoumarinamide (MCA) by VIP. Reaction rates were measured by fluorimetry (λ_{ex}370 nm, λ_{em}460 nm) at 1 μM L chain and 25 μM (●), 15 μM (▲), or 7.5 μM (◆) substrate. VIP, His-Ser-Asp-Ala-Val-Phe-Thr-Asp-Asn-Tyr-Thr-Arg-Leu-Arg-Lys-Gln-Met-Ala-Val-Lys-Lys-Tyr-Leu-Asn-Ser-Ile-Leu-Asn-NH$_2$. Data are from *(8)*.

    Inclusion of a low-pH sodium formate wash (pH 3.8) permits removal of most of the β-lactamase from the column with minimal loss of recombinant protein. The second round of chelating Sepharose chromatography furnishes essentially homogeneous antibody fragments. The procedure described here yielded about 1 mg of recombinant protein (about 20% recovery) at 99% purity judged by SDS-PAGE and IEF-PAGE. The N-terminal sequence of recombinant L chain obtained by automated Edman's degradation is identical to the natural antibody L chain secreted by hybridoma cells *(10)*.

14. Modeling of the anti-VIP F$_v$ has identified a possible catalytic triad in the L chain arranged in an orientation similar to the active-site residues of subtilisin *(8)*.

15. The specific activity (CPM/h/μg protein) with which radiolabeled VIP was hydrolyzed by recombinant L chain purified by Superose-12 gel filtration and Mono-Q anion-exchange chromatography was essentially identical *(8)*, indicating catalyst purity. Initial rates observed at increasing VIP concentrations were consistent with Michaelis-Menten kinetics (K_m 0.2 μM; k_{cat} 0.011 min^{-1}). Hydrolysis of an alternate substrate, Pro-Phe-Arg-methylcoumarinamide, was inhibited competitively by VIP (K_i 0.3 μM, deduced from the intersection point of curves in Fig. 2) *(8)*.

References

1. Paul, S., Volle, D. J., Beach, C. M., Johnson, D. R., Powell, M. J., and Massey, R. J. (1989) Catalytic hydrolysis of vasoactive intestinal peptide by human autoantibody. *Science* **244,** 1158–1162.
2. Paul, S., Sun, M., Mody, R., Eklund, S. H., Beach, C. M., Massey, R. J., and Hamel, F. (1991) Cleavage of vasoactive intestinal peptide at multiple sites by autoantibodies. *J. Biol. Chem.* **266,** 16,128–16,134.
3. Sun, M., Mody, B., Eklund, S. H., and Paul, S. (1991) VIP hydrolysis by antibody light chains. *J. Biol. Chem.* **266,** 15,571–15,574.
4. Suzuki, H., Imanishi, H., Nakai, T., and Konishi, Y. K. (1992) Human autoantibodies that catalyze the hydrolysis of vasoactive intestinal polypeptide. *Biochem. (Life Sci. Adv.)* **11,** 173–177.
5. Shuster, A. M., Gololobov, G. V., Kvashuk, O. A., Bogomolova, A. E., Smirnov, I. V., and Gabibov, A. G. (1992) DNA hydrolyzing autoantibodies. *Science* **256,** 665–667.
6. Paul, S., Sun, M., Mody, R., Tewary, H. K., Mehrotra, S., Gianferrara, T., Meldal, M., and Tramontano, A. (1992) Peptidolytic monoclonal antibody elicited by a neuropeptide. *J. Biol. Chem.* **267,** 13,142–13,145.
7. Sun, M., Gao, Q.-S., Li, light., and Paul, S. (1994) Proteolytic activity of an antibody light chain. *J. Immunol.* **153,** 5121–5126.
8. Gao, Q.-S., Sun, M., Tyutyulkova, S., Webster, D., Rees, A., Tramontano, A., Massey, R., and Paul, S. (1994) Molecular cloning of a proteolytic antibody light chain. *J. Biol. Chem.* **269,** 32,389–32,393.
9. McCafferty, J., Fitzgerald, K. J., Earnshaw, J., Chiswell, D. J., Link, J., Smith, R., and Kenton, J. (1994) Isolation of murine antibody fragments which bind a transition state analogue by phage display. *Appl. Biochem. Biotechnol.* **47,** 157–174.
10. Sun, M., Li, light., Gao, Q. S., and Paul, S. (1994) Antigen recognition by an antibody light chain. *J. Biol. Chem.* **269,** 734–738.
11. Clackson, T., Hoogenboom, H. R., Griffiths, A. D., and Winter, G. (1991) Making antibody fragments using phage display libraries. *Nature* **352,** 624–628.
12. Hall, B. light., Zaghouani, H., Daian, C., and Bona, C. A. (1992) A single amino acid mutation in CDR3 of the 3-14-9 light chain abolished expression of the IDA 10-defined idiotope and antigen binding. *J. Immunol.* **149,** 1605–1612.
13. Xiang, J., Chen, Z., Delbaere, light. T. J., and Liu, E. (1993) Differences in antigen-binding affinity caused by a single amino acid substitution in the variable region of the H chain. *Immunol. Cell. Biol.* **71,** 239–247.
14. Deng, S. J., MacKenzie, C. R., Sadowska, J., Michniewicz, J., Young, N. M., Bundle, D. R., and Narang, S. A. (1994) Selection of antibody single-chain variable fragments with improved carbohydrate binding by phage display. *J. Biol. Chem.* **269,** 9533–9538.

CHAPTER 20

Cloning and Bacterial Expression of an Esterolytic sF$_v$

Rodger G. Smith, Mark T. Martin, Rosa Sanchez, and John H. Kenten

1. Introduction

In 1988 the first report on the expression of a fully functional recombinant Fab in *E. coli (1)* was one of the initiating events in the development of the field of antibody engineering. Shortly after came the report of the cloning and expression of antibody-variable domains as single-chain F$_v$ or sF$_v$ *(2)*. This provided a method for rapid cloning of stable antibody domains from hybridoma cells into *E. coli* in a fully functional form. More recent developments in the field, such as expression and selection of libraries of sF$_v$ or Fab on phage particles, have allowed the *de novo* generation of antibodies with binding properties equivalent to or, in some cases, better than those derived by traditional hybridoma methods *(3)*.

One of the chief benefits of antibody engineering is the ability to rapidly probe structure–function relationships as they relate to antibody–antigen-binding interactions. Initially, much of the work was focused on sequencing of heavy and light chains cloned from panels of hybridomas. Comparison of amino acid sequences of antibodies with related binding properties provided some insight to which residues in the binding pocket can participate in antigen binding. With the ability to clone and express antibody domains in *E. coli* rapidly, antibody structure–function relationships can now be explored using a number of different sophisticated methods, such as site-directed mutagenesis, alanine-scanning mutagenesis, heavy- and light-chain shuffling, CDR shuffling, and CDR randomization *(4)*.

From: *Methods in Molecular Biology, Vol. 51: Antibody Engineering Protocols*
Edited by: S. Paul Humana Press Inc., Totowa, NJ

Antibody engineering has been particularly useful in the catalytic antibody field. The study of the binding properties of catalytic antibodies is inherently more complex, and perhaps more interesting, since the antibody has the combined properties of both binding and catalysis similar to enzymes. A recently published report described the use of site-directed mutagenesis of a catalytic antibody to elucidate the key residues in the binding pocket required for both substrate binding and catalysis *(5)*. The ability to clone and express the catalytic antibody in *E. coli* was essential to allow rapid construction and evaluation of a variety of different mutants. In addition to probing structural properties of catalytic antibodies, antibody engineering can be used to alter the antibody-binding pocket directly to improve or change catalytic properties. For example, metal coordination sites have been introduced into an antibody-binding pocket in an attempt to mimic cofactor enhanced catalysis *(6)*. Finally, the ability to display large repertoires of antibody domains on the surface of phage can be used, along with an appropriate selection and screening methods, to isolate new and useful antibody catalysts.

1.1. Rapid PCR Cloning of Mouse (or Human) Antibody-Variable Domains as Single-Chain F_vs (sF_v)

The polymerase chain reaction (PCR) provides a rapid method for directly amplifying heavy- and light-chain antibody-variable domains from immunoglobulin RNA *(7)*. Using the existing data base of mouse and human antibody sequences, repertoire primer sets have been designed to allow cloning of virtually any mouse or human V_H or V_L domain. (For further discussion of primer design for antibody cloning, *see* ref. *8*.) Additional sequences encoding a linker are placed in the primers to link the antibody domains prior to cloning and expression. A variety of antibody domain configurations have been successfully expressed in *E. coli*, including F_v, sF_v, and Fab *(9)*.

This chapter will focus exclusively on monovalent sF_v cloning and expression, using by way of example, the cloning of an esterolytic catalytic antibody, 20G9. A typical sF_v gene construct consists of V_L and V_H antibody domains connected in frame with a 28–51 bp nucleotide linker. In the expressed sF_v protein, the DNA linker fragment encodes a 14–27 residue flexible peptide, tethering the two antibody domains together and facilitating interchain interaction to form a monovalent binding pocket.

The order of the antibody domains in the sF_v construct does not appear to be important and can be either V_H-linker-V_L or V_L-linker-V_H. Linkers of a variety of different lengths and amino acid compositions have been successfully used in making sF_vs. The linker sequence consisting of three repeating units of $(Gly)_4Ser$ is one of the most common sequences reported in the literature (for review of sF_v structure and cloning, *see* ref. *10*).

A number of methods have been developed for linking the V_H and V_L gene segments to form a clonable sF_v gene fragment. One approach is to generate a linker fragment, either by PCR from an existing sF_v clone or by oligonucleotide synthesis, in which 20–30 bp at the 5'- and 3'-ends of the linker are complements of the 3'- and 5'-ends of the corresponding variable domains. A three-fragment splice overlap extension linking reaction is done using the two outside priming sites of the variable domains *(4)*. In another method, two of the PCR primers, one for V_H and one for V_L, have complementary sequences at their termini, which encode the linker sequence. PCR amplification of hybridoma-derived cDNA is first done in a single tube with all four V_H and V_L primers followed by a second PCR amplification with only the two outside primers *(11)*. A similar method, and one that will be described in more detail in this chapter, was first reported by Chaudhary et al. *(12)*. In this linking protocol, the entire linker sequence was incorporated at the 3'-end of a 3' V_L primer. A small portion of complementary sequence was added to the 3'-end of the 5' V_H primer. Following PCR of the V_H and V_L domains from hybridoma cDNA, the two products are combined and a second PCR done using only the outside PCR primers.

A final consideration for sF_v PCR assembly and cloning is the addition of restriction sites to the final assembled product. These sites are required for cloning of the sF_v into the appropriate vector for subsequent expression in *E. coli*. In addition to the restriction sites, short DNA tails of 6–15 bp are added after the site to increase the cutting efficiency of the restriction enzyme. Typically, the restriction sites are added to the final assembled sF_v product in a separate "pull-through" PCR reaction. One end of the pull-through oligonucleotide is complementary to either the 5'- or 3'-end of the sF_v with the remaining portion of the oligonucleotide encoding the restriction site and DNA tail. A set of mouse V_H- and V_L-specific PCR primers that was used to assemble the 20G9 sF_v using a method similar to that of Chaudhary et al. *(12)* is shown in Fig. 1.

5' VH PCR PRIMERS

VH1 - 5'CCAAAGTCGACGAGGTGCAGCTGCAGGAGTCTGGG/A 3'
VH2 - 5'CCAAAGTCGACGAGGTGCAGCTGCAGGAGTCAGGG/A 3'
VH3 - 5'CCAAAGTCGACGAGGTGCAGCTGCAGCAGCCTGGG/A 3'
VH4 - 5'CCAAAGTCGACGAGGTGCAGCTGCAGCAGTCTGGG/A 3'

3' JH-HIS(5) PCR PRIMERS

JH1 - 3'CCCTGGTGCCAGTGGCAGAGGAGTGTGGTAGTGGTAGTGATTACTCGCCGGCG 5'
JH2 - 3'CCGTGGTGCGAGTGTCAGAGGAGTGTGGTAGTGGTAGTGATTACTCGCCGGCG 5'
JH3 - 3'CCCTGAGACCAGTGACAGAGACGTGTGGTAGTGGTAGTGATTACTCGCCGGCG 5'
JH4 - 3'CCTTGGAGTCAGTGGCAGAGGAGTGTGGTAGTGGTAGTGATTACTCGCCGGCG 5'

HIS(5)

5' VL PCR PRIMERS

VL1 - 5'GCCCAACCAGCGATGGCCGAAATTGTGCTGACCCAGTCTCCA 3'
VL2 - 5'GCCCAACCAGCGATGGCCGAAATTGTGCTGACCCAGTCTCAA 3'
VL3 - 5'GCCCAACCAGCGATGGCCGAAATTGTGCTGACCCAAACTCCA 3'
VL4 - 5'GCCCAACCAGCGATGGCCGAAATTGTGCTGACCCAAACTCAA 3'

3' VL LINKER PCR PRIMERS

VL1-3'CCCTGGTTCGACCTCGACTTTCTCCCATTTAGGAGTCCTAGACCGAGGCTTAGGTTTC
AGCTGCTCCA 3'

VL2-3'CCGTGGTTCGACCTCGACTTTCTCCCATTTAGGAGTCCTAGACCGAGGCTTAGGTTTC
AGCTGCTCCA 3'

5' VL NHEI PT PRIMER		3' JH NOTI PT PRIMER

5'GCTATTGCTAGCTGCCCAACCAGCGATGGCC3'   3'GTAGTGATTACTCGCCGGCGTAAGAATACT5'
      NheI   NotI

Fig. 1. Sequences of primers used for PCR amplification of mouse V_H and V_L domains for subsequent cloning as functional sF_v. The sequences in bold in the 5' V_H primers and 3' V_L primers encode the 14 amino acid linker. The underlined portion within the linker sequence in the two sets of primers is complementary, which allows PCR linkage of the V_L and V_H domains. The sequence encoding the HIS(5) tag is incorporated into the 3' JH primers as indicated. The two pull-through primers shown (*Not*I and *Nhe*I PT primers) are used in the final PCR assembly reaction. These contain restriction sites and tail extensions to allow cloning of the sF_v into the expression vector.

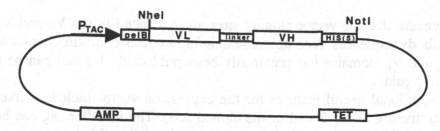

Fig. 2. *E. coli* vector, pIGEN1, used for expression and secretion of sF$_v$. The tetracycline resistance gene (TET) in the vector is nonfunctional.

1.2. Plasmid Vectors for Expression of sF$_v$

Functional sF$_v$ species have been successfully expressed in a wide variety of different host systems, including *E. coli*, yeast, plants, mammalian cells, and baculovirus *(10)*. The vast majority of published expression systems are in *E. coli*, and include vectors for both cytoplasmic expression *(2,13)* or secreted expression *(14)*. The best system for rapidly producing and purifying functional sF$_v$ for assay and characterization is secreted expression. The main drawback of secreted expression systems, in some instances, is a low level of secretion of the sF$_v$. Poor levels of sF$_v$ expression appear to be dependent on the nature of the antibody, and may be related to the ability of the antibody to fold properly in the periplasm. Cytoplasmic expression can provide much higher yields of functional sF$_v$ protein compared to secreted expression. However, the expressed protein typically forms an insoluble aggregate (inclusion body), requiring denaturation and refolding prior to purification of the sF$_v$ *(9)*.

The vector described in this chapter for expression of the 20G9 sF$_v$ catalytic antibody is shown in Fig. 2. The basic vector is commercially available (pKK233-2, Clontech Laboratories Inc., Palo Alto, CA) and utilizes the strong *tac* promoter originally described by Amann et al. *(15)*. The vector was modified for secreted expression of sF$_v$ by cloning in an oligo cassette that encodes the leader segment of the bacterial *pelB* gene (pectate lyase from *E. carotovora*). The leader peptide directs translocation of the expressed sF$_v$ to the *E. coli* periplasmic space and eventual secretion. The oligo cassette also contained two unique restriction sites, *Nhe*I and *Not*I, to allow cloning of the sF$_v$ gene in frame with the leader peptide. It is important when choosing or designing an expression vector to ensure that the vector cloning sites are not found in the V_H and V_L antibody sequences. A computer search for rare restriction sites in mouse V_L and V_H domains has previously been published *(12)* and can be a useful guide.

Additional useful features for the expression vector include a five-histidine tag at the 3'-end of the cloned scF_v. The histidine tag can be integrated into the vector by cloning or can simply be added to the 3'-end of the appropriate variable domain by incorporation into the 3' primary PCR primer (*see* Fig. 1). The histidine tag provides a simple and rapid means for subsequent purification of the sF_v, as will be described below. Alternatives to the histidine tag include various peptides, such as c-*myc* *(16)* and Flag *(17)*. Antibodies that specifically recognize these peptides can be used for subsequent detection of the sF_v by ELISA and for purification by affinity chromatography.

1.3. Purification of Expressed sF_v from E. coli

When using a secretion expression vector similar to the one described above, purification of expressed sF_v from the periplasmic space is achieved by osmotic shock followed by immobilized metal affinity chromatography or IMAC *(18)*. Short induction times are typically used (3–6 h) to achieve maximal levels of expressed sF_v in the periplasmic space. Some optimization of inducer concentrations and induction times may be required to determine appropriate conditions for maximal protein expression and accumulation in the periplasmic space. It has been demonstrated that if very long induction times are used, for example, 20 h or more, the expressed sF_v will accumulate to very high levels in the medium *(19)*. With the proper equipment, it is possible to concentrate and purify the sF_v from the culture supernatant, but in our experience, this is more difficult than purification from periplasmic extracts because of the large volumes that must be handled and processed. In addition, free metals in the culture medium appear to interfere with subsequent IMAC purification. Therefore, a dialysis or desalting step is required.

IMAC is a convenient method for purification of sF_v from periplasmic lysates or culture supernatants *(9)*. The extremely high capacity of the IMAC resin makes large-scale purification cost-effective and reasonably rapid. The chief advantage, however, is the fact that the sF_v can be eluted from the resin under nondenaturing conditions and neutral pH using either EDTA or imidazole. This is important, since it has been shown

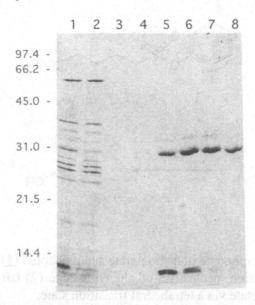

Fig. 3. Silver-stained SDS-PAGE of fractions from a large-scale IMAC purification of 20G9 sF$_v$ from an *E. coli* periplasmic lysate. Lane 1, total periplasmic lysate; lane 2, IMAC flow-through; lanes 3–8, IMAC column fractions 1–6 recovered by elution of bound sF$_v$ with 50 m*M* EDTA-0.5*M* NaCl. Migration of protein size markers in kDa units is shown on the left.

that many sF$_v$s are unstable at highly acidic or basic pH, conditions often encountered when purification is by affinity chromatography *(19)*. The level of purity of the sF$_v$ following IMAC is often as high as 90% or greater, which is acceptable for most uses (*see* Fig. 3). When one is screening sF$_v$ for catalytic activity, the issue of purity becomes more critical. In this case, a second purification using size-exclusion chromatography on a resin, such as Superdex-75, may be necessary. A catalytic assay of the column fractions is done to ensure the catalytic activity is at the same position as the sF$_v$ protein peak.

1.4. Activity Assay of 20G9, an Esterolytic Catalytic Antibody

Although many catalytic antibodies have been described since the first literature reports in 1986, the structural and mechanistic details of the vast majority are unknown. A notable exception is the esterolytic antibody, 20G9 (as well as the isoabzymes of 20G9; structurally and mecha-

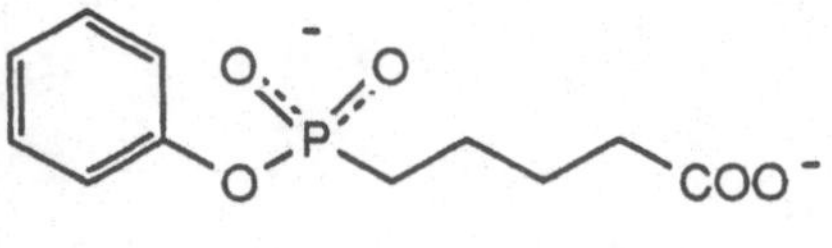

1

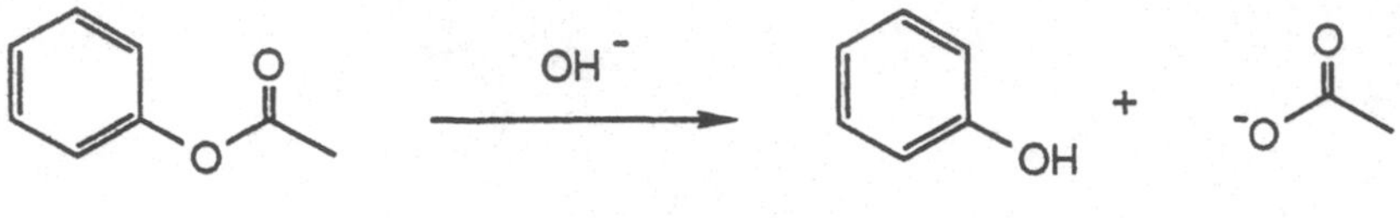

2

Fig. 4. Phenylphosphonate transition-state analog hapten (1) to which 20G9 was raised and reaction mechanism of phenyl acetate (2) base hydrolysis to form phenol and acetate via a tetrahedral transition state.

nistically similar catalytic antibodies generated from the same hybridoma fusion). 20G9 is an antiphosphonate monoclonal antibody (MAb) that catalyzes the hydrolysis of phenyl acetate to form acetate and phenol. The hapten to which the 20G9 antibody was raised, as well as the reaction catalyzed by the antibody, is shown in Fig. 4. The results of a typical catalytic assay comparing 20G9 whole IgG and 20G9 sFv are shown in Fig. 5.

Initially, 20G9 was used in pioneering studies to test the practical feasibility of catalytic antibodies in reverse micelles *(20)* and biosensors *(21)*. Soon thereafter, curiosity about 20G9's characteristic multiturnover presteady-state kinetic burst led to extensive mechanistic and structural studies *(22–24)*. A series of experiments indicated that the burst is caused by phenol binding to an *O*-acetyl-tyrosyl intermediate, inhibiting the rate of deacylation *(23)*. Further, structural and mechanistic evidence suggested that formation and/or breakdown of this acyl-intermediate is accelerated by hapten-elicited transition-state complementarity *(24)*. Other work demonstrated that catalysis by 20G9 is remarkably regulated by multiple molecules of substrate and product *(22;* and unpublished, T. S. Angeles and M. T. Martin) and that substrate-resembling inhibitors of 20G9 and its isoabzymes form stable acyl-tyrosyl antibodies via a Michaelis complex, and are hence mechanism-based inhibitors (or "sui-

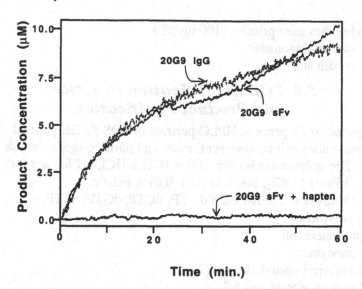

Time (min.)

Fig. 5. Spectrophotometric assay of phenylacetate hydrolysis by 20G9 IgG (whole antibody) or 20G9 sF$_v$ in the presence or absence of the phenyl-phosphonate hapten. Spectrophotometer tracing shows the UV absorbance change, converted to phenol concentration (in µM), corresponding to the product of phenylacetate hydrolysis.

cide substrates") *(25)*. Such in-depth catalytic antibody studies may not only lead to improved future catalysts, but also may provide insight into the basic principles of protein catalysis.

2. Materials
2.1. RNA Purification and Reverse Transcriptase cDNA Reaction

1. Kit for purification of mRNA (available from Invitrogen, San Diego, CA).
2. $3M$ sodium acetate, adjusted to pH 5.2 with glacial acetic acid.
3. Isopropanol.
4. DEPC-treated distilled water.
5. Microcentrifuge.
6. Superscript RNaseH⁻ Reverse Transcriptase (RT), 200 U/µL (Gibco/BRL, Gaithersburg, MD).
7. 5X RT buffer: $0.25M$ Tris-HCl, pH 8.3, $0.375M$ KCl, 15 mM MgCl$_2$.
8. $0.1M$ Diothiothreitol (DTT).
9. Placental ribonuclease inhibitor, 10 U/µL (Gibco/BRL).
10. 5 mM dNTPs: 1.25 mM each dATP, dCTP, dGTP, dTTP.

11. Random hexamer primers (100 ng/µL).
12. UV spectrophotometer.
13. Water bath at 37°C.

2.2. PCR Amplification Reactions and Product Purification

1. Oligonucleotide primers, HPLC-purified or SDS-PAGE purified. A number of companies will custom-synthesize and purify oligonucleotide primers.
2. 10X *Taq* polymerase buffer: 100 mM Tris-HCl, pH 8.3 at room temperature, 15 mM MgCl$_2$, 500 mM KCl, 0.01% gelatin.
3. 10 mM dNTPs: 2.5 mM each dATP, dCTP, dGTP, dTTP.
4. *Taq* polymerase.
5. Light mineral oil.
6. Thermocycler.
7. Chloroform:isoamyl alcohol (24:1).
8. 3M sodium acetate, pH 5.2.
9. Absolute ethanol (–20°C).
10. Agarose.
11. DNA electroelution buffer: 15% polyethylene glycol, TAE (0.04M Tris-acetate,.001M EDTA), 0.1 µg/mL ethidium bromide.
12. Phenol:chloroform:isoamyl alcohol (25:24:1).
13. Glycogen: 20 mg/mL, molecular-biology-grade.

2.3. Restriction Digestion and Vector Ligation

1. Cloning-grade agarose.
2. DNA size and concentration gel markers.
3. CsCl-purified plasmid vector DNA.
4. *Nhe*I restriction enzyme.
5. *Not*I restriction enzyme.
6. 10X *Nhe*I reaction buffer: 0.2M Tris-HCl, pH 7.5, 0.5M KCl, 50 mM MgCl$_2$.
7. 10X *Not*I reaction buffer: 0.5M Tris-HCl, pH 8.0, 0.1M MgCl$_2$, 1M NaCl.
8. T4 DNA ligase (400 U/µL).
9. 5X T4 DNA ligase buffer: 0.25M Tris-HCl, pH 7.6, 50 mM MgCl$_2$, 5 mM ATP, 5 mM DTT, 25% (w/v) polyethylene glycol 8000.
10. 7.5M Ammonium acetate.
11. Absolute ethanol.
12. Glycogen: 20 mg/mL (molecular-biology grade).

2.4. E. coli Transformation and Clone Screening by PCR

1. Electrocompetent or chemical competent *E. coli* XL1 Blue.
2. Electroporation apparatus and cuvets.

3. SOC broth: 20 g bacto-tryptone, 5 g yeast extract, 5 g NaCl/L dH$_2$O.
4. 2XYT/G/A agar plates: 17 g bacto-tryptone, 10 g yeast extract, 5 g NaCl, 2% glucose, 100 μg/mL ampicillin, 15 g agar/L dH$_2$O.
5. 30°C incubator.
6. 37°C shaking incubator.
7. Genereleaser (Bioventures, Inc. Murfreesboro, TN).
8. Oligonucleotide primers, HPLC-purified or SDS-PAGE purified.
9. 10X *Taq* polymerase buffer: 100 m*M* Tris-HCl, pH 8.3 at room temperature, 15 m*M* MgCl$_2$, 500 m*M* KCl, 0.01% gelatin.
10. 10 m*M* dNTPs: 2.5 m*M* each dATP, dCTP, dGTP, dTTP.
11. *Taq* polymerase.
12. Light mineral oil.
13. Thermocycler.

2.5. Analytical and Large-Scale Purification of sF$_v$ by IMAC

1. 2XYT/G/A broth: 17 g bacto-tryptone, 10 g yeast extract, 5 g NaCl, 2% glucose, 100 μg/mL ampicillin/L dH$_2$O.
2. Isopropylthio-β-galactoside (IPTG).
3. Periplasmic lysis buffer: 5 m*M* Na$_2$HPO$_4$, 1.7 m*M* KH$_2$PO$_4$, 1*M* NaCl, 1 m*M* EDTA.
4. Microcentrifuge.
5. Floor model centrifuge (Sorvall or equivalent).
6. 1*M* MgCl$_2$.
7. IMAC resin: Nickel-charged Sepharose (Probond resin, Invitrogen, San Diego, CA).
8. IMAC wash buffer: 5 m*M* Na$_2$HPO$_4$, 1.7 m*M* KH$_2$PO$_4$, 1*M* NaCl.
9. IMAC elution buffer: 50 m*M* EDTA, 0.5*M* NaCl.
10. Rotator or shaking table.
11. 13% SDS-polyacrylamide gel.
12. 4X SDS-PAGE sample buffer: 0.25*M* Tris-HCl, pH 6.8, 2.8*M* β-mercaptoethanol, 40% glycerol, 10% SDS, 0.1% bromophenol blue.
13. SDS-PAGE silver-staining kit (Bio-Rad, Hercules, CA).
14. Centricon microconcentrator, 10-kDa cutoff (Amicon, Beverly, MA).

2.6. Assay of Phenyl Acetate Hydrolysis

1. Substrate preparation: A solution of phenyl acetate (226 mL) and DMSO (900 mL) is suspended in deionized water to make a total volume of 50.0 mL. This suspension is inverted repeatedly to give a 50.0-m*M* aqueous phenyl acetate stock solution. A 5.0-m*M* working solution is made by further dilution in deionized water. The working solution is kept on ice, and used or discarded on the day of preparation.

2. Assay buffer: The standard buffer for the assay is 10 mM Tris-HCl, pH 8.8, containing 140 mM NaCl.
3. Antibody 20G9.
5. UV spectrophotometer.

3. Methods (*see* Notes 1–4)

3.1. RNA Purification and cDNA Reaction

1. Purify mRNA from hybridoma cells using a commercially available RNA purification kit following manufacturer's protocol (*see* Note 1). For this example, a hybridoma cell line, 20G9, which produced an antibody with an esterase catalytic activity, was used.
2. Following elution from oligo dT cellulose, precipitate RNA for 1 h at –80°C by adding 0.1 vol of sodium acetate and 2.5 vol of isopropanol. If the RNA is not to be used immediately, it is best stored in the isopropanol precipitation at –80°C. Otherwise, proceed to step 3.
3. Centrifuge at 12,000g for 20 min at 4°C. Dry pellet briefly under vacuum, or invert the tube and keep in a laminar flow hood until dry.
4. Resuspend pellet in DEPC-treated H$_2$O (15–25 μL). Dilute 1 or 2 μL of the RNA into 400 μL of DEPC H$_2$O, and measure the absorbance at 260 and 280 nM (*see* Note 2).
5. Set up a 100-μL (final volume) cDNA reaction with 20 μL 5X reverse transcriptase reaction buffer, 10 μL 5 mM dNTPs, 10 μL 0.1M DTT, 3 μL random hexamer primer (100 ng/μL), and 30 μL DEPC-H$_2$O (*see* Note 3).
6. Dilute 0.5 μg of mRNA from step 4 into 20 μL final volume of DEPC H$_2$O. Heat at 65°C for 3 min, and place on ice.
7. Add the RNA from step 6 to the reaction tube from step 5. Add 2 μL of RNaseH⁻ Superscript Reverse Transcriptase or any other commercially available reverse transcriptase, and 4 μL of RNase inhibitor. Incubate at 37°C for 60 min and then at 94°C for 5 min. Store at –20°C (*see* Note 4).

3.2. PCR Amplification of Antibody-Variable Domains (see Notes 5 and 6)

1. Separate V$_H$ and V$_L$ primary PCR amplification reactions are done in 50-μL reactions containing 5-μL 10X PCR buffer, 3 μL of 10 mM dNTPs, 150 ng each 5' PCR primer and 3' PCR primer pool, 3 μL of cDNA, 0.5 μL *Taq* polymerase, and H$_2$O to 50 μL (*see* Note 5). Overlay reactions with two drops of light mineral oil.
2. PCR amplify at 94°C for 1 min; at 55°C for 1 min; at 72°C for 1 min for 25 cycles.
3. Analyze 3 μL of each PCR reaction by running on an analytical agarose gel. At this point, one can make two separate pools of the V$_H$ and V$_L$ reactions that yield sufficient quantities of amplified PCR product (*see* Note 6).

4. Extract each V_H and V_L PCR reaction pool with an equal volume of chloroform:isoamyl alcohol (24:1). Remove the aqueous phase to a new tube, and add 0.1 vol of $3M$ potassium acetate and 2.5 vol of ethanol. Chill at −80°C followed by centrifugation at 12,000g. Wash the pellet with 80% ethanol, recentrifuge, and dry pellet under vacuum.

3.3. Linkage PCR to Generate 20G9 sF_v DNA

1. Gel-purify each V_H and V_L PCR product by running each product pool on a 1.2% preparative agarose gel using a wide-slotted comb. After staining the gel with ethidium bromide, the product DNA band is purified from the gel slice using a trough electroelution procedure (*see* Note 7).
2. Analyze V_H and V_L PCR products on an analytical gel to determine recovery and purity.
3. Set up a 50-μL PCR reaction containing 5 μL of 10X PCR buffer, 3 μL 10 mM dNTPs, 50 ng each of gel pure V_H- and V_L-linker PCR products, 150 ng each 5' V_L *Nhe*I PT and 3' JH *Not*I PT primers (*see* Fig. 1), and 0.5 μL *Taq* DNA polymerase.
5. PCR as follows: 94°C for 1 min; 42°C for 1 min; 65°C for 2 min for three cycles followed by 94°C for 1 min; 50°C for 1 min, 30 s; 72°C for 1 min, 30 s for 20 cycles.
6. Run 3 μL of the linkage PCR reaction product on an analytical gel to verify presence of linked sF_v cDNA.
7. Extract and precipitate each PCR reaction as described in Section 3.2., step 4.
8. Gel-purify the linked sF_v product using trough electroelution as described (*see* Notes 7 and 8).

3.4. Restriction Digestion of sF_v and E. coli Expression Vector

1. The linked sF_v PCR product (200–1000 ng) and CsCl purified pIGEN1 vector (20 to 100 μg) are digested in separate digestion reactions containing 10 μL 10X *Nhe*I buffer, 5 μL *Nhe*I, and H_2O to 100 μL. Incubate at 37°C for 12 h (or overnight).
2. Extract the reactions once with phenol:chloroform:isoamyl alcohol (25:24:1) and once with chloroform:isoamyl alcohol (24:1). Add 0.1 vol of $3M$ potassium acetate and 2.5 vol of ethanol. Chill at -80°C. Centrifuge at 12,000g. Wash pellet with 80% ethanol, recentrifuge, and dry pellet under vacuum.
3. Pellets are redissolved in a 100 μL *Not*I restriction digestion reactions containing 10 μL of 10X *Not*I buffer, 1 μL BSA (10 mg/mL), 5 μL *Not*I, and H_2O to 100 μL. Incubate at 37°C 12 h (or overnight).

4. The sF$_v$-*Not*I digestion mixture is extracted and ethanol-precipitated as in step 2 above. The digested sF$_v$ DNA is then repurified on a preparative agarose gel using protocol described in Section 3.3., step 8 (*see* Note 9).
5. The pIGEN1-*Not*I digestion mixture is loaded directly onto a Chromspin 1000 column (Clontech Laboratories, Palo Alto, CA), and spin column purification is performed following the manufacturer's protocol (*see* Note 10).

3.5. Ligation of sF$_v$ DNA into the Expression Vector

1. Quantitate the digested and purified sF$_v$ DNA and vector DNA by running small aliquots on an analytical agarose gel with DNA markers of known concentration (*see* Note 11).
2. Set up a ligation reaction containing 4 µL of 5X ligation buffer, 100 ng *Nhe*I- and *Not*I-digested vector, 50 ng of *Nhe*I- and *Not*I-digested sF$_v$ DNA, 2 µL T4 DNA ligase, and H$_2$O to 20 µL final volume. Incubate at 16°C overnight. A vector-only control ligation is typically set up to determine the vector self-ligation and transformation efficiency.
3. Ethanol-precipitate the ligation reactions by adding 3 µL of glycogen, 10 µL of 7.5M ammonium acetate, and 2.5 vol of ethanol. Store at –80°C for 30–60 min, centrifuge at 12,000g for 15 min, wash pellet with 80% ethanol, vacuum dry pellet, and resuspend in 10 µL of dH$_2$O.

3.6. Transformation of E. coli with sF$_v$-pIGEN1 Ligation Mixture

1. Obtain electrocompetent (or chemically competent) *E. coli* strain XL1 Blue or any other strain suitable for transformation with a bacterial expression plasmid similar to pIGEN1 (*see* Note 12).
2. Electroporate 40 µL of cells with 1 µL of ethanol-precipitated ligation reactions from Section 3.5., step 3, following electroporation parameters specified by manufacturer of the electrocompetent cells (*see* Note 13).
3. Following electroporation, cells are grown in 1 mL of SOC at 37°C for 1 h.
4. Plate various concentrations of cells on 2XYT/G/A plates. Incubate plates at 30°C for 24–48 h until colonies are visible (*see* Note 14).
5. Screen individual colonies for the presence of sF$_v$ insert using a PCR screening protocol (*see* Note 15).

3.7. Screening of sF$_v$ Clones for Protein Expression

1. Inoculate 50 mL of 2XYT/G/A medium with clones containing sF$_v$ inserts identified by PCR (Section 3.6, step 5). Grow overnight with shaking at 30°C to stationary phase.
2. Determine OD$_{600}$ for each culture. Reinoculate fresh 2XYT/A medium (no glucose) with the overnight culture to a starting OD$_{600}$ of 0.05. Grow with shaking for several hours at 30°C until OD$_{600}$ is 1.0–1.5.

3. Add IPTG to a final concentration of 1 m*M*. Reduce temperature of incubation to 25°C, and continue growth for 3 h.
4. Harvest cells in a 50-mL conical tube by centrifugation at 2000*g*. Pour off supernatant, and resuspend pellet in ice-cold periplasmic lysis buffer. Vortex vigorously to resuspend cell pellet. Incubate on ice for 30 min.
5. Transfer lysate to an Eppendorf tube, and centrifuge at 12,000*g* for 10 min. Remove cleared lysate to a new Eppendorf tube. Add MgCl$_2$ to 1.5 m*M* final concentration.
6. Add 75 μL of IMAC resin (Probond resin, washed three times with 10 vol of IMAC wash buffer) to each lysate. Incubate on rotator for 30 min at room temperature.
7. Pellet the resin by briefly spinning in a microcentrifuge. Wash resin 3X with 1 mL of IMAC wash buffer.
8. Elute bound sF$_v$ by washing IMAC resin 2X with 75 μL IMAC elution buffer. Combine two washes into a new Eppendorf tube.
9. Analyze the IMAC eluate by transferring 20 μL of eluate to a tube containing 7 μL of 4X SDS-PAGE sample buffer. Boil sample for 10 min, and load on a 13% SDS-polyacrylamide gel.
10. Silver stain gel using a Bio-Rad Silver Stain kit following manufacturer's protocol. Clones that express sF$_v$ will produce a 31-kDa protein band.

3.8. Large-Scale Purification of sF$_v$ by IMAC

1. Grow 50–100 mL overnight culture of an sF$_v$-expressing clone in 2XYT/ G/A medium at 30°C.
2. Inoculate 1–2 L of 2XYT/A (no glucose) with overnight culture to a starting OD$_{600}$ = 0.1.
3. Grow at 30°C to final OD$_{600}$ of between 1.5 and 2.0. Add IPTG to 1 m*M* final concentration and induce culture for 2.5 h. If possible, reduce temperature to 25°C during induction.
4. Harvest cells by centrifugation for 10 min at 4000*g* (*see* Note 16).
5. Resuspend the cell pellets in ice-cold periplasmic lysis buffer. Use 1.2 mL of lysis buffer/50 mL of starting culture volume.
6. Incubate on ice for 30 min and then centrifuge at 4°C for 30 min at 7000*g*.
7. Prepare a 2–3 mL (packed volume) column of IMAC resin. Wash column with 15–20 column volumes of IMAC wash buffer.
8. Add MgCl$_2$ to the lysate to a final concentration of 1.5 m*M* just prior to loading on the column. Pass lysate through the IMAC resin at a flow rate of 1–2 mL/min.
9. Wash column with 20 column volumes of IMAC wash buffer.
10. Elute bound sF$_v$ with 6 mL of IMAC elution buffer, collecting 12 individual 0.5-mL fractions.

11. Analyze 5–10 μL of each fraction by SDS-PAGE, followed by silver staining. An example of the results of a typical large-scale IMAC purification of 20G9 sF$_v$ is shown in Fig. 3.
12. Pool the sF$_v$-containing fractions, and concentrate and dialyze the protein using a 2-mL Amicon Centricon microconcentrator with 10-kDa cutoff (*see* Note 17).

3.9. Assay of Phenyl Acetate Hydrolysis by 20G9 sF$_v$

1. Hydrolysis of phenyl acetate is monitored spectrophotometrically at 270 nm using an instrument equipped with a thermostated cuvet holder set to 25°C. A typical assay concentration of antibody-combining sites is 1.0 mM (*see* Note 18).
2. In the sample cuvet, buffer and antibody are mixed and allowed to equilibrate to 25°C before the reaction is initiated by addition of phenyl acetate to 200–300 mM (*see* Note 19).
3. The typical length of an assay is 20–30 min. The results of a typical catalytic assay of 20G9 whole antibody and sF$_v$ are shown in Fig. 5.

4. Notes

1. Owing to the time and care that must be taken in preparing RNase-free reagents and plasticware, we find it is cost-effective to purchase a kit for preparing the mRNA. If one chooses not to use a kit, a detailed protocol for mRNA purification can be found in the Maniatis cloning manual *(26)*.
2. The amount of RNA recovered can be determined from the value of OD$_{260}$, assuming an OD$_{260}$ of 1.0 equals an RNA concentration of 40 μg/mL. The ratio of the absorbance 260/280 should be 1.5 to 2. Lower ratios indicate possible contamination of the RNA with protein, which may interfere with subsequent PCR reactions.
3. Some protocols suggest setting up two cDNA reactions using specific heavy- or light-chain cDNA primers that anneal 3' of the variable region of the target mRNA. We prefer to use a random hexamer as primer, since only one cDNA reaction needs to be done, and one does not need a set of different cDNA primers if working with hybridomas from other species, such as human. The quality of the subsequent PCR is not affected by the use of the random primer and in our experience appears to work better.
4. Because of the extreme sensitivity of the subsequent PCR step and its ability to amplify minute quantities of DNA, extreme caution must be used to avoid contaminating reagents for RNA preparation and cDNA reactions with exogenous DNA. This is especially important if one is working with previously cloned sF$_v$ or Fab in the same lab environment. One should try

to work in a laminar flow hood, especially when working with the purified mRNA and setting up the cDNA reaction.

5. Four PCR reactions are set up for V$_H$, each with a separate 5' V$_H$ primer in combination with a pool of 3' JH 1, 2, 3, 4-HIS(5) primers (*see* Fig. 1). For V$_L$, four reactions are set up for each 5' V$_L$ in combination with a pool of 3' V$_L$1/2 Linker PCR primers (Fig. 1). Reactions are set up in a laminar flow hood to prevent contamination by exogenous DNA. Control reactions, which are identical to the standard reaction, but without added cDNA, are set up for each primer set. Reactions are chilled on ice prior to the addition of *Taq* polymerase. The reaction tubes are then placed in the thermocycler block preheated to 94°C, and held for 4 min prior to thermocycling.

6. Depending on the degree of specificity of the PCR primers and the annealing temperature of the PCR reaction, not all the V$_H$ and V$_L$ PCR primers will yield a product when amplifying cDNA prepared from a hybridoma clone.

7. If only a single V$_H$ or V$_L$ product band of 350–400 bp is observed with little or no nonspecific product bands, it may be possible to eliminate the gel-purification step. In this case, the V$_H$ and V$_L$ PCR reaction pools can be filtered through a microconcentrator with a 30-kDa mol-wt cutoff filter (e.g., Suprec-02 filter, PanVera Corp., Madison, WI). This will effectively remove >90% of the PCR primers. The filtered samples can then be directly added to the sF$_v$-linking PCR reaction described below. If there are a number of different product bands, purify the product band by trough electroelution as follows (27). Excise the correct size product band (350–400 bp) from gel, and recast in a second agarose gel. Cut a trough slightly larger and wider than the excised gel slice. Fill trough with DNA electroelution buffer, and reapply current to the gel until DNA from gel slice is completely in the trough. Progress of DNA can be monitored by UV light. Remove DNA containing solution from trough and extract once with equal volume of phenol:chloroform:isoamyl alcohol (25:24:1). Remove aqueous phase, and extract once with chloroform:isoamyl alcohol (24:1). Remove aqueous phase, and precipitate the DNA by adding 0.1 vol of 3*M* potassium acetate, 3 μL of glycogen, and 2.5 vol of absolute ethanol. Chill at –80°C, then centrifuge at 12,000*g* for 15 min. Wash pellet with 80% ethanol, recentrifuge, and then dry pellet under vacuum. Resuspend pellets in 10–20 μL of dH$_2$O.

8. One should use a high-quality, molecular-biology-grade agarose for the linked sF$_v$ gel-purification step, since contaminants in the agarose may interfere with subsequent steps required for cloning. Agaroses, such as Seakem GTG (FMC Corp., Rockland, ME), are quality-control-tested for restriction enzyme digestion and ligation.

9. Repurification of the digested sF$_v$ is required to remove the small DNA "tails" liberated by the restriction enzymes. If not removed, these will interfere with the subsequent ligation reaction. If one is working with small quantities of DNA, one can remove the small fragments by filter purification using a 30-kDa cutoff microconcentrator (*see* Note 7).

10. Digestion of the vector pIGEN1 liberates a 10-bp fragment between the *Nhe*I and *Not*I restriction sites. As with the sF$_v$, this must be removed by use of a spin column prior to adding to the ligation reaction.

11. Several companies (i.e., BioVentures Inc., Gibco-BRL) provide DNA marker ladders of various sizes in which the ladder bands have defined DNA concentrations. Visual comparison of the sample bands with the ladder can provide a reasonably accurate quantitation of the DNA.

12. Electroporation in general yields 10-fold or more transformants compared to use of chemically competent cells, and is the preferred transformation method. A number of companies sell a wide variety of chemically competent and electrocompetent *E. coli* strains that are suitable for transformation with expression plasmids similar to pIGEN1. The main requirement is an F' that carries the *lac*I^q repressor gene allowing more stringent repression of the *tac* promotor. Strong repression is required, since some sF$_v$s are toxic to *E. coli* and are therefore difficult or impossible to clone into expression plasmid with a leaky promotor. In certain cases, the *lac*I^q gene may have to be cloned directly into the expression vector to provide an even tighter control of expression.

13. Typical electroporation conditions using a 0.1-cm gap cuvet are 1.8 kV, 200 Ω (resistance), and 25 µF (capacitance). Typical time constants observed ranged from 4.2 to 4.8 ms.

14. Like *lac*I^q, the addition of glucose to the plates and 30°C incubation provide additional repression of the *tac* promotor, which will aid in the recovery of transformants. XL1 Blue and related strains grow extremely slowly at 30°C, and may require 2 d or more of incubation to obtain visible colonies.

15. In order to quickly identify transformants containing plasmid that carries the sF$_v$ insert, a PCR screening protocol is used as follows. Place 10 µL Genereleaser into a 0.5-mL PCR reaction tube. Pick individual colonies with a sterile toothpick first to a masterplate (2XYT/G/A), and then swirl vigorously in the Genereleaser. Vortex the tubes briefly, and then microwave for 6 min on high power in a polypropylene Eppendorf tube rack. Set up a PCR master mix containing 5 µL 10X PCR buffer, 3 µL 10 m*M* dNTPS, 150 ng each 5' and 3' PCR primers (complementary to DNA sequence in the vector flanking the sF$_v$ insert), 0.5 µL *Taq* DNA polymerase, and H$_2$O to 40 µL. Preheat microwaved Genereleaser PCR reaction tubes at 94°C for 4 min in thermocycler block, add 40 µL of PCR

master mix, and overlay with two drops of mineral oil. PCR at 94°C for 1 min; 55°C for 1 min; 72°C for 2 min for 28 cycles. Run 5 µL of each PCR reaction on a 1.2% agarose gel with appropriate DNA size markers. Positive sF$_v$ clones will yield a PCR product band of about 900 bp.

16. To reduce the number of centrifuge bottles required, one can perform multiple harvests (two or three spins) in the same bottle. For convenience, the pellets can be frozen in the bottles at –20°C prior to the lysis step. Freeze-thawing may improve the lysis.

17. In the case of 20G9 sF$_v$, the sample is dialyzed into a buffer suitable for subsequent catalytic assay analysis. Buffers like PBS are suitable for binding assays. Typical yields of 20G9 sF$_v$ are 0.5 mg/2 L prep. Purity of the protein is 90% or better (*see* Fig. 3). The amount of sF$_v$ recovered will vary with different clones.

18. The concentration of combining sites in a pure sample of antibody or antibody-derived protein can be estimated spectrophotometrically. A 1.0 mg/mL solution of antibody or antibody-derived protein will have an absorbance of 1.30 at 280 nm. If a more rigorous determination of functional antibody is desired, the combining site concentration can be determined by active site titration *(22)*.

19. Although phenyl acetate is quite stable in water, there is measurable uncatalyzed hydrolysis in the assay buffer (pH 8.8). For this reason, a reference cuvet is routinely used containing the same solution as the sample cuvet, except lacking antibody.

References

1. Better, M., Chang, C. P., Robinson, R. R., and Horwitz, A. H. (1988) *Escherichia coli* secretion of an active chimeric antibody fragment. *Science* **240,** 1041–1043.
2. Bird, R. E., Hardman, K. D., Jacobsen, J. W., Johnson, S., Kaufman, B. M., Lee, S. W., Lee, T., Pope, S. H., Riordan, G. S., and Whitlow, M. (1988) Single-chain antigen-binding proteins. *Science* **242,** 423–426.
3. Chiswell, D. J. and McCafferty, J. (1992) Phage antibodies: will new "coliclonal" antibodies replace monoclonal antibodies? *TIBTECH* **10,** 80–84.
4. Hoogenboom, H. R., Marks, J. D., Griffiths, A. D., and Winter, G. (1992) Building antibodies from their genes. *Immunol. Rev.* **130,** 41–68.
5. Stewart, J. D., Roberts, V. A., Thomas, N. R., Getzoff, E. D., and Benkovic, S. J. (1994) Site-directed mutagenesis of a catalytic antibody: an arginine residue and a histidine residue play key roles. *Biochemistry* **33,** 1994–2003.
6. Iverson, B. L., Iverson, S. A., Roberts, V. A., Getzoff, E. D., Tainer, J. A., Benkovic, S. J., and Lerner, R. A. (1990) Metalloantibodies. *Science* **249,** 659–662.
7. Orlandi, R., Gussow, D. H., Jones, P. T., and Winter, G. (1989) Cloning immunoglobulin variable domains by the polymerase chain reaction. *Proc. Natl. Acad. Sci. USA* **86**, 3833–3837.

8. Marks, J. D., Hoogenboom, H. R., Bonnert, T. P., McCafferty, J., Griffiths, A. D., and Winter, G. (1991) By-passing immunization. Human antibodies from V-gene libraries displayed on phage. *J. Mol. Biol.* **222,** 581–597.

9. Plückthun, A. (1991) Stratagies for the expression of antibody fragments in *Escherichia coli. Methods: Companion to Methods Enzymol.* **2,** 88–96.

10. Whitlow, M. and Filpula, D. (1991) Single-chain F_v proteins and their fusion proteins. *Methods: Companion to Methods Enzymol.* **2,** 97–105.

11. Davis, G. T., Bedzyk, W. D., Voss, E. W., and Jacobs, T. W. (1991) Single-chain antibody (SCA) encoding genes. One-step construction and expression in eukaryotic cells *Bio/Technology* **9,** 165–169.

12. Chaudhary, V. K., Batra, J. K., Gallo, M. G., Willingham, M. C., Fitzgerald, D. J., and Pastan, I. (1990) A rapid method of cloning functional variable-region antibody genes in *Escherichia coli* as single-chain immunotoxins. *Proc. Natl. Acad. Sci. USA* **87,** 1066–1070.

13. Huston, J. S., Levinson, D. A., Mudgett-Hunter, M., Tai, M. S., Novotny, J., Margolies, M. N., Ridge, R. E., Bruccoleri, G., Haber, E., Crea, R., and Opperman, H. (1988) Protein engineering of antibody binding sites: recovery of specific activity in an anti-digoxin single-chain F_v analogue produced in *Escherichia coli. Proc. Natl. Acad. Sci. USA* **85,** 5879–5883.

14. Glockshuber, R., Malia,M., Pfitzinger, I., and Pluckthun, A. (1990) A comparison of strategies to stabilize immunoglobulin F_v-fragments. *Biochemistry* **16,** 1362–1367.

15. Amann, E., Brosius, J., and Ptashne, M. (1983) Vectors bearing a hybrid *trp-lac* promotor useful for regulated expression of cloned genes in *Escherichia coli. Gene* **25,** 167–178.

16. Hoogenboom, H. R., Griffiths, A. D., Johnson, K. S., Chiswell, D. J., Hudson, P., and Winter, G. (1991) Multi-subunit proteins on the surface of filamentous phage: methodologies for displaying antibody (Fab) heavy and light chains. *Nucleic Acids Res.* **19,** 4133–4137.

17. Power, B. E., Ivancic, N., Harley, V. R., Webster, R. G., Kortt, A. A., Irving, R. A., and Hudson, P. J. (1992) High-level temperature-induced synthesis of an antibody V_H-domain in *Escherichia coli* using the *pelB* secretion signal. *Gene* **113,** 95–99.

18. Hochuli, E., Bannwarth, W., Dobeli, H., Gentz, R., and Stuber, D. (1988) Genetic approach to facilitate purification of recombinant proteins with a novel metal chelate absorbent. *Bio/Technology* 1321–1325.

19. Takkinin, K., Laukkanen, M. L., Sigmann, D., Alfthan, K., Immonen, T., Vanne, L., Kaartinen, M., Knowles, J. K. C., and Teeri, T. T. (1991) An active single-chain antibody containing a cellulase linker domain is secreted by *Escherichia coli. Protein Eng.* **4,** 837–841.

20. Durfor, C. N., Bolin, R. J., Sugasawara, R. J., Massey, R. J., Jacobs, J. W., and Schultz, P. G. (1988) Antibody catalysis in reverse micelles. *J. Am. Chem. Soc.* **110,** 8713,8714.

21. Blackburn, G. F., Talley, D. B., Booth, P. M., Durfor, C. N., Martin, M. T., Napper, A. D., and Rees, A. R. (1990) Potentiometric biosensor employing catalytic antibodies as the molecular recognition element. *Anal. Chem.* **62,** 2211–2216.

22. Martin, M. T., Schantz, A. R., Schultz, P. G., and Rees, A. R. (1991) Characterization of the mechanization of action of a catalytic antibody, in *Catalytic Antibodies* (Chadwick, D. and Marsh, J., eds.), Wiley, Chichester, UK, pp. 188–200.
23. Martin, M. T., Napper, A. D., Schultz, P. G., and Rees, A. R. (1991) Mechanistic studies of a tyrosine-dependent catalytic antibody. *Biochemistry* **30,** 9757–9761.
24. Angeles, T. S., Smith, R. G., Darsley, M. J., Sugasawara, R. J., Sanchez, R. I., Kenten, J., Schultz, P. G., and Martin, M. T. (1993) Isoabzymes: structurally and mechanistically similar catalytic antibodies from the same immunization. *Biochemistry* **32,** 12,128–12,135.
25. Angeles, T. S. and Martin, M. T. (1993) Mechanism-based catalytic antibody inactivation. *Biochem. Biophys. Res. Commun.* **197,** 696–701.
26. Sambrook, J., Fritsch, E., and Maniatis, T. (1989) *Molecular Cloning; A Laboratory Manual,* vol. 2. Cold Spring Harbor Laboratory, Cold Spring Harbor, NY.
27. Zhen, L. and Swank, R. T. (1993) A simple and high yield method for recovering DNA from agarose gels. *BioTechniques* **14,** 894–898.

CHAPTER 21

Site-Directed Mutagenesis of Antibody-Variable Regions

Qing-Sheng Gao and Sudhir Paul

1. Introduction

Introduction of mutations in antibody combining sites provides a powerful means to assess the functional role of individual residues and segments of the combining sites in interactions with antigen. Once cloned antibody fragments are available, several methods can be utilized to introduce mutations. Commonly used methods include those of Kunkel et al. *(1)* involving the use of a uracil-labeled template, and Kramer and Fritz *(2)* in which gapped duplex DNA is used to construct oligonucleotide-directed mutants. Several polymerase chain reaction-based mutagenesis techniques have been described *(3–5)*. However, available thermostable polymerases are error-prone, leading to undesired sequence changes. For example, *Taq* polymerase has an average error rate of 0.8% *(6,7)*. In this chapter, we described an efficient method for mutagenesis of cloned antibody fragments in which mutant oligonucleotides are utilized to initiate the synthesis of a phosphorothioate nucleotide containing DNA strands using single-stranded phage or phagemid DNA as template. The original strand is removed by exonuclease digestion, the nonmutant strand is nicked with a restriction enzyme, gapped with exonuclease III, and mutant double-stranded DNA is generated using polymerase and ligase enzymes *(8–10)*. The method has been applied to generate point mutations and deletion mutations in an anti-VIP light (L) chain in the example described here. Insertion mutations can also be performed using appropriate oligonucleotides. In addition, oligonucleotides

From: *Methods in Molecular Biology, Vol. 51: Antibody Engineering Protocols*
Edited by: S. Paul Humana Press Inc., Totowa, NJ

synthesized using mixtures of nucleotide phosphoramidites in individual cycles can be used to produce libraries of random mutants. A major advantage of this approach is the high mutation efficiency. pCANTAB5-his6, a phagemid vector derived from pUC119, was used in the present example. In principle, any M13 vector can be employed. An easy-to-use kit with excellent instructions is supplied by Amersham (Sculptor). In combination with appropriate strategies to select mutant clones (*see* Tramontano, Chapter 16, and Huang et al., Chapter 27), new constructs can be prepared rapidly and clones with the desired activity isolated.

2. Materials
2.1. Preparation of Single-Stranded Phagemid DNA

1. *E. coli* TGI: K12,Δ(1ac-pro), supE, thi, hsdD5/F'traD36, proA + B, lacI^q, lacZΔM15.
2. 100 mg/mL ampicillin in water: Filter-sterilize and store at –20°C.
3. 50 mg/mL kanamycin in water: Filter-sterilize and store at –20°C.
4. 2YT medium-2% glucose: Mix 16 g bacto-tryptone (Difco, Detroit, MI), 10 g bacto-yeast extract (Difco), 5 g NaCl, and water to 1 L. Autoclave. When the medium cools, add ampicillin to 100 μg/mL and glucose to 2% w/v (glucose stock solution, 20% w/v).
5. 2YT-ampicillin plates: Prepare and autoclave 1.5% bacto-agar (Difco) in 2YT medium as in step 11. Cool to about 45°C, add ampicillin to 100 μg/mL and glucose to 2% w/v, and pour into Petri dishes.
6. M13K07 helpe ir phage: These are available commercially at concentrations >1 × 10^{11} PFU/mL (Pharmacia, Piscataway, NJ).
7. TE buffer: 10 m*M* Tris-HCl, pH 8.0, 1 m*M* EDTA.
8. PEG solution: 20% polyethylene glycol 6000, 2.5*M* sodium chloride.
9. Phenol saturated with TE buffer.
10. Chloroform/isoamyl alcohol: 24:1(v/v) mixture.
11. 3*M* sodium acetate, pH 5.2.
12. Microcentrifuge and microfuge tubes.
13. Heating blocks.
14. TAE buffer: 4 9 m*M* Tris-acetate, pH 8.0, 1 m*M* EDTA. A 50X TAE stock solution can be prepared by mixing 242 g Tris base, 57.1 mL acetic acid, 100 mL 0.5*M* EDTA, and water to 1 L.
15. 0.6% agarose gel in TAE buffer containing 50 ng/mL ethidium bromide (EtBr).
16. 6X agarose gel electrophoresis sample buffer: 40% (w/v) sucrose, 0.1% Bromophenol blue, and 0.1% xylene cyanol FF in water.

17. 1 kb DNA ladder (BRL, Gaithersburg, MD).
18. GeneClean II DNA purification kit (Bio 101, La Jolla, CA).
19. UV transilluminator.
20. Spectrophotometer.

2.2. Oligonucleotide Phosphorylation

1. Water bath an heating block.
2. Bio-Spin 6 chromatography column (Bio-Rad, Hercules, CA).
3. Mutagenic oligonucleotide primers: 0.025 OD_{260}/mL/base in TE buffer (equivalent to 1.6 pmol/µL).
4. T4 polynucleotide kinase and 10X kinase buffer (700 mM Tris-HCl, pH 7.6, 100 mM $MgCl_2$, 50 mM DTT; New England BioLab, Beverly, MA).
5. 10 mM ATP.

2.3. Site-Directed Mutagenesis

1. Sculptor in vitro mutagenesis system (Amersham, RPN 1526.5, Arlington Heights, IL). The system contains: Native T7 DNA polymerase; T4 DNA ligase; T5 exonuclease; *Nci*I restriction endonuclease; Exonuclease III; DNA polymerase; buffer A (1.4M MOPS, pH 8, and 1.4M NaCl); buffer B (70 mM Tris-HCl, pH 8, 10 mM $MgCl_2$, 45 mM NaCl); buffer C (700 mM Tris-HCl, pH 8, 350 µM EDTA, 20 mM DTT), buffer D (250 mM Tris-HCl, pH 8, 150 mM NaCl, and 500 µM EDTA); dNTP mix A (1.01 mM dATP, dCTPαS, dGTP, dTTP, 2.02 mM ATP, and 20 mM $MgCl_2$); dNTP mix B (1.25 mM dATP, dCTP, dGTP, dTTP, 2.5 mM ATP, and 25 mM $MgCl_2$); water; lyophilized *E. coli*. TG1 host cells; M13 mp8 RF control DNA; control template (single-stranded); control mutagenic oligonucleotide (phosphorylated).
2. Water bath and heating block.
3. 0.6% agarose gel in TAE buffer containing 50 ng/mL EtBr.
4. UV transilluminator.
5. GeneClean II: DNA purification kit (Bio 101).
6. Competent *E. coli* HB2151 cells for electroporation: Harvest 500 mL of the bacteria in midlog-phase growth (OD_{600} = 0.4–0.6; 1 OD_{600} = 5 × 10^8 cells/mL) by centrifugation at 4000g for 15 min at 4°C. Wash the cells three times with 500 mL ice-cold 10% glycerol. Resuspend cells gently in 10% glycerol at a density of 3 × 10^{10} cells/mL. Freeze 100-µL aliquots on dry ice, and store at –80°C.
7. Gene Pulser electroporation apparatus (Bio-Rad).
8. SOC medium: 2% bacto-tryptone (Difco), 0.5% bacto-yeast extract (Difco), 10 mM sodium chloride, 2.5 mM potassium chloride, 10 mM magnesium chloride, 10 mM magnesium sulfate, and 10 mM glucose. Make up

20 g tryptone, 5 g yeast extract, and 0.5 g NaCl to 1 L with water, and autoclave. Add filter-sterilized 1M MgCl$_2$ (1 mL), 1M MgSO$_4$ (1 mL), and 20% glucose (5 mL)/100 mL medium (after cooling).
9. 2YT-ampicillin plates.

2.4. Identification and Expression of Mutants

The required materials and reagents are listed in the accompanying chapter (Gao and Paul, Chapter 19).

3. Methods

3.1. Preparation of Single-Stranded Template DNA (see Note 1)

Single-stranded DNA to be used as template should be free from degraded DNA and RNA. These molecules can act as primers during mutagenesis. In the protocol described here, mutagenesis of cloned antibody fragments was done using single-stranded DNA prepared from pmk18, which is a phagemid vector containing antibody L-chain cDNA cloned in pCANTAB*his6*.

1. Inoculate 5 mL 2YT-100 µL/mL ampicillin–2% glucose medium with a single colony of *E. coli* TG1 cells harboring the pmk18 vector. Incubate at 37°C overnight with shaking.
2. Inoculate 15 mL 2YT-100 µg/mL ampicillin–2% glucose medium with 0.5 mL of the overnight culture in a 50-mL sterile disposable centrifuge tube. Incubate at 37°C vigorous shaking until the culture reaches A$_{600}$ = 0.5.
3. Add M13K07 helper phage at a 10- to 20-fold excess, computed as the ratio PFU phage: bacterial cell number (e.g., 250 µL of 1 × 10^{11} PFU/mL phage solution/15 mL of the culture grown to A$_{600}$ = 0.5).
4. Incubate at 37°C with slow shaking for 30 min and then for 30 min with vigorous shaking.
5. Spin at 3000g for 15 min. Resuspend the cells in 100 mL of 2YT medium containing 100 µg/mL ampicillin and 50 µg/mL kanamycin.
6. Incubate at 37°C overnight with vigorous shaking.
7. Spin the overnight culture at 8000g for 15 min. Filter the supernatant through 0.45-µm filter. Add 0.2 vol of 20% PEG–2.5M NaCl, mix, and leave on ice for 30 min.
8. Spin at 8000g for 20 min at 4°C. Carefully discard the supernatant, and resuspend the pellet in 1 mL TE buffer.
9. Add 200 µL 20% PEG–2.5M NaCl to the phage solution. Mix well and leave on ice for 10 min.

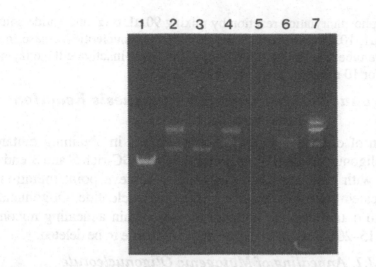

Fig. 1. EtBr-stained agarose gel showing the migration patterns of reaction products at various stages of the mutagenesis procedure. Lane 1, single-stranded template DNA; lane 2, DNA polymerized with T7 DNA polymerase (sample 1); lane 3, T5 exonuclease digested reaction mixture (sample 2); lane 4, *Nci*I nicked DNA (sample 3); lane 5, exonuclease III gapped DNA (sample 4); lane 6, repolymerized DNA (sample 5); lane 7, double-stranded pmk 18 DNA.

10. Spin at 16,000g in a microfuge for 10 min. Resuspend the pellet in 1 mL TE buffer.
11. Extract twice with TE buffer–saturated phenol, three times with phenol–chloroform–isoamyl alcohol (25:24:1), and once with chloroform–isoamyl alcohol (24:1). Add 0.1 vol of 3M sodium acetate and 2.5 vol of ethanol to precipitate the DNA.
12. Spin at 16,000g for 15 min. Wash the pellet DNA with 75% ethanol and then dissolve in 100 μL water. Dilute 5 μL DNA solution to 0.5 mL with water and measure A_{260} (1 A_{260} =30 μg/mL single-stranded DNA).
13. Load 2 μL DNA solution on a 0.6% agarose gel containing 50 ng/mL EtBr to check the quality of the preparation. The phagemid single-stranded DNA (5 kb) migrates close to the 3.4-kbp double-stranded DNA marker (Fig. 1). Helper phage single-stranded DNA migrates close to the 5.5-kbp marker. Typical yields of single-stranded DNA are 20–50 μg.

3.2. Oligonucleotide Phosphorylation

1. Desalt synthetic oligonucleotides primers by passage through a desalting spin column (e.g., Bio-Spin 6). Measure A_{260} to determine the oligonucleotide concentration and adjust to 0.025 OD_{260}/mL/base (equivalent to 1.6 pmol/μL).

2. Perform phosphorylation reaction by mixing 90 μL oligonucleotide solution, 10 μL 10X kinase buffer, and 10 U T4 polynucleotide kinase in a microfuge tube. Incubate at 37°C for 20 min. Heat-inactivate the enzyme at 70°C for 10 min and then store at –20°C.

3.3. Oligonucleotide-Directed Mutagenesis Reaction (see Notes 2 and 3)

The design of oligonucleotide primers is critical in obtaining mutant clones. The oligonucleotides should preferably have GC-rich 5' and 3' ends. Mismatches with template DNA designed to achieve point mutations should be located toward the middle of the oligonucleotide. Oligonucleotides used to obtain deletion mutants should contain annealing regions composed of 15–20 bases on either side of the sequence to be deleted.

3.3.1. Annealing of Mutagenic Oligonucleotide

1. Mix 2 μg single-stranded template DNA, 1 μL phosphorylated oligonucleotide (1.6 pmol/μL), and 1 μL buffer A supplied with the Sculptor kit in a 500-μL sterile microfuge tube, and adjust the volume to 10 μL with water.
2. Incubate the reaction tube at 75°C for 3 min, followed by 30 min at 37°C in a water bath (*see* Note 4).
3. Spin the tube briefly to collect the condensate, and then place on ice.

3.3.2. Extension and Ligation of Mutant Strand (see Note 4)

1. Add 10 μL of dNTP mix A (1.01 m*M* dATP, dCTPαS, dGTP, dTTP, 2.02 m*M* ATP in 20 m*M* MgCl₂), 2.5 U of T4 ligase and 0.8 U of T7 DNA polymerase to the reaction mixture from step 3, Section 3.3.1.
2. Incubate for 10 min at room temperature, followed by 30–60 min at 37°C.
3. Heat-inactivate at 70°C for 10 min. Save a 2-μL aliquot labeled sample 1 for electrophoresis.

3.3.3. Removal of Single-Stranded Template DNA (see Note 5)

1. Add 50 μL buffer B and 2000 U of T5 exonuclease to the reaction mixture of step 3, Section 3.3.2.
2. Mix and incubate at 37°C for 30 min. Heat-inactivate for 20 min at 70°C (*see* Note 5). Save a 5-μL aliquot labeled sample 2 for electrophoresis.

3.3.4. Nicking the Nonmutant Strand (see Note 6)

1. Add 5 μL buffer C and 5 U of *Nci*I to the T5 exonuclease digest (step 2, Section 3.3.3.).
2. Mix and incubate at 37°C for 90 min. Save a 10-μL aliquot labeled sample 3 for electrophoresis.

3.3.5. Digestion of the Nonmutant Strand

1. Add 20 µL buffer D and 160 U of exonuclease III to the reaction mixture of step 2, Section 3.3.4.
2. Mix and incubate at 37°C for 30 min. Then heat-inactivate for 20 min at 70°C. Save a 10-µL aliquot labeled sample 4 for electrophoresis.

3.3.6. Repolymerization of Gapped DNA

1. Add 20 µL dNTP mix B (1.25 mM of dATP, dCTP, dGTP, dTTP, 2.5 mM ATP in 25 mM MgCl$_2$), 3.5 U T4 ligase, and 3.5 U DNA polymerase I to the reaction mixture of step 2, Section 3.3.5.
2. Mix and incubate at 37°C for 60 min. Save a 15-µL aliquot labeled sample 5 for electrophoresis.

3.3.7. Product Analysis by Agarose Gel Electrophoresis

Electrophorese samples 1–5 collected at various stages of the mutagenesis protocol on a 0.6% agarose gel. Include single-stranded and double-stranded phagemid DNA as size markers. see Fig. 1 for typical migrations patterns.

3.3.8. Sequencing and Expression of Mutants

1. Use GeneClean DNA purification kit to purify the mutant phagemid DNA according to the protocol supplied by the manufacturer (Bio 101). Resuspend the DNA in 35 µL water.
2. Transform *E. coli* HB2151 with phagemid DNA by electroporation, grow transformed cells, purify phagemid DNA, and sequence mutant DNA as described in the accompanying chapter (Gao and Paul, Chapter 19). *See* Fig. 2 for details of anti-VIP mutants.
3. Induce mutant protein expression with 1 mM IPTG for 3 h at 30°C. Confirm expression by dot-blotting for c-*myc* (*see* Note 7).

4. Notes

1. TG1 cells shoud be maintained in M9 minimal medium prior to transformation with phagemid DNA to retain the F' episome.
2. The phosphorothioate-based site-directed mutagenesis procedure has been used to make mutants for cloned anti-VIP antibody fragments (*see* Fig. 2). The method is notable for high mutagenesis efficiencies, around 90% for point mutations and 40% for a CDR1 deletion mutation. The entire mutagenesis procedure can be completed in 1 d.
3. Optimal temperatures and times for annealing can differ widely, especially for construction of deletion mutants. Initial attempts can be made at annealing temperatures estimated as (T_m −10°C). If the nonspecific

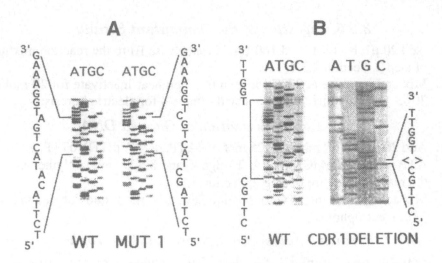

Fig. 2. Segments of DNA sequencing gels showing wild-type (WT) nucleotides 86–105 (A) and nucleotides 65–122 (B) of an anti-VIP L chain cloned in
pCANTAB*his6*. Mutated nucleotides in MUT 1 are indented (A → C, A → C,
C → G). MUT 1 contains Ala^{27D} and Ala^{28} instead of His^{27D} and Asp^{28}, respectively, in the wild-type L chain (Kabat numbering). (B) Shows the deletion of
CDR1 (< >; corresponding to nucleotides 70–117). MUT 1 was prepared using the
mutagenic primer TGTCTTTCCAGCAGTAGCTAAGAGGCTCTGACT (mis-
match nucleotides underlined), and the deletion mutant, using GCCTCTG-
TAACAACCA < > GCAAGAGATGGAGGC (sequences designed to anneal
segments flanking the deleted region are separated by < >).

annealing is a problem, annealing temperatures are increased. A primer
that can be used successfully for sequencing of template DNA is also suitable for mutagenesis. Careful sequencing is not necessary for this preliminary test. Clean bands on a sequencing gel show that the mutagenic
primer is satisfactory.

4. T7 DNA polymerase synthesizes DNA more rapidly at 37°C than the
   Klenow fragment at room temperature. Polymerization with Klenow fragment can be done using 5 U enzyme at 16°C for 14–18 h. We monitor
   completion of the extension step by agarose gel electrophoresis of an aliquot of the reaction mixture.

5. Failure to inactivate T5 exonuclease completely will result in loss of DNA
   during the nicking step.

6. *Nci*I supplied with the Sculptor kit is suitable for nicking the phosphor-
   othioate-containing nonmutant strand, except when the mutagenic oli-

gonucleotide primer also contains *Nci*I site *(10)*. In this case, the nonmutant strand can be nicked with *Ava*I or *Pvu*I. Detailed instructions for the use of these enzymes are provided with the kit.

7. A 10-residues c-*myc* peptide sequence close to the C-terminus of the recombinant proteins permits detection using anti-c-*myc* antibody.

References

1. Kunkel, T. A., Robert, J. D., and Zakour, R. A. (1987) Rapid and efficient site-specific mutagenesis without phenatypic selection. *Methods Enzymol.* **154,** 367–382.
2. Kramer, W. and Fritz, H. J. (1987) Oligonucleotide-directed construction of mutations via gapped duplex DNA. *Methods Enzymol.* **154,** 350–367.
3. Hemsley, A., Arnheim, N., Toney, M. D., Cortopassi, G., and Galas, D. J. (1989) A simple method for site directed mutagenesis using the polymerase chain reaction. *Nucleic Acids Res.* **17,** 6545–6551.
4. Kadowaki, H., Kadowaki, T., Wondisford, F. E., and Taylor, S. I. (1989) Use of polymerase chain reaction catalyzed by *Taq* polymerase for site-specific mutagenesis. *Gene* **76,** 161–166.
5. Landt, O., Grunert, H. P., and Hahn, U. (1990) A general method for rapid site-directed mutagenesis using the polymerase chain reaction. *Gene* **96,** 125–128.
6. Keohavong, P. and Thilly, W. G. (1989) Fidelity of DNA polymerase in DNA amplification. *Proc. Natl. Acad. Sci. USA* **86,** 9253–9257.
7. Leung, D. W., Chen, E., and Goeddel, D. V. (1989) A method for random mutagenesis of a defined DNA segment using a modified polymerase chain reaction. *J. Methods Cell Mol. Biol.* **1,** 11–15.
8. Sayers, J. R., Krekel, C., and Eckstein, F. (1992) Rapid high-efficiency site-directed mutagenesis by the phosphorothioate approach. *Biotechniques* **13,** 592–596.
9. Taylor, J. W., Ott, J., and Eckstein, F. (1985) The rapid generation of oligo-nucleotide-directed mutations at high frequency using phosphorothioate-modified DNA. *Nucleic Acids Res.* **13,** 8765–8785.
10. Nakamaye, K. and Eckstein, F. (1986) Inhibition of restriction endonuclease Nci I cleavage by phosphorothioate groups and its application to oligonucleotide-directed mutagenesis. *Nucleic Acids Res.* **14,** 9679–9698.

CHAPTER 22

Synthetic Antibody Gene Libraries for In Vitro Affinity Maturation

Su-jun Deng, C. Roger MacKenzie, and Saran A. Narang

1. Introduction

The application of phage display to the screening of antibody V-gene libraries promises to replace animal immunization and hybridoma technology as a means of antibody generation (1,2). Synthetic libraries offer the potential for expanding the immune system repertoire and designing libraries for particular sets of antigens. We have developed a method for the generation of synthetic antibody gene libraries by which spiked oligonucleotides are assembled by a ligase chain reaction protocol (3). This is a synthetic adaptation of a reaction that was previously used as a diagnostic tool (4,5).

This technique has been successfully applied to the in vitro affinity maturation of an scFv version of an antibody, Se155-4, specific for the *Salmonella* serogroup B *O*-polysaccharide (6). This antibody offers the advantages of a well-refined crystal structure (7) and an efficient *Escherichia coli* expression system (8–10). Anticarbohydrate antibodies are obvious candidates for affinity improvement, since they normally exhibit relatively low affinities that do not meet the requirements of diagnostic and therapeutic applications (11).

In the examples given here, the experimental procedures describe Se155-4 CDR randomization to a degree that resembles the somatic

From: *Methods in Molecular Biology, Vol. 51: Antibody Engineering Protocols*
Edited by: S. Paul Humana Press Inc., Totowa, NJ

hypermutation component of the in vivo affinity maturation process *(12)*. The equation:

$$P = n!/[k! \, (n-k) \,!] \, m^k \, (1-m)^{n-k} \tag{1}$$

where P = probability of a specified number of residue substitutions, m = mutation frequency of each amino acid at a selected spiking level, ignoring unequal triplet redundancy, k = number of amino acid substitutions obtained, and n = number of randomized residues, is used to predict the probabilities of residue substitutions at different spiking levels. At a spiking level of 10%, mutants with one to four independent point mutations in the CDRs should dominate randomized V_H and V_L libraries (Fig. 1). This approximates the mutation rate resulting from somatic hypermutation during the affinity maturation stage of the immune response *(12)*.

The procedures described here could be readily adapted to the improvement of other low-affinity antibodies, such as those isolated by phage display from naive repertoires. Also, the technique should have general applicability in one-step gene assembly and randomized library approaches to protein engineering.

2. Materials

2.1. Vector Construction

1. Plasmid ptsFvLH(el) encoding Se155-4 scFv *(8)*.
2. M13mp18 RF DNA (Life Technologies, Gaithersburg, MD).
3. PCR primers: 5'-GCGAGATCTGGTGGCGGTGGATCCCCATTC-GTTTGTGAATATCAA and 5'-AACAAGCTTCTAATAATAACGG-AATACCCAAAAGAACTGG.
4. Plasmid pBluescriptII SK(+) (Stratagene, La Jolla, CA).

2.2. Deoxyoligonucleotide Synthesis

1. Phosphoramidite derivatives (Applied Biosystems, Foster City, CA) of dA, dC, dG, T, and dI (deoxyinosine).
2. Standard reagents for oligonucleotide synthesis.

2.3. Assembly of V_H and V_L Deoxyoligonucleotides

2.3.1. Ligase Chain Reaction (LCR)

2.3.1.1. V_H Sense Deoxyoligonucleotides

1. 5'-CTAGCGGTTACACCTTCACC<u>AACTACTGGATGCAC</u>TGGATC-AAACAGCGGCCGGGT.

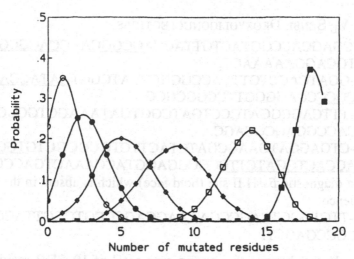

Fig. 1. Predicted levels of amino acid substitutions at different spiking levels.
○—○, 5%; ●—●, 10%; ◇—◇, 20%; ◆—◆, 40%; □—□, 70%; ■—■, 100%.

2. 5'-p-CAGGGTCTCGAATGGATCGGCGCCATC<u>TATCCGGGTAA-
CAGCGCGACCTTC</u>TACAACCACAAATTCCGTGCTA.

3. 5'-p-AAACCAAACTGACCGCTGTTACTAGTACCATCACCGCG-
TACATGGAACTGAGCAGCCTGACCAACGAAGAT.

4. 5'-p-TCTGCGGTTTACTACTGCACGCGT<u>GGTGGTCATGGTTACTAC-
GGTGATTACTGGGGC**CAAGG**CGCGAGCCTGACCGTGTCCTCCA
containing a diagnostic *Sty*I site (bold face) which is absent in the wild-
type sequence.

The underlined sequences encoding a total of 19 CDR residues were
partially randomized by spiking, at a level of 10%, with a mixture containing equimolar amounts of each of the four DNA precursors. *See* Note 1.

2.3.1.2. V_H ANTISENSE DEOXYOLIGONUCLEOTIDES

1. 5'-p-ATTCGAGACCCTGACCCGGCCGCTGTTTGATCCA<u>IIIIIIIIIIIIIII</u>-
GGTGAAGGTGTAACCG.

2. 5'-p-CAGTTTGGTTTTAGCACGGAATTTGTGGTTGTA<u>IIIIIIIIIIIIII</u>-
<u>IIIIIIIIIII</u>GATGGCGCCGATCC.

3. 5'-p-AACCGCAGAATCTTCGTTGGTCAGGCTGCTCAGTTCCATG-
TACGCGGTGATGGTACTAGTAACAGCGGT.

4. 5'-GATCTGGAGGACACGGTCAGGCTCGCGCCTTGGCCCCA-
GTAATCACC<u>IIIIIIIIIIIIIIIIIIIIIII</u>ACGCGTGCAGTAGTA.

I denotes inosine. *See* Note 2.

2.3.1.3. V_L Sense Deoxyoligonucleotides

1. 5'-TCGAGCACCGGTACTGTTACC<u>AGCGGCAACCACGCG</u>AACTG-GGTGCAGGAAAAACC.
2. 5'-p-GGATCACCTGTTCACCGGGCTCATCGGT<u>GATACCAACAAC-CGCGCC</u>CCAGGGGTTCCGGCGCG.
3. 5'-p-TTTCAGCGGATCCCTGATCGGTGATAAAGCTGCGCTGACC-ATCACCGGAGCGCAGC.
4. 5'-p-CTGAGGATGAAGCGATCTACTTCTGCGCGCTG<u>**TGGTCTAA-CAACCACTGGATCTTC**</u>GGCGGAGGTACCAAACTGACCG contain-ing a diagnostic *Bss*H II site (bold face) which is absent in the wild-type sequence.
5. 5'-p-TTCTGGGTCAGCCGAAAAGCAGCCCGTCGGTTACCCTGTT-CCCGCCGAGCT.

The underlined sequences encoding a total of 19 CDR residues were partially randomized by spiking, at a level of 10%, with a mixture containing equimolar amounts of each of the DNA precursors.

2.3.1.4. V_L Antisense Deoxyoligonucleotides

1. 5'-p-GGTGATCCGGTTTTTCCTGCACCCAGTT<u>IIIIIIIIIIIIIII</u>GGTAA-CAGTACCGGTGC.
2. 5'-p-GGATCCGCTGAAACGCGCCGGAACCCCTGG<u>IIIIIIIIIIIIIIIII</u>-ACCGATGAGCCCGGTGAACA.
3. 5'-p-TCATCCTCAGGCTGCGCTCCGGTGATGGTCAGCGCAGC-TTTATCACCGATCAG.
4. 5'-p-CAGAACGGTCAGTTTGGTACCTCCGCC<u>IIIIIIIIIIIIIIIIIIIII</u>-CAGCGCGCAGAAGTAGATCGCT.
5. 5'-CGGCGGGAACAGGGTAACCGACGGGCTGCTTTTCGG-CTGACC.

2.3.1.5. Purification of Deoxyoligonucleotides

1. 12% Polyacrylamide gels containing $7M$ urea.
2. Gel elution buffer: 100 mM Tris, pH 8.0, 500 mM NaCl, 5 mM EDTA, pH 8.0.
3. Sep-Pak C18 Cartridges (Millipore, Bedford, MA).
4. TEAB buffer: 0.1M triethlyammonium bicarbonate, pH 7.3, 50% methanol.

2.3.1.6. Other LCR Reagents

1. Reaction buffer (10X): 200 mM Tris-HCl, pH 7.6, 100 mM KCl, 100 mM MgCl$_2$, 1% Triton X-100, 1 mM ATP, 10 mM DTT.
2. *Pfu* DNA ligase (Stratagene).
3. pSK4 template DNA.
4. GeneClean (B10 101, La Jolla, CA).

2.3.2. Polymerase Chain Reaction (PCR)

1. V_H upstream primer: 5'-AGCTGCAAAGCTAGCGGTTACACCTTCACC.
2. V_H downstream primer: 5'-CGCCACCAGATCTGGAGGACACGGTCA-GGCTCGCGCCTTGG.
3. V_L upstream primer: 5'-GCCGCTCGAGCACCGGTACTGTTAC.
4. V_L downstream primer 5'-CCGTTGGAGCTCGGCGGGAACAGGGTA.
5. *Taq* DNA polymerase and 10X PCR buffer (Perkin Elmer, Norwalk, CT).

2.4. Phage Display and Biopanning

1. Suitable restriction and DNA-modifying enzymes (N. E. Biolabs, Beverly, MA).
2. *E. coli* XL1-Blue cells (Stratagene).
3. SOC medium (Life Technologies).
4. SB medium (35 g/L tryptone, 20 g/L yeast extract, 5 g/L NaCl) containing 50 or 100 μg/mL ampicillin and 75 μg/mL tetracycline.
5. M13K07 helper phage (Life Technologies).
6. 20% Polyethylene glycol (PEG; Sigma, St. Louis, MO), containing 2.5M NaCl.
7. *Salmonella* serogroup B lipopolysaccharide (LPS).
8. Microtiter plates.
9. Phosphate-buffered saline (PBS): 16.5 mL 0.2M NaH$_2$PO$_4$·H$_2$O and 33.5 mL 0.2M Na$_2$HPO$_4$/L.
10. 0.1M sodium acetate buffer, pH 2.8, containing 0.5M NaCl.
11. 2M Tris-HCl, pH 9.5.
12. Isopropylthiogalactopyranoside (IPTG; Sigma).
13. Lysis buffer: 50 mM Tris-HCl, pH 8.0, containing 150 mM NaCl, 5 mM MgCl$_2$, 400 μg/mL lysozyme, and 1 U/mL DNase.
14. PBST: PBS (*see* Section 2.4.) containing 0.05% Tween-20.
15. Antimouse λ chain–biotin conjugate (Caltag, San Francisco, CA), diluted 1:10,000 in PBST.
16. Streptavidin/horseradish peroxidase (HRP) conjugate (Kirkegaard and Perry, Gaithersburg, MD) diluted 1:1000 in PBST.
17. HRP substrates: TMB (3,3',5,5'-tetramethylbenzidine) system (Kirkegaard and Perry).
18. HRP stopping solution: 1M phosphoric acid.

2.5. DNA Sequencing

1. dsDNA cycle sequencing kit (Life Technologies).
2. V_H primers: 5'-TGCGAGCGTTAAAATGAGCTGC and 5'-CGATTGGC-CTTGATATTCACAAACC.
3. V_L primers: 5'-CCGCTCTGCTGAACCTGAACTTG and 5'-ACCGCTA-TCGCGATCGCAG.

2.6. Production and Isolation of scFv

1. Termination sequence: 5'-GATCTTAATAGTGATCACTATTAA.
2. M-9 medium: 0.6 g Na_2HPO_4, 0.3 g $KH_2 PO_4$, 0.1 g $NH_4 Cl$, 0.1 g NaCl, 1 mM $MgCl_2$, 0.1 mM $CaCl_2$, 5 µg vitamin B-1, and 2 g glucose/L.
3. IPTG: *see* Section 2.4.
4. TB nutrients (12 g tryptone, 24 g yeast extract, and 4 mL glycerol/100 mL).
5. Sucrose buffer: 10 mM Tris-HCl, pH 8.0, containing 25% sucrose, 1 mM EDTA.
6. Shock buffer: 10 mM Tris-HCl, pH 8.0, containing 0.5 mM $MgCl_2$.
7. Affinity gel: *Salmonella essen O*-chain coupled to epoxy Sepharose.
8. Equilibration buffer: 50 mM Tris-HCl, pH 8.0, containing 0.15M NaCl.
9. Elution buffer: 100 mM Na acetate buffer, pH 4.5, containing 0.5M NaCl.
10. 1M Tris-HCl, pH 9.5.
11. PBS: *see* Section 2.4.

2.7. Affinity Measurements

1. Purified single-chain Fvs.
2. BSA-*O*-polysaccharide conjugate *(6)*.
3. 10 mM Na acetate buffer, pH 4.5.
4. HBS buffer: 10 mM HEPES, pH 7.4, 100 mM NaCl, 3.3 mM EDTA.
5. 10 mM HCl.
6. BIAcore sensor chips (research-grade or CM5; Pharmacia Biosensor, Piscataway, NJ).
7. Amine coupling kit (Pharmacia Biosensor).

3. Methods

3.1. Vector Construction

1. Amplify the gene III sequence-encoding residues 198–406 from M13mp18 RF DNA by PCR with primers that incorporate *Bgl*II and *Hind*III sites.
2. Using the *Bgl*II and *Hind*III sites, insert the amplified sequence after the scFv gene in plasmid ptsFvLH(el), which encodes Se155-4 scFv with a V_L-V_H domain orientation with Val106L and Glu1H linked by a sequence (LGQPKSSPSVTLFPPSSNG) derived from the L-chain elbow region *(8)*.
3. Digest the resulting plasmid with *Pvu*II, and ligate the fragment containing scFv-gIII with the *Pvu*II large fragment of pBluescript II SK (+). Confirm the insertion orientation by *Hind*III-*Nae*I digestion. Phagemid expressing the highest level of fusion protein was used as wild-type scFv-gIII construct for mutation studies (pSK4 for the Se155-4 example given here).

3.2. Deoxyoligonucleotide Synthesis

1. Synthesize sense deoxyoligonucleotides with desired regions (Fig. 2) spiked at a level of 10% with an equimolar mixture of each of the four bases using an automatic DNA/RNA synthesizer model 394 (Applied

CDR-1H

Nhe I
25 Ser Gly Tyr Thr Phe Thr | Asn Tyr Trp Met His | Trp Ile Lys Gln Arg Pro Gly Gln Gly 44
   CTAGC GGT TAC ACC TTC ACC | AAC TAC TGG ATG CAC | TGG ATC AAA CAG CGG CCA GGT CAG GGT
   G   CCA ATG TTT AAG | III III III | ACC TAG TTT GTC GCC GCC CCA GTC CCA

CDR-2H

45 Leu Glu Trp Ile Gly Ala Ile | Tyr Pro Gly Asn Ser Ala Thr Phe | Tyr Asn His Lys Phe 64
   CTC GAA TGG ATC GGC GCC ATC | TAT CCG GGT AAC AGC GCT TTC | TAC AAC CAC AAA TTC
   GAG CTT ACC TAG CCG CGG TAG | III III III III III III III III | ATG TTG GTG TTT AAG

65 Arg Ala Lys Thr Lys Leu Thr Ala Val Thr Ser Thr Ile Thr Ala Tyr Met Glu Leu Ser 84
   CGT GCT AAA ACC AAA CTG ACC GCT GTT ACT AGT TCA TAC ATC ACC GCG TAC ATG GAA CTG AGC
   GCA CGA TTT TGG TTT GAC TGG CGA CAA TGA TCA AGT ATG TAG TGG CGC ATG TAC CTT GAC TCG

CDR-3H

85 Ser Leu Thr Asn Glu Asp Ser Ala Val Tyr Tyr Cys Thr Arg | Gly Gly His Gly Tyr Tyr 104
   AGC CTG ACC AAC GAA GAT TCT GCG GTT TAC TAC TGC ACG CGT | GGT GGT CAT GGT TAC TAC
   TCG GAC TGG TTG CTT CTA AGA CGC CAA ATG ATG ACG TGC GCA | III III III III III III
                                              Sty I site

105 Gly Asp Tyr Trp Gly Gln Gly Ala Ser Leu Thr Val Ser Ser 118
    GGT GAT TAC TGG GGC CAA GGC GCG AGC CTG ACC GTG TCC TCC A
    CCA CTA ATG ACC CCG GTT CCG CGC TCG GAC TGG CAC AGG TCCTAG
                                              Bgl II site

Fig. 2. Nucleotide and amino acid sequences of Se155-4 V_H showing CDR sequences (boxed) that were targeted for mutation. Boxed regions were spiked at a level of 10% with the other three nucleotides. I = inosine.

335

Biosystems Inc.). Synthesis of spiked oligos is performed essentially as described by Hutchison et al. *(13)*.

2. Synthesize antisense deoxyoligonucleotides with 100% inosine in the regions that base pair with the spiked regions in the sense oligonucleotides (Fig. 2).

3.3. Synthetic LCR Assembly of V Genes

3.3.1. V_H Domain

1. Purify oligonucleotides by electrophoresis in polyacrylamide-urea gels. Soak gel slices containing oligonucleotides overnight in elution buffer (3 mL) at 37°C.

2. Pass oligonucleotides through Sep-Pak C18 cartridges that had been previously washed once with 5 mL HPLC-grade methanol and twice with 5 mL distilled water. Following sample application, wash column cartridges four times with 5 mL distilled water. Elute DNA with 3 mL TEAB buffer. Dry samples in a savant SpeedVac centrifuge, and dissolve in sterile distilled water.

3. Prepare a synthetic LCR mixture containing 4 pmol of each of eight oligonucleotide building blocks in a total volume of 8 µL, 5 µL 10X reaction buffer, 4 µL *Pfu* DNA ligase, 5 µL (20 ng) template DNA (pSK4 encoding wild-type Se155-4 scFv), and 28 µL distilled water. *See* Note 3.

4. Perform LCR in a thermocycler (Perkin Elmer Cetus GeneAmp PCR System 9600) by running step I (92°C for 3 min, 60°C for 3 min) for 1 cycle, step II (92°C for 45 s, 60°C for 30 s) for 30 cycles and step III (92°C for 4 min, 60°C for 3 min) for 1 cycle.

5. Purify the 300-bp LCR product by agarose gel electrophoresis, and isolate using Geneclean.

6. Kinase 50% of LCR product and ligate between the *Nhe*I and *Bgl*II sites of the wild-type phagemid vector, pSK4 (Fig. 3).

7. Amplify the remaining LCR product by PCR using *Taq* DNA polymerase in a GeneAmp 9600 system at 94°C for 3 min (1 cycle), 94°C for 35 s, 50°C for 45 s, 72°C for 30 s (15 cycles), and 72°C for 5 min for the final extension. The PCR product is digested with *Nhe*I and *Bgl*II, and cloned between the *Nhe*I and *Bgl* II sites of the phagemid vector pSK4 (Fig. 3).

8. Combine the ligation products from steps 6 and 7, and electroporate 2–3 µL aliquots into 80 µL *E. coli* XL1-Blue cells at 50 µF, 1800 V_{max}, and 150 Ω to give approx 2×10^7 transformants.

3.3.2. V_L Domain

1. Assemble V_L oligonucleotides by LCR using 5 pmol of each of the 10 oligonucleotides, one of which contains a diagnostic *Bss*HII site. Reaction

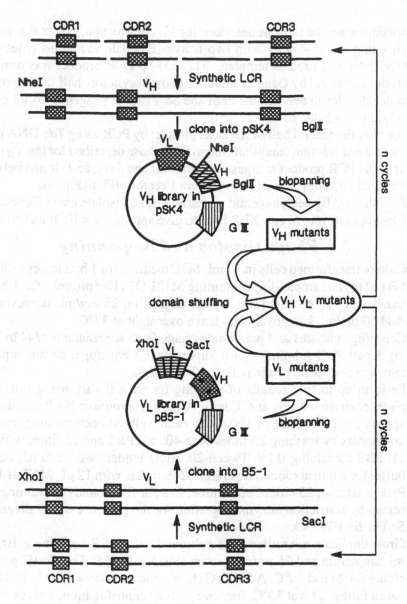

Fig. 3. Library generation strategy showing the LCR assembly of eight oligonucleotides encoding the CDR randomized V$_H$ library and LCR assembly of ten oligonucleotides encoding the CDR randomized V$_L$ library using the wild-type (WT) scFv gene as the template DNA for the V$_H$ library and the mutant B5-1, isolated from the first stage library, scFv gene as the template DNA for the V$_L$ library.

conditions are the same as described for V_H construction, except that pB5-1, encoding Se155-4 scFv with two heavy (H)-chain mutations (Met34Ile, Gly109Ser), is used as template. The 300-bp LCR product was removed from agarose gel by Geneclean. After phosphorylation, half of the product is directly cloned between the *Xho*I and *Sac*I sites of phagemid vector pB5-1 (Fig. 3). *See* Note 4.

2. Amplify the second half of the LCR product by PCR using *Taq* DNA polymerase and reaction conditions identical to those described for the V_H product. The PCR product is digested with *Xho*I and *Sac*I, and cloned between the *Xho*I and *Sac*I sites of the phagemid vector pB5-1 (Fig. 3).

3. Pool the two ligated phagemid preparations, and isolate using GeneClean. Electroporate into *E. coli* XL1-Blue to give approx 1.2×10^7 transformants.

3.4. Phage Display and Biopanning

1. Culture transformed cells in 17 mL SOC medium for 1 h, transfer to 30 mL SB (50 µg/mL ampicillin) containing M13KO7 (10^{12} pfu/mL) for 1 h, and transfer to 200 mL SB (100 µg/mL ampicillin, 25 mg/mL tetracycline). Add 50 mg/mL kanamycin and leave overnight at 37°C.

2. Centrifuge cultures and precipitate phage from supernatants *(14)* by adding 1 part PEG solution/4 parts supernatant. Centrifuge, decant supernatant, and resuspend phage pellet in 2 mL PBS.

3. Perform up to five rounds of panning for each library using microtiter plates coated overnight at 4°C with 10 µg/mL serogroup B LPS, and apply approx 2×10^{11} phage in 100 µL to each well. At each panning, remove nonbinders by washing 25 times with 400 µL PBS and 25 times with 400 µL PBS containing 0.1% Tween-20. Elute binders with 200 µL acetate buffer for 8 min at room temperature. Neutralize with 12 µL 2*M* Tris-base.

4. Pick at random 25 clones after three, four, or five rounds of panning, and screen by restriction enzyme digestion for the presence of the diagnostic *Sty*I or *Bss*HII sites.

5. Grow duplicate microtiter plate cultures (200 µL SB containing 100 µg/ mL ampicillin and 25 µg/mL tetracycline/well) of *Sty*I or *Bss*HI positive clones for 24 h at 30°C. Add IPTG (final concentration = 1 m*M*), and incubate a further 24 h at 30°C. Remove cells by centrifugation, and resuspend in 100 µL lysis buffer. After 1 h, remove cell debris by centrifugation and retain supernatants.

6. Coat microtiter plates overnight at 4°C with 10 µg/mL serogroup B LPS in 0.1*M* sodium carbonate buffer, pH 9.8. Wash plates three times with PBS, and add blocking solution. Leave for 1 h, wash three times with PBS and apply 100-µL aliquots of supernatants (diluted 1:1 with PBS) from lysed microtiter plate cultures. Leave for 3 h, wash three times with PBST,

and add 100-µL aliquots of anti L-chain conjugate to wells. After 1 h, wash three times with PBST, and add 100-µL aliquots of streptavidin conjugate to wells. Wash plates three times with PBST, and add peroxidase substrate. Stop the reactions by acid addition, and measure A_{280}. Unless stated otherwise, procedures are carried out at room temperature.

3.5. DNA Sequencing

1. Pick, at random, 20 clones from each library before biopanning, screen for the presence of the diagnostic *Sty*I and *Bss*HII sites, and sequence the scFv genes in each direction. *See* Note 5.
2. Sequence clones showing activity levels above that of the wild-type or B5-1 by ELISA screening.

3.6. scFv Production and Isolation

1. On the basis of ELISA screening, digest V_H mutants and V_L mutants with improved binding with *Bgl*II, and insert self-complementary terminator sequence between the scFv and gIII regions using standard ligation conditions. *See* Note 6.
2. Grow 1-L cultures of selected mutants in M-9 at 25°C for 24 h. Add 100 mL TB nutrients and IPTG to give a final concentration of 1 m*M*. Incubate a further 72 h at 25°C.
3. Centrifuge cultures, wash cells twice with wash buffer, and suspend cells from 1 L in 50 mL sucrose buffer (room temperature). Leave 10 min and resuspend in 50 mL ice-cold shock buffer. Leave 10 min and centrifuge. Retain supernatants as periplasmic extracts.
4. Dialyze periplasmic extracts against column equilibration buffer, and apply to affinity column equilibrated in the same buffer. Wash out unbound material with the equilibration buffer, and recover bound scFv with elution buffer.
5. Neutralize eluted fraction with 1*M* Tris, and dialyze against PBS prior to affinity measurements.

3.7. Affinity Measurements

1. Immobilize, using the amine coupling kit, the BSA-*O*-polysaccharide on sensor chips in 10 m*M* Na acetate, pH 4.5 (using the amine coupling kit), at concentrations and contact times that give approx 200 response units (RU) of immobilized conjugate.
2. Perform measurements at 25°C in HBS at a flow rate of 5 µL/min. Regenerate surfaces with 10 m*M* HCl. Using an appropriate range of concentrations for each mutant, determine the kinetics of scFv binding to the BSA-*O*-polysaccharide conjugate from association and dissociation rate constants calculated using BIAevaluation 2.0 software. *See* Notes 7–9.

4. Notes

1. The main objective in the examples described here was to introduce diversity in the CDRs at a relatively low level that would exert a fine-tuning effect on antigen binding. The main advantage of the technique is the flexibility that it provides in targeting different levels of randomization to selected regions of a molecule. Spiking at higher levels would generate libraries encoding more diverse structures with possible specificities for a wide variety of antigens. Targeting the introduction of diversity to selected framework regions could be used to restore full activity to antibodies in which murine CDRs had been grafted on human frameworks.

2. The antisense strand oligonucleotides are synthesized such that the spiked regions of the sense oligonucleotides are paired with inosine in the antisense strands. This is done to facilitate annealing of complementary strands, since inosine acts as a general base-pairing partner. Assuming this strand is replicated in vivo and can be PCR-amplified in vitro, this would introduce completely randomized CDR sequences into the library, but only two clones from 20 sequenced unpanned clones showed a run of Gs in VH CDR3, thought to be the result of inosine incorporation.

3. Although template DNA was employed in the examples given here, we have successfully performed synthetic LCR in the absence of template. In the latter case, oligonucleotides corresponding to the complete sequence of the desired gene are synthesized and permitted to form DNA duplexes via annealing of overhangs sufficiently long (approx 15 bases) to allow for stable base-pairing with adjacent DNA duplexes. Diphosphate ester bonds are formed by heat-stable *Pfu* DNA ligase.

4. It should be possible to achieve further affinity improvements by repeated cycles of CDR randomization/phage selection (Fig. 3).

5. DNA sequencing showed all possible substitutions: A → T, C, G; T → C, A, G; C → T, A, G; G → T, C, A. Some deletion and frameworks mutations, thought to result from DNA synthesis errors or *Taq* DNA polymerase infidelity, were also observed.

6. The self-complementary sequence gives the same reading frame, regardless of orientation.

7. These assays are performed using a BIAcore™ biosensor system (Pharmacia Biosensor). BIAcore is an automated surface plasmon resonance-based instrument that permits real-time biospecific analysis of unlabeled reactants. One of the interacting molecules (BSA-*O*-chain in the examples described here) is coupled covalently to the sensor chip surface, where the interactions and detection occur. The second interacting molecule (scFv in the examples described here) is passed over the sensor chip surface using an integrated fluidics system, and the interaction is recorded

as a sensorgram by an on-line computer. Kinetic and affinity constants can be calculated from sensorgrams using software supplied by the manufacturer.

8. Other techniques, including standard ELISA procedures, could be used to monitor affinity changes.

9. Amino acid substitutions were limited to a relatively small number of positions in the mutants selected from the libraries described here. Frequently occurring mutations included Met34HIle, Ser56HGly, Ala57HGly, Ile77H-The, and Gly109HSer. Several factors such as removal of steric clashes between the extended epitope and H-chain CDR2, improved scFv production in *E. coli* and increased scFv dimerization formed the basis of selection.

Acknowledgments

The authors thank Doris Bilous for synthesizing the deoxyoligonucleotides and Joe Michniewicz for help with the DNA sequencing. They also acknowledge the assistance of Tomoka Hirama and Joanna Sadowska with the screening assays. This is NRCC publication no. 37431.

References

1. Marks, J. D., Hoogenboom, H. R., Bonnert, T. P., McCafferty, J., Griffiths, A. D., and Winter, G. (1991) By-passing immunization: human antibodies from V-gene libraries displayed on phage. *J. Mol. Biol.* **222,** 581–597.

2. Griffiths, A. D., Malmqvist, M., Marks, J. D., Bye, J. M., Embleton, M. J., McCafferty, J., Baier, M., Holliger, K. P., Gorick, B. D., Hughes-Jones, N. C., Hoogenboom, H. R., and Winter, G. (1993) Human anti-self antibodies with high specificity from phage display libraries. *EMBO J.* **12,** 725–734.

3. Deng, S.-J., MacKenzie, C. R., and Narang, S. A. (1993) Simultaneous randomization of antibody CDRs by a synthetic ligase chain reaction strategy. *Nucleic Acids Res.* **21,** 4418–4419.

4. Landegren, U., Kaiser, R., Sanders, J., and Hood, L. (1988) A ligase-mediated gene detection technique. *Science* **241,** 1077–1080.

5. Barany, F. (1991) Genetic disease detection and DNA amplification using cloned thermostable ligase. *Proc. Natl. Acad. Sci. USA* **88,** 189–193.

6. Bundle, D. R., Eichler, E., Gidney, M. A. J., Meldal, M., Ragauskas, A., Sigurskjold, B. W., Sinnott, B., Watson, D. C., Yaguchi, M., and Young, N. M. (1994) Molecular recognition of a *Salmonella* trisaccharide epitope by monoclonal antibody Se155-4. *Biochemistry* **33,** 5172–5182.

7. Cygler, M., Rose, D. R., and Bundle, D. R. (1991) Recognition of a cell-surface oligosaccharide of pathogenic *Salmonella* by an antibody fragment. *Science* **253,** 442–445.

8. Anand, N. N., Mandal, S., MacKenzie, C. R., Sadowska, J., Sigurskjold, B., Young, N. M., Bundle, D. R., and Narang, S. A. (1991) Bacterial expression and secretion of various single-chain Fv genes encoding proteins specific for a *Salmonella* serotype B *O*-antigen. *J. Biol. Chem.* **266,** 21,874–21,879.

9. Brummell, D. A., Sharma, V. P., Anand, N. N., Bilous, D., Dubuc, G., Michniewicz, J., MacKenzie, C. R., Sadowska, J., Sigurskjold, B. W., Sinnott, B., Young, N. M., Bundle, D. R., and Narang, S. A. (1993) Probing the combining site of an anti-carbohydrate antibody by saturation-mutagenesis: role of the heavy-chain CDR3 residues. *Biochemistry* **32,** 1180–1187.
10. Deng, S.-J., MacKenzie, C. R., Sadowska, J., Michniewicz, J., Young, N. M., Bundle, D. R., and Narang, S. A. (1994) Selection of antibody single-chain variable fragments with improved carbohydrate-binding by phage display. *J. Biol. Chem.* **269,** 9533–9538.
11. Schlom, J., Eggensperger, D., Colcher, D., Molinolo, A., Houchens, D., Miller, L. S., Hinkle, G., and Siler, K. (1992) *Cancer Res.* **53,** 1067–1072.
12. Berek, C. and Milstein, C. (1987) Mutation drift and repertoire shift in the maturation of the immune response. *Immunol. Rev.* **96,** 23–41.
13. Hutchison, C. A., Nordeen, S. K., Vogt, K., and Edgell, M. H. (1986) A complete library of point substitution mutants in the glucocorticoid response element of mouse mammary tumor virus. *Proc. Natl. Acad. Sci. USA* **83,** 710–714.
14. Cwirla, S. E., Peters, E. H., Barrett, R. W., and Dower, W. S. (1990) Peptides on phage: a vast library of peptides for identifying ligands. *Proc. Natl. Acad. Sci. USA* **87,** 6378–6382.

CHAPTER 23

Chaperonins in Phage Display of Antibody Fragments

Eskil Söderlind, Marta Dueñas, and Carl A. K. Borrebaeck

1. Introduction

The display of antibody fragments on the surface of filamentous bacteriophages (1–7) constitutes a powerful system for the selection of molecules with desired specificities. In phage display, the antibody fragment is coupled to the minor coat protein (protein3) of bacteriophage M13 phage and is, in this way, both anchored in the phage capsid and exposed on the phage surface, linking specificity and genetic information. This permits direct isolation and sequence determination of the gene encoding the antibody fragment. The gene can subsequently be exposed to further engineering and selection in order to improve affinity and specificity.

The procedure of selecting antibody fragments with phage-display methodology entails several steps. The V region genes in B-cells are amplified, ligated into a phagemid vector, and electroporated into the *Escherichia coli* host. Any gene coding for the V regions can be amplified using the polymerase chain reaction and degenerate primers (8,9). Antibody gene libraries cloned in *E. coli* can then be rescued by infecting the *E. coli* cells with a helper phage, resulting in the packaging of phage particles with antibody fragments displayed on their surface. Natural gene libraries derived from different B-cell populations have served as sources for various antibody specificities, selected using phage-display methodology. Semisynthetic gene libraries have been constructed in which one or several CDR regions of pre-existing V-region genes have

From: *Methods in Molecular Biology, Vol. 51: Antibody Engineering Protocols*
Edited by: S. Paul Humana Press Inc., Totowa, NJ

been mutagenized in vitro to produce new antibody specificities *(10,11)*. Furthermore, completely synthetic antibody gene repertoires have also been constructed, opening the way for selection and design of synthetic antibody fragments *(12)*.

To tap the vast potential of antibody libraries further, new selection systems have been developed in which the selection of specificity of the antibody fragment is directly linked to the replication of the genes encoding the specificity, thus mimicking the humoral immune response *(13)*. These systems are based on engineered bacteriophages, where a portion or the entire gene3 in the helper phage has been deleted.

Here, we review the use of the GroE molecular chaperonins in antibody engineering. Molecular chaperonins are proteins that assist in the folding of polypeptides into their functional forms *(14)*. ATP is consumed in this process, and the chaperonins themselves are released after assisting in polypeptide folding.

2. Chaperonin-Assisted Phage Display

The size of a phage antibody gene library is determined by two factors. First, the transformation frequency determines the number of individual clones in the library. Second, the amplification of the bacteriophages determines the copy number of each individual clone. Both these parameters are important for successful selection of antibody fragments.

Transformation into *E. coli* with phagemid yields around 10^8 different clones/μg electroporated DNA. This number is only a fraction of the total number of different antibody genes in the human immune system, which can be as high as 10^{12} *(11)*. Thus, only a small fraction of the human antibody gene repertoire is displayed on the phage surface in any particular transformation experiment.

The limitation of the electroporation technique for transformation has been partly overcome with the development of so-called extended libraries. Such libraries offer an increased representation of individual clones and, therefore, an increased probability of finding the desired specificity. The use of the *lox*-Cre site-specific recombination system *(15)* has been successful in producing libraries containing up to 6.5×10^{10} different members *(11)*. Several high affinity antibody fragments have been selected from these large libraries.

A large number of individual clones is not enough, however, for successful selection and cloning of antibody fragments with desired specificities. If phages encoding such specificities are represented only in a few copies, it will be difficult to find these specificities. One possible way to increase the copy number of individual clones is to grow large quantities of the phage and then concentrate the solution several-fold *(11)*. For example, if a 1-L culture with a phage titer of 10^{11} cfu/mL is concentrated 100-fold, the final titer would be 10^{13} cfu/mL. Thus, the representation of individual clones is elevated 100-fold.

We have examined the use of the molecular chaperonins GroES and GroEL (Hsp10, Hsp60) as an alternative approach to increase the phage titer. The GroES/L chaperonins have been found to take part in the assembly of the bacteriophage λ, T4, T5, and 186 *(16)*. Based on this rationale, we investigated the role of these chaperonins on the assembly of bacteriophage M13. Overexpression of the chaperonins GroES and GroEL from the pGroE-vector in *E. coli* assists in the assembly of foreign heterologous proteins in vivo *(17)* and folding of foreign proteins in vitro *(18)*. The pGroE plasmid carried a chloramphenicol-resistance marker and a p15A origin of replication. *E. coli* were coinfected with the pGroE plasmid and the phagemid vector pEXmide3 *(7)*, which carries an ampicillin resistance gene and a ColE1 origin of replication. When XL1-Blue cells harboring both these plasmids were infected with a helper phage, the pEXmide3 vector was exported into the medium as DNA packed in the M13 capsid. When equal volumes of phage supernatant were plated on bacteria grown in ampicillin, increased colony formation was observed from supernatants of bacteria harboring both vectors, compared to bacteria harboring a control vector (Fig. 1). Clearly, expression of GroE resulted in an improved phage titer (by nearly 200-fold; from ~4 $\times 10^{11}$ cfu/mL to ~7 $\times 10^{13}$ cfu/mL). As control, the bacteria were infected with the empty vector pTG10, which does not contain the genes for GroES/L chaperonins. No amplification of the phage titer could be detected using the empty vector.

The increase in the phage titer is beneficial only if the proportion of particles with displayed antibody fragments is not affected. Therefore, it was important to examine the presence of functional antibody fragments on the phage surface in the chaperonin-assisted phage preparations compared to the nonassisted phage preparations. At equivalent infectivity titers, the two phage preparations displayed identical antigen binding in an ELISA, indicating approximately equivalent display of the antibody fragments.

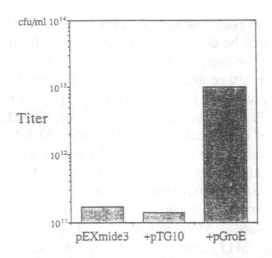

Fig. 1. Increased phage titer (expressed in colony-forming units, cfu) of ampicillin resistant pEXmide3 phagemid by the GroES/L chaperonin assisted assembly. pEXmide3, without coexpression of chaperonins; +TG10, coexpressed pEXmide3 and TG10 (empty vector); +pGroE, coexpressed pEXmide3 and pGroE.

3. Chaperonins in Intracellular Expression of Antibody Fragments in *E. coli*

Expression of antibody fragments in bacteria is a prerequisite for facile production of these proteins for their application as biosensors and their analysis by X-ray crystallography or NMR. The V_L and V_H subunits can be expressed in the form of noncovalent associated F_v fragments, single-chain F_v *(13,19,20)*, or Fab-fragments *(21,22)*, and their affinity parameters can be examined directly *(23)*. However, such heterologous expression systems in *E. coli* are not always successful. Factors like mRNA secondary structure *(24)* or misfolding of the protein in *E. coli (25)* are hurdles for successful antibody fragment expression. In the case of problems with secondary structure of mRNA, no protein is produced, probably because the structure of the nucleic acid hinders correct translation at ribosomes. On the other hand, misfolding of the protein yields a polypeptide with no biological activity, which accumulates in denatured form inside the host bacterium. It is possible to refold intracellularly expressed inactive antibody fragments in vitro into active proteins. The approach adopted here is first to allow high levels of protein accumulation inside the cell, with no regard to the folding of the protein into an active conformation. Accordingly, we have investigated the effect of GroES/L chaperonins on the levels of intracellularly produced antibody fragments.

A single-chain F_v fragment (scF$_v$) specific for carcinoembryonic antigen (CEA) was chosen as a model system *(25)*. The fragment was expressed intracellularly from the vector pIL-2f derived from the plasmid pFP-15 *(26)*. The scF$_v$ contains an N-terminal extension consisting of 26 residues of human interleukin-2, which probably stabilizes the molecule to proteolysis. The expression is under the control of the tryptophan promotor. A soluble, denatured scF$_v$ that is not aggregated is produced. Active scF$_v$ fragments can be obtained after refolding by dialysis, assessed using an ELISA to determine the antigen-binding activity. When the GroES/L chaperonins were coexpressed in this expression system, the concentration of intracellular anti-CEA scF$_v$ was upregulated from 0.6 to 1.2 mg/mL, determined by SDS-PAGE and Western blot analysis. The total yield of active refolded protein was increased in direct proportion to the amount of intracellularly expressed protein. Thus, in this system, the GroES/L chaperonins significantly increased the total amount of active protein recovered from the bacteria.

4. Effects of Chaperonins on Engineered Bacteriophages

The selection of a desired antibody specificity in vivo is followed by activation and proliferation of the antigen-specific B-cells. In contrast, selection of phage-displayed antibody fragments is performed by panning the phage preparation with immobilized antigens. After panning is completed, the eluted phages are reinfected into *E. coli* in order to clone and amplify the genes encoding the selected antibody specificity. This is an antigen-independent process.

We have designed a phage-display system in which the recognition of the antigen and amplification of the DNA encoding this specificity is linked, thus directly mimicking the clonal selection of cells during the immune response in vivo *(13)*. This system is called Selection and Amplification of Phages (SAP) and is based on the use of a helper phage that does not express protein3 in its capsids and, consequently, is unable to infect *E. coli* cells through the sex pili. Restoration of infectivity is obtained using a fusion protein composed of an N-terminus derived from protein3 and a C-terminus corresponding to the antigen against which antibodies are desired. When this fusion protein is presented to noninfectious phages displaying antibodies, only those phages that recognize the antigen will be capable of infecting *E. coli* and undergoing clonal expansion (Fig. 2). Clonal enrichment of specific antibody displaying phage by 10^{10}-fold has been achieved, which represents an important selection advantage when screening naive or synthetic libraries.

A portion of or the entire gene coding for protein3 was deleted in the helper phage used in the SAP system. The two truncated versions of M13K07 were constructed and assembled by PCR *(13)*. The first version is M13MDΔ3, which has a deletion between bases 1525 and 2646 of gene3, leaving behind a small C-terminal part of protein3. This truncated phage was used as a helper phage for superinfection of *E. coli*. Protein3 was produced by infection with a separate plasmid. Consequently, the packaged helper phage carries protein3 in the phage capsid, but does not carry the DNA encoding functional protein3 in its genome. This type of phage can only infect host cells once. Using the M13MDΔ3 helper phage, we obtained phage stocks with an infectivity titer of ~10^5 cfu/mL (kanamycin resistant). A second generation of M13 (M13MDΔ3.2) was then constructed carrying a deletion between nucleotides 1579 and 2851, resulting in removal of the entire gene3 sequence. When M13MDΔ3.2 was packaged as helper phage, titers as high as 10^9 cfu/mL were obtained (Table 1). This suggests an important role for the intergenic region in regulation of phage packaging *(27)*.

Control M13MDΔ3, M13MDΔ3.2, and two derivatives of bacteriophage Fd tet (fKN 16 and fCA 55; these contain 507- and 930-bp deletions in gene III, respectively; ref. *28*) exhibited low phage titers. As noted above, when these phages were produced in *E. coli* together with a plasmid that provided protein3 in trans-complementation to the phage particle, increased infectivity and increased titers were evident. Table 1 shows the different helper phage titers obtained with or without the coexpression of protein3. Although incorporation of protein3 in the phage capsid did restore the infection potential in every case, different phage titers were observed using different vectors. In *E. coli* TG1 host cells, the M13MDΔ3 phage formed only 4×10^5 cfu/mL (kanamycin resistant) when complemented with protein3, in contrast to M13MDΔ3.2 and fCA 55, which yielded titers of 3×10^8 and 5×10^8 cfu/mL, respectively.

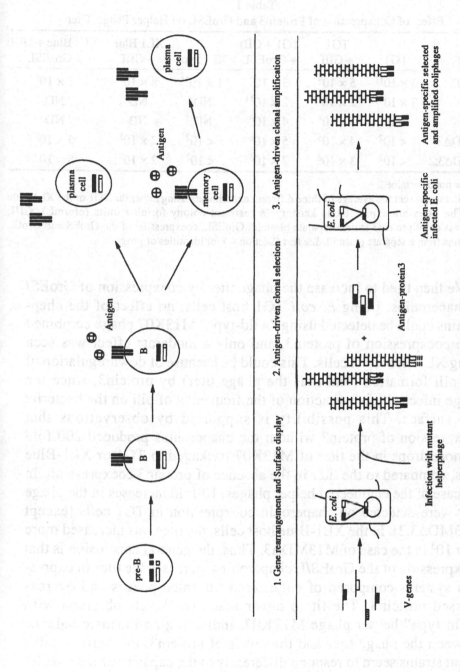

Fig. 2. A schematic representation of the analogy between the immune system and a bacteriophage based system. The principle of selection and amplificaton of phages (SAP) is illustrated (13).

Table 1
Effect of Coexpression of Protein3 and GroESL on Helper Phage Titer

PHAGE	TG1	TG1 + GIII	TG1 + GIII + GroESL	XL1 Blue	XL1 Blue + GIII	XL1 Blue + GIII + GroESL
M13 K07	3×10^{11}	5×10^9	3×10^9	1×10^{11}	8×10^8	1×10^9
fKN 16	3×10^4	2×10^{10}	2×10^{11}	ND[a]	ND	ND
fCA 55	$< 10^2$	5×10^8	4×10^9	ND	ND	ND
M13 MDΔ3	$< 10^2$	4×10^5	5×10^6	$< 10^2$	2×10^5	5×10^8
M13 MDΔ3.2	$< 10^2$	3×10^8	2×10^8	$< 10^2$	2×10^9	5×10^9

[a]ND = not determined.
The titers represent the average of three different experiments using either the TG1 or the XL1-blue strain. The titers are expressed as kanamycin resistant colony-forming units (cfu/mL). GIII, overexpression of protein3 from a separate plasmid; GroESL, coexpression of the GroES and GroEL chaperonins from a separate plasmid. *See text* (Section 4.) for identities of phage.

We then tried to increase the phage titer by coexpression of GroES/L chaperonins. Using *E. coli* TG1 host cells, no effect of the chaperonins could be detected using "wild-type" M13K07 phage combined with coexpression of protein3, and only a moderate effect was seen using XL1-Blue host cells. This could be because of downregulation of sex pili formation (and thus the phage titer) by protein3, since the phage infectivity is a function of the frequency of pili on the bacterial cell surface. This possibility is supported by observations that coexpression of protein3 without the chaperonins produced 200-fold or more drops in the titer of M13K07 packaged in TG1 or XL1-Blue cells, compared to the titer in the absence of protein3 coexpression. In the case of the engineered helper phages, 10-fold increases in the phage titer were detected on chaperonin coexpression in TG1 cells (except M13MDΔ3.2). In the XL1-Blue host cells, the titer was increased more than 10^3 in the case of M13MDΔ3. Thus, the general conclusion is that coexpression of the GroES/L chaperonins increases the titer in expression systems composed of engineered truncated phages and overexpressed protein3. The titers never reach the levels obtained with "wild-type" helper phage M13K07, indicating an intrinsic balance between the phage titer and the levels of protein3. Furthermore, different strains seem to respond differently to the capacity of the GroES/L chaperonins to assist in phage assembly.

5. Conclusions

The chaperonins GroES/L can be used in phage display of engineered antibodies. The coexpression of chaperonins increased the titer of packed phagemid vector, i.e., the copy number of individual clones. This is useful when high-phage titers are required, as in the screening of large extended libraries. When the chaperonins were coexpressed with scF$_v$ fragments, the intracellular expression of the antibody fragment was increased twofold, and the yield of the refolded fragment was also increased by the same factor. Finally, coexpression of the chaperonins increased the titer of truncated helper phages, as demonstrated with several different versions of helper phages containing gene3 deletions.

Acknowledgment

This investigation was supported by the Swedish Research Council for Engineering Sciences.

References

1. Parmley, S. F. and Smith, G. P. (1988) Antibody-selectable filamentous fd phage vectors affinity purification of target genes. *Gene* **73,** 305–318.
2. McCafferty, J., Griffiths, A. D., Winter, G., and Chiswell, D. J. (1990) Phage antibodies: filamentous phage displaying antibody variable domains. *Nature* **348,** 552–554.
3. Barbas, C. F., III, Kang, A. S., Lerner, R. A., and Benkovic, S. J. (1991) Assembly of combinatorial antibody libraries on phage surfaces: the gene III site. *Proc. Natl. Acad. Sci. USA* **88,** 7978–7982.
4. Chang, C. N., Landolfi, N. F., and Queen, C. (1991) Expression of antibody Fab domains on bacteriophage surfaces. Potential use for antibody selection. *J. Immunol.* **147,** 3610–3614.
5. Garrard, L. J., Yang, M., O'Conell, M. P., Kelley, R. F., and Henner, D. J. (1991) Fab assembly and enrichment in a monovalent phage display system. *Bio/Technology* **9,** 1373–1377.
6. Hoogenboom, H. R., Griffiths, A. D., Johnson, K. S., Chiswell, D. J., Hudson, P., and Winter, G. (1991) Multi-subunit proteins on the surface of filamentous phage: methodologies for displaying antibody (Fab) heavy and light chains. *Nucleic Acids Res.* **19,** 4133–4137.
7. Söderlind, E., Simonsson Lagerkvist, A.-C., Dueñas, M., Malmborg, A.-C., Ayala, M., Danielsson, L., and Borrebaeck, C. A. K. (1993) Chaperonin assisted phage display of antibody fragments on filamentous bacteriophage. *Bio/Technology* **11,** 503–507.
8. Larrick, J. W., Danielsson, L., Brenner, C. A., Abrahamsson, M., Fry, K. E., and Borrebaeck, C. A. K. (1989) Rapid cloning of rearranged immunoglobulin genes from human hybridoma cells using mixed primers and polymerase chain reaction. *Biochem. Biophys. Res. Commun.* **160,** 1250–1256.

9. Campbell, M. J., Zelenetz, A. D., Levy, S., and Levy, R. (1992) Use of family specific leader region primers for PCR amplification of the human heavy chain variable region gene repertoire. *Mol. Immunol.* **29,** 193–203.
10. Barbas, C. F., III, Bain, J. D., Hoekstra, D. M., and Lerner, R. A. (1991) Semisynthetic combinatorial libraries: a chemical solution to the diversity problem. *Proc. Natl. Acad. Sci. USA* **89,** 4457–4461.
11. Griffiths, A. D., Williams, S. C., Hartley, O., Tomlinson, I. M., Waterhouse, P., Crosby, W. L., Kontermann, R. E., Jones, P. T., Low, N. M., Allison, T. J., Prospero, T. D., Hoogenboom, H. R., Nissim, A., Cox, J. P. L., Harrison, J. L., Zaccolo, M., Gherardi, E., and Winter, G. (1994) Isolation of high affinity human antibodies directly from large synthetic repertoires. *EMBO J.* **13,** 3245–3260.
12. Söderlind, E., Vergeles, M., and Borrebaeck, C. A. K. (1995) Domain libraries: synthetic diversity for de novo design of antibody V-regions. *Gene,* in press.
13. Dueñas, M. and Borrebaeck, C. A. K. (1994) Clonal selection and amplification of phage displayed antibodies by linking antigenic recognition and phage replication. *Bio/Technology* **12,** 999–1002.
14. Ellis, R. J. (1994) Molecular chaperones. Opening and closing the Anfinsen cage. *Curr. Biol.* **4,** 633–635.
15. Waterhouse, P., Griffiths, A. D., Johnson, K. S., and Winter, G. (1993) Combinatorial infection and in vivo recombination: a strategy for making large phage antibody repertoires. *Nucleic Acids Res.* **21,** 2265,2266.
16. Zeilstra-Ryalls, J., Fayet, O., and Georgopoulos, C. (1991) The universally conserved GroE (Hsp60) chaperonins. *Annu. Rev. Microbiol.* **45,** 301–325.
17. Goloubinoff, P., Gatenby, A. A., and Lorimer, G. H. (1989) GroE heat shock proteins promote assembly of foreign procaryotic ribulose bisphosphate carboxylate in *Escherichia coli. Nature* **337,** 44–47.
18. Goloubinoff, P., Christeller, J. T., Gatenby, A. A., and Lorimer, G. H. (1989) Reconstitution of active ribulose bisphosphate carboxylase from an unfolded state depends on two chaperonin proteins and MG-ATP. *Nature* **342,** 884–889.
19. Huston, J. S., Levinson, D., Mudgett-Hunter, M., Tai, M.-S., Novotny, J., Margolies, M. N., Ridge, R. J., Bruccoleri, R., Haber, E., Crea, R., and Opperman, H. (1988) Protein engineering of antibody binding sites: recovery of specific activity in an anti-digoxin single-chain Fv analogue. *Proc. Natl. Acad. Sci. USA* **85,** 5879–5883.
20. Skerra, A. and Plückthun, A. (1988) Assembly of a functional immunoglobulin Fv fragment in *Escherichia coli. Science* **240,** 1038–1041.
21. Plückthun, A. and Skerra, A. (1989) Expression of functional antibody Fv and Fab fragments in *Escherichia coli. Methods Enzymol.* **178,** 497–515.
22. Ward, E. S., Güssow, D., Griffiths, A. D., Jones, P. T., and Winter, G. (1989) Binding activities of a repertoire of immunoglobulins secreted from *Escherichia coli. Nature* **341,** 544–546.
23. Borrebaeck, C. A. K., Malmborg, A.-C., Furebring, C., Michaelsson, A., Ward, S., Danielsson, L., and Ohlin, M. (1992) Kinetic analysis of recombinant antibody-antigen interactions: relation between structural domains and antigen binding. *Bio/Technology* **6,** 697,698.

24. Dueñas, M., Ayala, M., Vázguez, J., Ohlin, M., Söderlind, E., Borrebaeck, C. A. K., and Gavilondo, J. V. (1995) A point mutation in a murine immunoglobulin V-region strongly influences the antibody yield in *Escherichia coli*. *Gene*, in press.
25. Dueñas, M., Vázquez, J., Ayala, M., Söderlind, E., Ohlin, M., Perez, L., Borrebaeck, C. A. K., and Gaviolondo, J. V. (1994) Intra-and extracellular expression of a scFv antibody fragment in *E. coli:* Effect of bacterial strains and pathway engineering using GroES/L chaperoniris. *BioTechniques* **16,** 476–483.
26. Novoa, L. I., Madrazo, J., Fernandez, J. R., Benitez, J., Narciandi, E., Rodriquez, J. C., Estrada, M. P., Garcia, J., and Herrera, L. (1991) Method for the expression of heterologous protein produced in fused fon-n in *E. coli*, use thereof, expression vectors and recombinant strains. European Patent Application 416673 A1.
27. Dueñas, M. and Borrebaeck, C. A. K. (1995) Novel helper phage design: intergenic region affects the assembly of bacteriophages and the size of antibody libraries. *FEMS Microbiol. Lett.* **125,** 317–322.
28. Crissman, J. W. and Smith, G. P. (1984) Gene-III protein of filamentous phages: evidence for carboxy-terminal domain with a role in morphogenesis. *Virology* **132,** 445–455.

CHAPTER 24

Phage-Display Libraries of Murine and Human Antibody Fab Fragments

Jan Engberg, Peter Sejer Andersen, Leif Kofoed Nielsen, Morten Dziegiel, Lene K. Johansen, and Bjarne Albrechtsen

1. Introduction

This chapter describes efficient systems for construction, expression, and screening of comprehensive libraries of murine or human antibody Fab fragments displayed monovalently on the surface of filamentous (fd) phage. Both systems use phagemid vectors that co-express combinations of randomly assembled pairs of light (L) and heavy (H) coding regions under transcriptional control of the *lacZ* promoter. The combinatorial Fab gene cassette is inserted in-frame with a truncated version of the phage surface protein pIII (ΔpIII), which results in the positioning of the assembled Fab molecule at one tip of the phage particle.

The PCR-amplified murine Fd (composed of V_H and C_H1 domains) and L-chain coding regions are assembled into a bicistronic operon by a PCR-based technique before cloning, whereas the PCR-amplified human V_H and L-chain coding regions are cloned directly into a specially designed phagemid vector. This vector contains the remaining coding parts necessary for the generation of a bicistronic mRNA encoding the complete Fab molecule. Expression of the L and H chains as soluble periplasmic proteins permits Fab assembly within the periplasmic space. On infection with helper phage, the Fab-ΔpIII fusion proteins become displayed on the phage surface by displacing some of the wild-type pIII proteins (1–6). Enrichment of Fab phages with affinity for a specific

From: *Methods in Molecular Biology, Vol. 51: Antibody Engineering Protocols*
Edited by: S. Paul Humana Press Inc., Totowa, NJ

antigen is done by successive rounds of affinity purification on antigen-coated microtiter wells and reinfection of *E. coli* cells by the bound phages.

2. Materials

2.1. Extraction of Total RNA from Mouse Spleen or Human Blood Lymphocytes and Production of cDNA

1. Buffer A: Add 0.36 mL β-mercaptoethanol to 50 mL buffer B just before use.
2. Buffer B: 4*M* guanidinium thiocyanate, 25 m*M* sodium citrate, pH 7.0, 0.5% sarcosyl (filter-sterilized, stable at room temperature for 3 mo).
3. 2*M* sodium acetate (NaOAc), pH 4.1: Mix 41 mL 2*M* CH₃COOH and 9 mL 2*M* NaOAc.
4. Chloroform:isoamyl alcohol (49:1): 49 volumes chloroform and 1 vol isoamyl alcohol.
5. Diethylpyrocarbonate (DEPC) water: Double-distilled water containing 0.1% DEPC is incubated at 37°C for 60 min followed by autoclaving.
6. Water-saturated (DEPC) phenol: Phenol is extracted three times with DEPC-treated water.
7. 5 m*M* dNTP: 5 m*M* dTTP, 5 m*M* dATP, 5 m*M* dGTP, and 5 m*M* dCTP (100 m*M* lithium salt solutions, pH 7.0, from Boehringer Mannheim [Mannheim, Germany] are diluted with DEPC-treated water).
8. 5X first-strand buffer (Gibco/BRL, Gaithersburg, MD): 0.25*M* Tris-HCl, pH 8.3 at room temperature, 0.375*M* KCl, 15 m*M* MgCl₂.
9. Superscript reverse transcriptase (200 U/μL; Gibco/BRL).

2.2. PCR-Assembly Method for Constructing Murine Antibody Fab Libraries

1. Murine H-chain-variable region primers (*see* Notes 1 and 2 and Fig. 1):

```
MVH-1:  G CCG GCC ATG GCC GAG GTR MAG CTT CAG GAG TCA GGA C
MVH-2:  G CCG GCC ATG GCC GAG GTS CAG CTK CAG CAG TCA GGA C
MVH-3:  G CCG GCC ATG GCC CAG GTG CAG CTG AAG SAS TCA GG
MVH-4:  G CCG GCC ATG GCC GAG GTG CAG CTT CAG GAG TCS GGA C
MVH-5:  G CCC GCC ATG GCC GAR GTC CAG CTG CAA CAG TCY GGA C
MVH-6:  G CCC GCC ATG GCC CAG GTC CAG CTK CAG CAA TCT GG
MVH-7:  G CCG GCC ATG GCC CAG STB CAG CTG CAG CAG TCT GG
MVH-8:  G CCC GCC ATG GCC CAG GTY CAG CTG CAG CAG TCT GGR C
MVH-9:  G CCG GCC ATG GCC GAG GTY CAG CTY CAG CAG TCT GG
MVH-10: G CCG GCC ATG GCC GAG GTC CAR CTG CAA CAA TCT GGA CC
MVH-11: G CCG GCC ATG GCC CAG GTC CAC GTG AAG CAG TCT GGG
MVH-12: G CCG GCC ATG GCC GAG GTG AAS STG GTG GAA TCT G
MVH-13: G CCG GCC ATG GCC GAV GTG AAG YTG GTG GAG TCT G
```

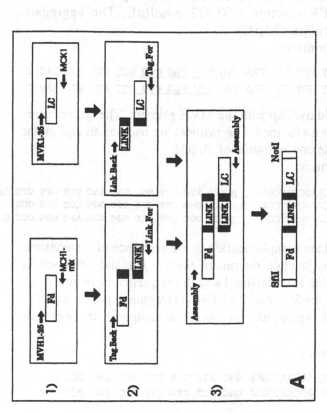

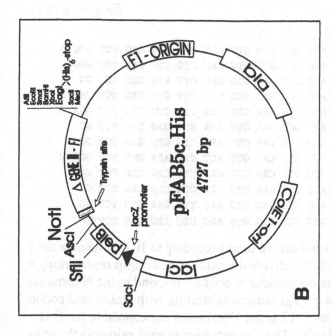

Fig. 1. Overview of the primers and the steps involved in the PCR assembly of murine Fab gene fragments and a map of the expression vector pFab5c. (A) Strategy for "Jumping-PCR" assembly. Diagram exemplifying the primary amplification PCR (1), the linker assembly (2), and the final assembly (3), respectively. The boxes show different gene segments included in the construction of the Fab expression cassette: Fd, includes the H chain from the N-terminal amino acid to the cysteine residue of the hinge region, which forms the disulfide bridge to the C-terminal cysteine of the L chain; Light chain, corresponds to the entire variable and constant parts of the L (κ) chain; LINK, a 117-bp fragment containing a translational stop codon for Fd translation, a ribosome-binding site for L-chain expression and the coding region corresponding to the N-terminal part of the *PelB* leader. Primers depicted below the boxes are forward primers and complementary to mRNA. Primers above the boxes are back-primers and complementary to first strand cDNA. Stippled zones within boxes represent regions of overlapping complementarity. (B) Expression vector pFAB5c.His. Phagemid vector used for expression of murine antibody Fab fragments. The Fab antibody cassette is introduced as a *SfiI-NotI* fragment and is expressed from the inducible *lacZ* promoter (*see* ref. 6).

```
MVH-14:  G CCG GCC ATG GCC GAG GTG CAG SKG GTG GAG TCT GGG G
MVH-15:  G CCG GCC ATG GCC GAK GTG CAM CTG GTG GAG TCT GGG
MVH-16:  G CCG GCC ATG GCC GAG GTG AAG CTG ATG GAR TCT GG
MVH-17:  G CCG GCC ATG GCC GAG GTG CAR CTT GTT GAG TCT GGT G
MVH-18:  G CCG GCC ATG GCC GAR GTR AAG CTT CTC GAG TCT GGA
MVH-19:  G CCG GCC ATG GCC GAA GTG AAR STT GAG GAG TCT GG
MVH-20:  G CCG GCC ATG GCC GAA GTG ATG CTG GTG GAG TCT GGG
MVH-21:  G CCG GCC ATG GCC CAG GTT ACT CTR AAA GWG TST GGC C
MVH-22:  G CCG GCC ATG GCC CAG GTC CAA CTV CAG CAR CCT GG
MVH-23:  G CCG GCC ATG GCC CAG GTY CAR CTG CAG CAG TCT G
MVH-24:  G CCG GCC ATG GCC GAT GTG AAC TTG GAA GTG TCT GG
MVH-25:  G CCG GCC ATG GCC GAG GTG AAG GTC ATC GAG TCT GG
```

(One-letter nucleotide symbols are used according to IUB nomenclature.) These primers consist of 25 individually synthesized oligos representing a total of 88 variants. The nucleotides in bold correspond to the N-terminal part of the variable heavy (V_H) sequences starting with amino acid codon number one. Nucleotides 1–13 at the 5'-terminus correspond to the C-terminal part of the *pel*B leader. The concentration of each primer in the mixture used for the PCR reaction is 0.227 pmol/µL. The aggregate concentration is 20 pmol/µL (20 µ*M*).

2. Secondary extension primers:

```
Tag.Back1:  CA GTC ACA GAT CCT CGC GAA TTG GCC CAG CCG GCC ATG GCC SAN G
Tag.Back2:  CA GTC ACA GAT CCT CGC GAA TTG GCC CAG CCG GCC ATG GCC SAN C
```

The nucleotides in bold overlap with the MVH primers. The *Sfi*I recognition site (*see* Fig. 1) is underlined. The primers are used as an equimolar mixture at an aggregate concentration of 20 µ*M*.

3. Murine C_H1 chain primers:

```
MCH1-G1:   CGACTAGTTTAGAATTCAAGCTGTCGAC TCA ACA ATC CCT GGG CAC AAT TTT CTT GTC CAC
MCH1-G2A:  CGACTAGTTTAGAATTCAAGCTGTCGAC TCA ACA GGG CTT GAT TGT GGG CCC TCT GGG
MCH1-G2B:  CGACTAGTTTAGAATTCAAGCTGTCGAC TCA ACA GGG GTT GAT TGT TGA AAT GGG CCC G
```

Nucleotides in bold are complementary to the sequence of the constant heavy (C_H1) and hinge junction regions of the γ1, γ2a, and γ2b H-chain isotypes. The stop codon is underlined and the sequence positions 1–26 are complementary to the 5'-end of the LINK-D fragment, positions 1–26. The primers were used as an equimolar mixture at an aggregate concentration of 20 µ*M*.

4. Murine κ L-chain primers:

```
MVK-1:  TTGGCTGCACAACCAGCAATGGCA GAC ATT GTT CTC ACC CAG TCT CC
MVK-2:  TTGGCTGCACAACCAGCAATGGCA GAC ATT GTG CTS ACC CAG TCT CC
```

```
MVK-3:  TTGGCTGCACAACCAGCAATGGCA GAC ATT GTG ATG ACT CAG TCT CC
MVK-4:  TTGGCTGCACAACCAGCAATGGCA GAC ATT GTG CTM ACT CAG TCT CC
MVK-5:  TTGGCTGCACAACCAGCAATGGCA GAC ATT GTG YTR ACA CAG TCT CC
MVK-6:  TTGGCTGCACAACCAGCAATGGCA GAC ATT GTR ATG ACA CAG TCT CC
MVK-7:  TTGGCTGCACAACCAGCAATGGCA GAC ATT MAG ATR ACC CAG TCT CC
MVK-8:  TTGGCTGCACAACCAGCAATGGCA GAC ATT CAG ATG AMC CAG TCT CC
MVK-9:  TTGGCTGCACAACCAGCAATGGCA GAC ATT CAG ATG ACD CAG TCT CC
MVK-10: TTGGCTGCACAACCAGCAATGGCA GAC ATT CAG ATG ACA CAG ACT AC
MVK-11: TTGGCTGCACAACCAGCAATGGCA GAC ATT CAG ATG ATT CAG TCT CC
MVK-12: TTGGCTGCACAACCAGCAATGGCA GAC ATT GTT CTC AWC CAG TCT CC
MVK-13: TTGGCTGCACAACCAGCAATGGCA GAC ATT GTT CTC TCC CAG TCT CC
MVK-14: TTGGCTGCACAACCAGCAATGGCA GAC ATT GWG CTS ACC CAA TCT CC
MVK-15: TTGGCTGCACAACCAGCAATGGCA GAC ATT STG ATG ACC CAR TCT C
MVK-16: TTGGCTGCACAACCAGCAATGGCA GAC ATT KTG ATG ACC CAR ACT CC
MVK-17: TTGGCTGCACAACCAGCAATGGCA GAC ATT GTG ATG ACT CAG GCT AC
MVK-18: TTGGCTGCACAACCAGCAATGGCA GAC ATT GTG ATG ACB CAG GCT GC
MVK-19: TTGGCTGCACAACCAGCAATGGCA GAC ATT GTG ATA ACY CAG GAT G
MVK-20: TTGGCTGCACAACCAGCAATGGCA GAC ATT GTG ATG ACC CAG TTT GC
MVK-21: TTGGCTGCACAACCAGCAATGGCA GAC ATT GTG ATG ACA CAA CCT GC
MVK-22: TTGGCTGCACAACCAGCAATGGCA GAC ATT GTG ATG ACC CAG ATT CC
MVK-23: TTGGCTGCACAACCAGCAATGGCA GAC ATT TTG CTG ACT CAG TCT CC
MVK-24: TTGGCTGCACAACCAGCAATGGCA GAC ATT GTA ATG ACC CAA TCT CC
MVK-25: TTGGCTGCACAACCAGCAATGGCA GAC ATT GTG ATG ACC CAC ACT CC
```

These primers consist of 25 individually synthesized oligos representing a total of 50 variants. The concentration of each variant in the mixture used for the PCR reactions is 0.4 pmol/µL. Aggregate concentration is 20 pmol/µL (20 µM). Nucleotides in bold correspond to the 5'-end of the κ chain sequences starting with amino acid codon number one. Sequence positions 1–24, corresponding to the C-terminal part of the *pel*B leader, overlap the LINK-D fragment, positions 94–117.

5. Murine C_K chain primer:

MCK1: TGC GGC CGC ACA CTC ATT CCT GTT GAA GCT CTT GAC

Sequences in bold are complementary to the C-terminus of the constant part of the κ chain. The *Not*I recognition site (*see* Fig. 1) is underlined.

6. Extension primer:

Tag.For: CAG TCA CAG ATC CTC GCG AAT TGG TGC GGC CGC ACA CTC ATT CCT G

The sequence in bold corresponds to that of MCK1, positions 1–22. The *Not*I site is underlined.

7. Linker primers:

Link.Forw: GTC TGC CAT TGC TGG TTG TGC AGC CAA

This sequence is complementary to the 3'-end of the LINK-D fragment.

Link.Back: CGA CAG CTT GAA TTC TAA ACT AGT CGA AGG CGC GCC AAG GAG ACA GTC AT

This sequence overlaps the 5'-end of the LINK-D fragment.

8. LINK-D fragment:

CGACAGCTTGAATTCTAAACTAGTCGAAGGCGCGCC<u>AAGGAG</u>ACAGTCATA <u>ATG</u> AAA
TAC CTA TTG CCT ACG GCA GCC GCT GGA TTG TTA TTA **TTG GCT GCA CAA
CCA GCA ATG GCA**

The bold-faced sequence at the 5'-end overlaps with the MCH1 primers, whereas the sequence in bold at the 3'-end is complementary to the MVK primers. The ribosome-binding site and the ATG triplet marking the start of the *pel*B leader sequence is underlined. The LINK-D fragment originates from the λc2 vector *(6)* and was taken through several PCR cloning steps using different sets of tagged primers in order to introduce the sequence changes necessary for the present assembly system. The LINK-D fragment was cloned into the Bluescript KS+ vector giving rise to pLINK-D as described in ref. *(6)*.

9. Assembly primer:

Assembly: CA GTC ACA GAT CCT CGC GAA TTG G.

This sequence is complementary to the 5' end of Tag.For and Tag.Back. The concentration of the working solution is 5 μM.

10. 10X *Taq* buffer I (Perkin-Elmer Cetus, Norwalk, CT).
11. AmpliTaq polymerase (Perkin-Elmer Cetus, 5 U/μL).
12. GeneClean (Bio101 Inc., Vista, CA).
13. 10X buffer 3 (New England Biolabs, Beverly, MA).
14. 10X BSA (0.1%, Amersham, Buckinghamshire, UK).
15. *Sfi*I.
16. *Not*I.
17. Qiagen maxiprep columns (Qiagen GmbH, Hilden, Germany).
18. T₄ DNA ligase (Gibco, 1 U/μL).
19. 5X T₄ DNA ligase buffer (Gibco).
20. Genepulser and electroporation cuvets (Bio-Rad, Hercules, CA).
21. The vector pFAB5c.His, contains several improvements to the pFAB5c vector previously described by us *(6)*. In the polylinker region downstream of ΔgIII, an adaptor was introduced that contained an *Eag*I site followed by six histidine codons ending with a stop codon. This makes it possible to delete ΔgIII by *Eag*I digestion followed by religation, since *Eag*I recognizes a subset of the *Not*I recognition sequence *(see* Fig. 1). The latter site is regenerated. Additionally, the His and stop codons are in reading frame

with C_K, and the (His)$_6$ tail facilitates easy purification of free Fab molecules on metal affinity columns. (Johansen et al., manuscript submitted).

22. TE buffer, LB, 2X TY, and SOC media were prepared as described in ref. *(7)*.
23. Ampicillin is used at a concentration of 100 µg/mL and tetracycline at a concentration of 10 µL/mL.
24. *E. coli* strains used:

JM 103: *thi⁻,strA,supE,endA,sbcB,hsdR⁻Δ(lac-proAB), F'{traD36, proAB, lacI^q,lac-ZΔ15}*

TOP10F': *mcrA,Δ(mrr-hsdRMS-mcrBC)θ80ΔlacX74,deoR, recA1,araD1,Δ(ara.leu), 7697,galU,galK,λ⁻, rpsL, endA1,nupG,F'{tet^r}* (British Biotechnology).

XL-1 Blue: *recA1,endA1,gyrA96,thi,hsdR17(r_k^-,m_k^+),supE44, relA1.λ⁻, (lac), F'{proAB,l acI^q,laZΔM15,Tn10 (tet^r}* (Stratagene, La Jolla, CA).

2.3. Direct Cloning Method for Making Human Antibody Fab Libraries

1. Human H-chain V-region primers (*see* Fig. 2):

HVH-1: CAG CCA GCA ATG GCA **CAG GTN CAG CTG GTR CAG TCT GG**

HVH-2: CAG CCA GCA ATG GCA **CAG GTC CAG CTK GTR CAG TCT GGG G**

HVH-3: CAG CCA GCA ATG GCA **CAG GTK CAG CTG GTG SAG TCT GGG**

HVH-4: CAG CCA GCA ATG GCA **CAG GTC ACC TTG ARG GAG TCT GGT CC**

HVH-5: CAG CCA GCA ATG GCA **CAG GTG CAG CTG GTG GAG WCT GG**

HVH-6: CAG CCA GCA ATG GCA **CAG GTG CAG CTG GTG SAG TCY GG**

HVH-7: CAG CCA GCA ATG GCA **CAG GTG CAG CTG CAG GAG TCG G**

HVH-8: CAG CCA GCA ATG GCA **CAG GTG CAG CTG TTG SAG TCT G**

HVH-9: CAG CCA GCA ATG GCA **CAG GTG CAG CTG GTG CAA TCT G**

HVH-10: CAG CCA GCA ATG GCA **CAG GTG CAG CTG CAG GAG TCC GG**

HVH-11: CAG CCA GCA ATG GCA **CAG GTG CAG CTA CAG CAG TGG G**

HVH-12: CAG CCA GCA ATG GCA **CAG GTA CAG CTG CAG CAG TCA G**

These primers consist of 12 individually synthesized oligonucleotides representing a total of 31 variants. The nucleotides in bold correspond to the 5'-sequences of the V_H region starting with the codon for amino acid number one. Primers are invariant for the first five nucleotides from position +1 of the V-region. The first 15 nucleotides at the 5'-end of the primers correspond to the 3'-part of the *Pel*B leader gene. This gives a unique template for the primer, HVH.EXT, used in the secondary extension PCR (*see* step 3 *below*). The concentration of each variant in the solution used for the PCR is 0.65 pmol/µL. The total concentration is 20 pmol/µL.

2. Human H-chain J-region primers:

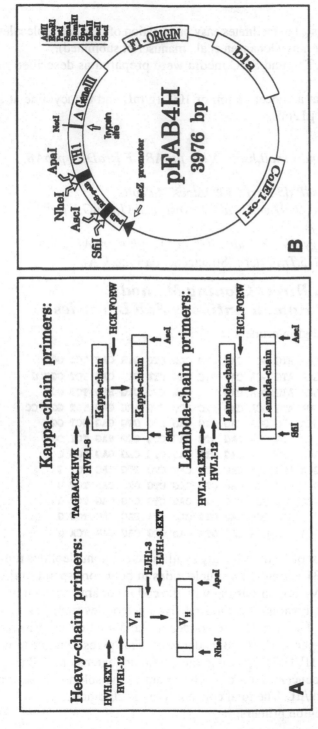

Fig. 2. Overview of the primers used to generate human F_v, κ, and λ fragments and a map of the expression vector pFab4H. (A) PCR overview (human Fab). Diagram exemplifying the primary PCR amplifications and extensions of the V_H, κ, and λ gene fragments. (B) Expression vector pFAB4H. Phagemid vector used for expression of antibody fragments. The V_H fragment is introduced as a NheI-ApaI fragment. The κ and λ chains are introduced as SfiI-AscI fragments. The region between the AscI and NheI sites consists of a 117-bp fragment containing a translational stop codon for κ and λ translation, a ribosome-binding site for Fd expression, and the coding region corresponding to the N-terminal part of the PelB leader. The region between the ApaI and NotI sites consists of the C_H1-γ1 region.

HJH1: GGC TGA GGA GAC RGT GAC CAG GGT
HJH2: GGC TGA AGA GAC GGT GAC CAT TGT
HJH3: GGC TGA GGA GAC GGT GAC CGT GGT

The J-region primers consist of three individually synthesized oligonucleotides representing a total of four variants. All nucleotides are complementary to the J-region, and the first codon at the 5'-end corresponds to the amino acid residue 114 of C_H1 *(8)*. The concentration of each variant in the solution used for the PCR is 5 pmol/µL (5 µM).

3. Secondary H-chain extension primers:

HVH.EXT: GCA GCC GCT GGA TTG TTA TT<u>G CTA GC</u>A GCA **CAG CCA GCA ATG GCA CAG GT**
HJH.EXT: CAG TCA CAG ATC CTC GCG AAT T<u>GG GCC C</u>TT GGT GGA **GGC TGA RGA GAC RGT GAC C**

Nucleotides in HVH.EXT corresponding to sequences in HVH1-12 are in bold, and the *Nhe*I site is underlined. Nucleotides in HVJ.EXT corresponding to sequences in HJH1-3 are in bold, and the *Apa*I site is underlined. The aggregate concentration of variants in each primer solution used for PCR is 20 pmol/µL (20 µM).

4. Human κ-chain V-region primers:

HVK-1: G CCG GCC ATG GCC **GAC ATC CAR WTG ACC CAG TCT CC**
HVK-2: G CCG GCC ATG GCC **GAC ATC CRG ATG ACC CAG TCT CCW TC**
HVK-3: G CCG GCC ATG GCC **GAC ATC GTG MTG ACC CAG TCT CC**
HVK-4: G CCG GCC ATG GCC **GAC ATC GTG TTG ACS CAG TCT CCR GG**
HVK-5: G CCG GCC ATG GCC **GAC ATC GTG ATG ACY CAG WCT CCA C**
HVK-6: G CCG GCC ATG GCC **GAC ATC GTG ATG AYR CAG TCT CCA GC**
HVK-7: G CCG GCC ATG GCC **GAC ATC GTG MTG ACW CAG TCT CCA GA**
HVK-8: G CCG GCC ATG GCC **GAC ATC GTA ATG ACA CAG TCT CCA CC**

These primers consist of eight individually synthesized oligonucleotides representing 27 variants. Nucleotides in bold correspond to the 5'-sequences of the V_K gene starting with the codon for amino acid number one. The N-terminal two amino acids of the V-region are invariant. The sequences upstream of the V-region represent the 3'-part of the *Pel*B leader gene (located between the *Asc*I and *Nhe*I sites). This constitutes a unique template for the primers used in the secondary extension PCR (*see* step 6 *below*). The concentration of each variant in the solution used for the PCR is 0.74 pmol/µL. The aggregate concentration is 20 pmol/µL (20 µM).

5. κ-chain constant-region primer:

HCK.FORW: GTC TCC TTC TCG A<u>GG CGC GCC TCA CTA</u> **ACA CTC TCC CCT GTT GAA GCT**

This primer is complementary to codons for the seven carboxy-terminal amino acid residues of the κ-constant domain, indicated by bold letters. The tandem stop codons and the *Asc*I site are underlined. Concentration of working solution is 20 pmol/μL.

6. Secondary κ-chain extension primers:

TAGBACK.HVK: CA GTC ACA GAT CCT CGC GAA TT<u>G GCC CAG CCG GCC</u> **ATG GCC GAC ATC**

HCK.FORW: GTC TCC TTC TCG A<u>GG CGC GCC</u> TCA <u>CTA</u> ACA CTC TCC CCT GTT GAA GCT

The bold-faced part of the TAGBACK.HVK sequence overlaps with the 5'-end of the primary PCR primers. The *Sfi*I site introduced into the secondary V$_K$ PCR products is underlined. The concentration of the working solution is 20 pmol/μL. The HCK.FORW primer is used for both the primary and secondary amplifications.

7. Human λ-chain V-region primers:

HVL-1: G CCG GCC ATG GCC **CAG TCT GYC CTG ACT CAG CCT G**
HVL-2: G CCG GCC ATG GCC **CAG TCT GCC CTG ACT CAG CCT C**
HVL-3: G CCG GCC ATG GCC **CAG TCT GTG CTG ACT CAG CCG TC**
HVL-4: G CCG GCC ATG GCC **CAG TCT ATG CTG ACT CAG CCC CAC TC**
HVL-5: G CCG GCC ATG GCC **CAG TCT GTG CTG ACT CAG CCA CCC TC**
HVL-6: G CCG GCC ATG GCC **CAG TCT GAG CTG ACT CAG GAC CCT GC**
HVL-7: G CCG GCC ATG GCC **CAG TCT GAG GTG ACT CAG GAG CC**
HVL-8: G CCG GCC ATG GCC **CAG TCT GTG ATG ACY CAG TCT CMA**
HVL-9: G CCG GCC ATG GCC **CAG TCT GTG CTG ACT CAG CCA CC**
HVL-10: G CCG GCC ATG GCC **CAG TCT GTS BTG ACG CAG CCG CC**
HVL-11: G CCG GCC ATG GCC **CAG TCT CAG CTG ACG CAG CCT GC**
HVL-12: G CCG GCC ATG GCC **CAG TCT TTA YTG ACT CAA YCG CCC TC**

These primers consist of 12 individually synthesized oligonucleotides representing a total of 24 variants. Nucleotides in bold correspond to the 5'-sequences of the V$_λ$ genes starting with the codon for amino acid number one. The remaining nucleotides are identical to the similarly positioned nucleotides in the κ primers. The concentration of each variant in the solution used for PCR is 0.83 pmol/μL. The aggregate concentration is 20 pmol/μL.

8. Human λ-chain constant region primer:

HCL.FORW: GTC TCC TTC TCG A<u>GG CGC GCC</u> TCA <u>CTA</u> **TGA ACA TTC YGT AAG GGC MAC**

HCL.FORW contains four variants and is complementary to codons for the seven carboxy-terminal amino acid residues of the λ-constant domain, indicated by bold letters. The tandem stop codons and the *Asc*I site are underlined. Concentration of working solution is 20 pmol/μL.

9. Secondary extension primers:

TAGBACK.HVL: CA GTC ACA GAT CCT CGC GAA TTG GCC CAG CCG GCC ATG GCC CAG TCT
HCL.FORW: GTC TCC TTC TCG AGG CGC GCC TCA CTA TGA ACA TTC YGT AAG GGC MAC

The features of the extension primer, TAGBACK.HVL, are analogous to those of the V_K extension primer, TAGBACK.HVK, described above. The HCL.FORW primer is used for both primary and secondary amplifications. The concentration of the working solution is 20 pmol/μL.

10. The vector, pFAB4H, has the general features depicted in Fig. 2 and is described in more detail in a separate publication *(9)*.
11. 10X *Taq* buffer (HT Biotech, Cambridge, UK).
12. Super*Taq* polymerase (HT Biotech).

2.4. Superinfection of Libraries

1. Phage-precipitation buffer: 20% polyethylene glycol (PEG$_{6000}$) in 2.5M NaCl.
2. PBS buffer: 8.1 mM Na$_2$HPO$_4$, 1.47 mM KH$_2$PO$_4$, 2.68 mM KCl, 137 mM NaCl, pH 7.4.
3. Helper phage R408 (approx 7.5×10^{10} PFU/mL obtained from Stratagene).
4. IPTG stock solution: 100 mM isopropyl-β-D-thiogalactopyranoside in sterile water.

2.5. Selection of Antigen Binders by Panning

1. Washing buffer: 0.5 % Tween-20 in PBS buffer.
2. Blocking buffer: 2% skimmed milk powder (Difco, Detroit, MI) in PBS buffer.
3. Trypsin elution buffer: 1 mg trypsin (Worthington, Freehold, NJ)/mL PBS buffer.
4. Glycine elution buffer: 0.1M glycine-HCl, pH 2.2, containing 1 mg/mL BSA.
5. Microtiter plates (Maxisorp, NUNC, Soskilde, Denmark).

3. Methods

3.1. Extraction of Total RNA from Mouse Spleen or Human Blood Lymphocytes and Production of cDNA

1. Add 10 mL of buffer A to a freshly dissected spleen from an immunized mouse (about 0.5–1 g), and transfer to a glass homogenizer (*see* Note 3). Spleen tissue is homogenized with repeated strokes of a Teflon™-coated pestle for 1 min in an ice-water bath. In the case of human blood, centrifuge 100 mL at 2000g for 10 min, collect 1 mL of the upper layer of the blood cell pellet (the "buffy coat" containing about 10^8 lymphocytes), and mix with 10 mL buffer A.

2. Transfer homogenate or lymphocytes to a chloroform/phenol-resistant centrifuge tube, and immediately add 1 mL 2*M* NaOAc, pH 4.1, 10 mL water-saturated phenol, and 2 mL chloroform:isoamyl alcohol (49:1). Whirlmix vigorously for 30 s.

3. Centrifuge at 10,000*g* for 20 min at 4°C.

4. Transfer upper phase to a fresh centrifuge tube, mix with 10 mL isopropanol, and let stand at −20°C for 30 min or longer.

5. Pellet the RNA by centrifugation at 12,000*g* for 30 min.

6. Discard the supernatant, resuspend the wet pellet in 0.5 mL buffer A, and repeat steps 2–5 above using appropriately scaled-down volumes. Resuspend final pellet in 0.5 mL buffer A, mix with 0.5 mL isopropanol, and keep at −20°C (*see* step 4 above).

7. Collect the RNA as in step 5 above, and resuspend the wet pellet in 0.5 mL DEPC-treated water.

8. Whirlmix for 1 min, spin for 5 min at 15,000*g*, transfer supernatant to a fresh microfuge tube, add 0.5 mL water-saturated phenol, whirlmix, spin for 1 min at 15,000*g*, and transfer upper phase to a fresh microfuge tube.

9. Add 0.5 mL chloroform, extract as described in step 8, and continue with phenol/chloroform extractions until no visible protein interphase is present.

10. Add 50 µL 3*M* NaOAc, pH 5.2 (0.1 vol), mix with 1.1 mL 96% ethanol (2 vol), and keep at −20°C until use.

11. When making cDNA, whirlmix the RNA/alcohol solution before transferring 200 µL to a fresh microfuge tube, and pellet the RNA by centrifugation at 15,000*g* for 15 min.

12. Wash the RNA pellet with 1 mL 70% ethanol before drying lightly in a SpeedVac centrifuge.

13. Resuspend pellet in 26 µL of DEPC-treated water, remove a 1-µL aliquot, and determine the concentration and purity. The RNA concentration should be about 2 µg/µL with an $A_{260/280}$ ratio of about 2.0.

14. Mix in an ice-cold sterile microfuge tube:

DEPC-treated water	2.5 µL
5 m*M* dNTP	5.0 µL
5X first-strand buffer	10.0 µL
0.1*M* DDT	5.0 µL

15. Add 2.5 µL poly(dT)$_{12-18}$ (500 µg/mL) to the remainder of the RNA solution from step 13 (25 µL), and incubate at 70°C for 10 min, cool on ice, centrifuge at 5000*g* for 5 s, and transfer supernatant to the cDNA mixture of step 14. The total volume is now 50 µL.

16. Incubate the mixture at 47°C for 2 min, add 3 µL SuperScript reverse transcriptase (200 U/µL) and continue incubation for 1 h at 47°C (*see* Note 4).

17. Following incubation, heat the reaction at 100°C for 3 min, centrifuge at 15,000g for 15 min, transfer supernatant to a fresh microfuge tube, and precipitate as in step 10. Resuspend pellet in 15 μL, DEPC-treated water.

3.2. PCR-Assembly Method for Constructing Murine Antibody Fab Libraries

The PCR-assembly method for making murine Fab antibody libraries consists of five steps:

1. Primary amplification of the Fd and κ L-chain genes.
2. PCR assembly of each of the primary PCR fragments with Link-D.
3. Final PCR assembly of pairs of Fd/LinkD and Link-D/L-chain fragments.
4. Cloning of the final PCR product into the expression vector pFAB5c.His.
5. Electroporation, plating, growth, and storage of library.

Figure 1 shows an overview of the PCR primers, the steps involved in the PCR assembly procedure, and the expression vector.

1. For primary amplification of the Fd gene fragment, mix in a PCR tube:

cDNA (*see* Section 3.1., step 17)	5 μL
10X *Taq* buffer I	10 μL
10X dNTP (1.25 m*M* each)	8 μL
MVH 1-25 (20 μ*M* mix)	2.5 μL
MCH1 mix (20 μ*M* mix)	2.5 μL
Sterile water	72 μL

   Top with two drops of mineral oil.

2. For primary amplification of the L-chain gene, mix in a PCR tube:

cDNA (*see* Section 3.1., step 17)	5 μL
10X *Taq* buffer I	10 μL
10X dNTP (1.25 m*M* each)	8 μL
MVK 1-25 (20 μ*M* mix)	2.5 μL
MCK 1 (20 μ*M*)	2.5 μL
Sterile water	72 μL

   Top with two drops of mineral oil.

3. For generation of the Link-D fragment, mix in a PCR tube:

Plasmid pLINK-D (1 ng/μL)	1 μL
10X *Taq* buffer I	10 μL
10X dNTP (1.25 m*M* each)	8 μL
Link.Back (20 μ*M*)	1 μL
Link.Forw (20 μ*M*)	1 μL
Sterile water	79 μL

   Top with two drops of mineral oil.

4. PCR program: 94°C 5 min, suspend, add 0.3 µL Ampli*Taq* polymerase (5 U/ µL); 94°C 1 min, 55°C 1 min, 72°C 1 min, 30 cycles, 72°C 10 min, refrigerate.
5. The primary amplification products are purified by 1 or 2% agarose gel electrophoresis in combination with GeneClean procedures according to the manufacturer's guidelines (Bio101 Inc.). Fd gene fragments are about 720 bp, L-chain genes about 650 bp, and the Link-D fragment is 117 bp (*see* Note 5).
6. For assembly of Fd gene fragments and the Link-D fragment, mix in a PCR tube (*see* Note 6).

1–50 ng purified Fd	5.00 µL
1–20 ng purified Link-D	2.00 µL
10X *Taq* buffer I	10.00 µL
10X dNTP (1.25 m*M* each)	8.00 µL
Tag.Back 1-2 (20 µ*M* mix)	1.25 µL
Link.For (20 µ*M*)	1.25 µL
Sterile water	72.50 µL

Top with two drops of mineral oil.
7. For assembly of L-chain gene fragments and the Link-D fragment, mix in a PCR tube:

About 5 ng purified L-chain	5.00 µL
About 1 ng purified Link-D	2.00 µL
10X *Taq* buffer I	10.00 µL
10X dNTP (1.25 m*M* each)	8.00 µL
Link.Back (20 µ*M*)	1.25 µL
Tag.For (20 µ*M* mix)	1.25 µL
Sterile water	72.50 µL

Top with 2 drops of mineral oil.
8. PCR program: 94°C 5 min, suspend, add 0.3 µL Ampli*Taq* polymerase (5 U/ µL); 94°C 1 min, 65°C 1 min, 72°C 1 min, 25 cycles, 72°C 10 min, refrigerate.
9. The assembled Fd/Link-D and Link-D/L-chain fragments, which have increased about 100 bp in size, are processed as described in step 5 above.
10. For final assembly, mix in a PCR tube (*see* Note 7):

1 ng purified Fd-Link-D	5 µL
1 ng purified L-chain-Link-D	5 µL
10X *Taq* buffer I	10 µL
10X dNTP (1.25 m*M* each)	8 µL
Assembly primer (5 µ*M*)	2 µL
Sterile water	70 µL

Top with two drops of mineral oil.

11. PCR program: 94°C 10 min, suspend, add 0.3 μL Ampli*Taq* polymerase (5 U/μL); 94°C 1.5 min, 69°C 1 min, 72°C 2 min, 25 cycles, 72°C 10 min, refrigerate.

12. The assembled Fd/Link-D/L-chain fragments (about 1.6 kb in size) are run on a 1.5% agarose gel and further purified using the GeneClean procedure.

13. Mix in a microcentrifuge tube:

About 0.5 μg of final assembly product	37.5 μL
10X buffer 3	5.0 μL
10X BSA (0.1%)	5.0 μL
*Sfi*I (50 U)	2.5 μL
Sterile water	7.5 μL

14. Incubate at 50°C for 3 h.

15. Add 3 μL *Not*I (25 U) and incubate at 37°C for three more hours (*see* Note 8).

16. Run the reaction mixture on a 1.5% agarose gel, and purify the DNA further using the GeneClean procedure. This step eliminates the small *Not*I and *Sfi*I fragments generated by cutting the ends off the final PCR assembly product. The purified fragment is resuspended in TE buffer at a final concentration of 50 ng/μL.

17. A plasmid maxipreparation of pFAB5c.His is made using Qiagen columns according to the manufacturer's recommendations. A portion is digested with *Sfi*I and *Not*I and processed as described in steps 13–16 above.

18. For ligation of insert to vector mix in a microfuge tube:

Insert DNA from 3.2.16. (50 ng/μL)	6.0 μL
Vector DNA from 3.2.17. (50 ng/μL)	6.0 μL
5X T$_4$ ligase buffer	10.0 μL
Sterile water	25.5 μL
T$_4$ DNA ligase (1 U/μL)	2.5 μL

and incubate over night at 16°C.

19. Add 80 μL TE buffer to the ligation mixture, extract once with phenol/chloroform (9:1), add 0.1 vol of 3*M* NaOAc, and precipitate with 2.5 vol ethanol. Collect precipitate by centrifugation at 15,000*g* for 30 min in a microfuge, rinse pellet with 70% alcohol, dry lightly in a SpeedVac centrifuge, and resuspend pellet in 10 μL sterile water.

20. Electrocompetent cells (TOP10F'Tc or XL-1 Blue; *see* Note 9) are prepared according to the protocol of the supplier of the *E. coli* electropulser (Bio-Rad) and stored at –80°C in 50-μL aliquots. The cells should preferably give 10^{10} transformants/μg DNA when tested with 10 pg of supercoiled pUC18.

21. Thaw cells on ice, transfer to an ice-cold cuvet (0.2 cm, Bio-Rad), and add 1 μL purified ligation mixture from step 19.

22. Apply a pulse at the setting of 25 μF, 2.5 kV, and 200 Ω, and add immediately thereafter 950 μL SOC medium supplemented with 10 mM MgCl$_2$.
23. Transfer the transformation mixture to a sterile 10-mL vial, and shake at 37°C for 1 h. Withdraw 1 μL, make dilutions, and spread on LB-ampicillin plates to obtain an estimate of the size of the total library.
24. For each 1 mL of transformation mixture, 40 mL LB-ampicillin/tetracycline medium supplemented with 1% glucose (*see* Note 10) are used, and the culture is incubated with shaking at 37°C until an OD$_{600}$ of 1–2 is reached. Five 8-mL aliquots are made into glycerol stocks (*7*), and plasmid DNA is prepared from the remainder of the culture to keep as a backup of the library.

3.3. Direct Cloning Method for Human Antibody Fab Libraries

The direct cloning method for constructing human antibody Fab libraries consists of five steps:

1. Primary PCR amplifications of the V$_H$, κ, and λ L-chains.
2. "Tagging" the primary amplification products with restriction enzyme sites.
3. Cloning of the V$_H$ cDNA fragments in pFAB4H (equivalent to the Fd library).
4. Cloning of the L-chain genes using the Fd library as vector material.
5. Electroporation, plating, growth, and storage of library.

Figure 2 shows an overview of the PCR primers and the expression vector.

1. For primary amplifications of F$_v$ gene fragments, mix in a PCR tube:

cDNA (*see* Section 3.1., step 17)	5 μL
10X *Taq* buffer	10 μL
10X dNTP (2 mM each)	10 μL
HVH 1-12 (20 μM mix)	1 μL
HJH 1-3 (20 μM mix)	1 μL
Sterile water	73 μL

   Top with two drops of mineral oil.
2. For primary amplification of κ-chain genes, mix in a PCR tube:

cDNA (*see* Section 3.1., step 17)	5 μL
10X *Taq* buffer	10 μL
10X dNTP (2 mM each)	10 μL
HVK 1-8 (20 μM mix)	1 μL
HCK.Forw (20 μM)	1 μL
Sterile water	73 μL

Top with two drops of mineral oil.
3. For primary amplification of lambda chain genes, mix in a PCR tube:

cDNA (*see* Section 3.1., step 17)   5 µL
10X *Taq* buffer   10 µL
10X dNTP (2 m*M* each)   10 µL
HVL 1-12 (20 µ*M* mix)   1 µL
HCL.Forw (20 µ*M*)   1 µL
Sterile water   73 µL

Top with two drops of mineral oil.
4. PCR program: 94°C 5 min, suspend, add 0.3 µL Super*Taq* polymerase (5 U/µL); 94°C 1 min, 55°C 1 min, 72°C 1 min, 30 cycles, 72°C 10 min, refrigerate (*see* Note 11).
5. Isolate the primary amplification products by preparative gel electrophoresis followed by GeneClean procedures (*see* Section 3.2., step 5). V_H gene fragments are about 380 bp, and κ and λ genes are about 680 bp.
6. For PCR extensions of the primary PCR products, use the methods described in the previous paragraphs with about 1 ng purified template material and 1 µL of 20-µ*M* solutions of the following primers:
For V_H extension: HVH.EXT and HJH.EXT
For κ extension: TAGBACK.HVK and HCK.FORW
For λ extension: TAGBACK.HVL and HCL.FORW
PCR program: 94°C 5 min, suspend, add 0.3 µL Super*Taq* polymerase (5 U/µL); 94°C 1 min, 55°C 1 min, 72°C 1 minute, 15 cycles, 72°C 10 min, refrigerate.
7. Cloning of human V_H gene fragments: In separate reactions, digest the extended and gel-purified V_H gene fragments and the plasmid pFAB4H with *Nhe*I and *Apa*I according to the manufacturer's recommendations, isolate the relevant fragments from agarose gels, and purify them further using the GeneClean procedure. This vector already contains the C_H1 domain. Insertion of V_H yields the Fd segment cDNA, corresponding to half of the H chain found in Fab.
8. Ligate, electroporate, and plate cells as described in steps 18–23, Section 3.2.
9. Harvest the cells at $OD_{600} = 1$ (*see* Section 3.2., step 24) and make a Qiagen maxiplasmid preparation according to the manufacturer's instructions. This DNA constitutes the Fd library and is used as vector material for the cloning of the L-chain genes.
10. Cloning of human L-chain genes: Digest the purified and extended κ and λ genes and the plasmid preparation containing the Fd-library with *Sfi*I and *Asc*I.
11. Ligate, electroporate, grow, and store cells as described in steps 18–24, Section 3.2. (*see* Note 9).

3.4. Superinfection of Libraries

1. Generation of Fab phages: 1 mL of a glycerol stock from step 24, Section 3.2. or step 11, Section 3.3. containing about 2×10^8 cells is used to inoculate 40 mL LB-medium containing ampicillin and tetracycline. Cells are grown at 37°C with shaking until OD_{600} of the culture reaches 0.5 (*see* Note 12).
2. Add 2×10^{11} R408 helper phage particles/40 mL of culture corresponding to a phage excess of about 50. The phage excess ensures that all cells become infected.
3. Incubate with gentle shaking for 20 min at 37°C.
4. Add IPTG to a final concentration of 100 μM (*see* Note 13), transfer the culture flask to a shaker at room temperature (*see* Note 14), and continue incubation with shaking at 300 rpm for a minimum of 10 and a maximum of 16 h (cell lysis occurs after 16 h).
5. Pellet the cells by centrifugation at 10,000g for 10 min.
6. Transfer supernatant to a fresh centrifuge tube, and add 1 vol of phage-precipitation buffer to 4 vol of phage supernatant. Mix the solution by shaking, and incubate at 4°C for 1 h or longer.
7. Pellet the phage particles by centrifugation at 15,000g for 30 min. Resuspend pellet in 1 mL of PBS buffer. Make a clearing spin at 15,000g for 15 min. Transfer supernatant to a fresh microfuge tube, and precipitate phages as above.
8. Resuspend pellet in 200 μL PBS buffer, make a clearing spin, and titrate Fab phages by counting ampicillin-resistant colonies formed by infection of a lawn of Top10/F'Tc cells. A Fab phage concentration of 5×10^{12} CFU/mL of the concentrated phages is typical. Store the phage stock at 4°C after filtration through a 0.45-μm Millipore filter.

3.5. Selection of Antigen Binders by Panning

1. Microtiter wells are coated with 100 μL of antigen solution (5–50 μg/mL in PBS) overnight at 4°C followed by two to three short rinses with washing buffer, and blocked for 2 h at room temperature with blocking buffer, using 300 μL/well.
2. Rinse the wells briefly two to three times in washing buffer, and transfer about 10^{11} Fab phages diluted in blocking solution (100 μL/well).
3. Incubate for 2–3 h with rocking at room temperature. After incubation, the wells are washed and rinsed with 200-μL solutions in the following manner (*see* Note 15):
   a. Five brief rinses in washing buffer.
   b. Incubation with blocking buffer for 10 min.
   c. Five incubations with washing buffer, each for 2 min.

d. Incubation with blocking buffer for 5 min.

e. Five incubations with washing buffer, each for 2 min.

f. Brief rinse in sterile water.

Bound phages are eluted by one of two methods: glycine-buffer treatment (steps 4 and 5) or digestion with trypsin (step 6).

4. Add 100 µL 0.1*M* glycine elution buffer/well. Incubate for 15 min at room temperature.

5. Transfer eluates to fresh microtiter wells containing 8 µL 2*M* Tris-base to neutralize the eluate.

6. Add 100 µL of trypsin elution buffer, and incubate for 30 min at room temperature.

7. The eluates from step 5 or 6 are transferred to vials containing 400 µL exponentially growing cells with an OD_{600} of 0.8–1.0 (*see* Note 16).

8. Incubate at 37°C for 20 min with gentle shaking.

9. Withdraw 5 µL from each culture, make serial dilutions, and spread on ampicillin plates to determine the number of ampicillin-transducing phages in the eluate.

10. Transfer each culture to 40 mL 2X TY-medium supplemented with 1% glucose, ampicillin, and tetracycline, and incubate at 37°C with shaking overnight.

11. Prepare glycerol stocks and plasmid DNA samples as described in step 24, Section 3.2.

12. For preparation of phages for the next round of panning, use 200 µL of the glycerol stock to inoculate 30 mL of TY medium containing ampicillin and tetracycline.

13. When the culture reaches an OD_{600} of 0.5–0.8, add 2×10^{11} R408 helper phages, and incubate at 37°C with gentle shaking for 20 min.

14. Add IPTG (final concentration 100 µ*M*), and grow overnight at room temperature with shaking.

15. Prepare phages for the next panning round as described in steps 5–8, Section 3.4.

16. Between each round of panning, determine the number of eluted bound phages relative to the amount of phages added to the wells. Likewise, the ELISA signal generated from a fixed amount of eluted bound phages should be monitored between each round of panning (we use peroxidase-conjugated anti-M13, Pharmacia Biotech [Sollentima, Sweden] as secondary antibody). An increase in these two parameters by a factor of 10 or more should be observed between each round of panning.

17. Following three or four rounds of panning, isolate individual clones and characterize their binding characteristics by ELISA assays.

4. Notes

1. All primers in the present study were synthesized on an Applied Biosystems oligonucleotide machine, model 394, and subsequently checked by electrophoresis on sequencing gels. Only high-quality preparations that predominantly contained full-size product were used for further applications.
2. The rationale behind the design of our rather extensive series of PCR primers for the variable H and L chains has been presented previously *(6)*. In short, we believe that the primer sets used should match all available sequence data for these regions, and we argue that highly degenerate primers for the variable regions are likely to generate biased libraries and to introduce amino acids not normally found in the variable regions.
3. We find it important to work with fresh biological material when isolating RNA *(see* Section 3.1., step 1). If immediate processing of samples is not possible, it is recommended to transport the sample to the laboratory as frozen material in an appropriate volume of buffer A, rather than to transport the sample as frozen material and then add buffer A upon arrival to the laboratory.
4. From previous experience working with reverse dideoxy sequencing of RNA *(10)*, we know that secondary structures in RNA can obstruct the processive action of reverse transcriptase, but that this can be overcome by increasing the reaction temperature. Because the GC content of the IgG mRNAs is relatively high *(8)* and will allow for extensive secondary structure formation, we recommend that cDNA synthesis be performed at 47°C *(see* Section 3.1., step 16).
5. If the yields of the primary PCR reactions are unsatisfactory, check the integrity of the RNA preparation by running a formaldehyde-agarose gel *(7)*. If the bands representing rRNA look distinct and are of the correct molecular size, assume that the mRNAs for H and L chains are intact, too. We recommend repeating the phenol/chloroform extractions described in Section 3.1., steps 8 and 9 to improve the success of the cDNA synthesis and subsequent PCR reactions.
6. This reaction sometimes needs optimization which is done by varying the relative concentrations of the two templates *(see* Section 3.2., step 6). We normally obtain the best results by using a 10-fold molar excess of the Link-D fragment to the Fd gene fragment.
7. It is important to use a relatively low concentration of the assembly primer (10 pmol/100 µL) in the final assembly reaction (Section 3.2., step 10).
8. Vectors prepared for ligation of inserts should always be checked for self-ligation as a measure of the extent of cleavage by *Sfi*I and *Not*I (Section 3.2., steps 13–15), *Nhe*I and *Apa*I (Section 3.3., step 8) and *Sfi*I and *Asc*I

(Section 3.3., step 10). Despite the fact that phage particles that do not have Fab molecules displayed on their surface will be mostly lost in the panning procedure, there will always be some nonspecific binding of the phage particles to the antigen coat of the microtiter plate. This may lead to an outgrowth of the specific binders because of the growth advantage of phage particles having a smaller genome size. This can be prevented by gel-purifying the entire library as phagemid DNA before each round of panning (Andersen et al., manuscript in preparation). As depicted in Fig. 1, pFab5c.His contains an *Asc*I site between the *Sfi*I and *Not*I sites. Additional cutting of the *Sfi*I and *Not*I-cleaved vector with *Asc*I will therefore reduce the chance of self-ligation effectively. Future versions of the pFab4H will include "stuffer" fragments between the cloning sites that contain recognition sites for restriction enzymes not found in known H- and L-chain sequences.

9. Since the pFab4H vector does not harbor the *lacI* gene, it is advisable to use XL-1 Blue (which contains the *lacI*q gene) when working with this vector.
10. Glucose is added to act as a catabolite repressor of *lacZ* promoter expression.
11. Super*Taq* (HT Biotechnology) and Ampli*Taq* (Perkin-Elmer Cetus), together with their cognate buffers, can be used interchangeably.
12. The stated conditions are suitable for libraries that contain about 10^7 or less members. If a larger library is used, scale-up correspondingly to ensure that all library members are represented in the inoculum. Tetracycline is added to ensure that all growing cells have sex pili.
13. We have varied the IPTG concentration used for induction of the *lacZ* promoter during superinfection between 0 and 2 m*M*, and found no increase in Fab phage production with IPTG concentration above 100 µ*M* (*see* Section 3.4., step 4).
14. It is important to incubate at 22 to 30°C following superinfection for two reasons: (a) It has been reported that folding of active Fab molecules proceeds more successfully at room temperature than at 37°C (*11*), and (b) Fab phages will not be lost as a result of reinfection at room temperature since sex pili are not generated at temperatures below 30°C (*12*).
15. The washing procedure outlined in step 3, Section 3.5. has been used successfully when screening for high-affinity binders (apparent K_d of about $10^{-9}M$) normally present in libraries generated from immunized animals. When dealing with low-affinity binders (apparent K_d of about $10^{-6}M$), washing procedures are reduced to three brief washes in washing buffer.
16. We have not systematically compared the two elution methods described in steps 4–6, Section 3.5., but we like the trypsin elution method since it is very reliable and removes all bound phages, measured by testing the eluted wells in ELISA assays using antiphage antibodies (peroxidase-conjugated

anti-M13, Pharmacia). The eluted phages maintain their infectivity even after hours of treatment with the specified amounts of trypsin.

Acknowledgments

The authors would like to thank Henrik Ørum, Anne Øster, and Mads Bjørnvad for their help during the initial phases of this work. This work was supported by the Danish Medical and Natural Science Research Councils, the Center of Medical Biotechnology, University of Copenhagen, the Velux Foundation, the Novo Nordisk Research Foundation, Danmarks Frivillige Bloddonorer, Direktør Ib Henriksens Fond, and The Danish Hospital Foundation for Medical Research; Region of Copenhagen, The Faroe Islands and Greenland.

References

1. Scott, J. K. and Smith, G. P. (1990) Searching for peptide ligands with an epitope library. *Science* **249**, 386–390.
2. Garrard, L. J., Yang, M., O'Connell, M. P., Kelly, R. F., and Henner, D. J. (1991) *Bio/Technology* **9**, 1373–1377.
3. Hoogenboom, R. H., Griffiths, A. D., Johnson, K. S., Chiswell, D. J., Hudson, P., and Winter, G. (1991) Multi-subunit proteins on the surface of filamentous phage: methodologies for displaying antibody (Fab) heavy and light chains. *Nucleic Acids Res.* **19**, 4133–4137.
4. Kang, A. K., Barbas, C. F., Janda, K. D., Benkovic, S. J., and Lerner, R. A. (1991) Linkage of recognition and replication functions by assembling combinatorial antibody Fab libraries along phage surfaces. *Proc. Natl. Acad. Sci. USA* **88**, 4363–4366.
5. Breitling, F., Dübel, S., Seehaus, T., Klewinghaus, I., and Little, M. (1991) A surface expression vector for antibody screening. *Gene* **104**, 147–153.
6. Ørum, H., Andersen, P. S., Riise, E., Øster, A., Johansen, L. K., Bjørnvad, M., Svendsen, I., and Engberg, J. (1993) Efficient method for constructing comprehensive murine Fab antibody libraries displayed on phage. *Nucleic Acids Res.* **21(19)**, 4491–4498.
7. Sambrook, J., Fritsch, E. F., and Maniatis, T. (1989) *Molecular Cloning. A Laboratory Manual*, 2nd. ed. Cold Spring Harbor Laboratory, Cold Spring Harbor, NY.
8. Kabat, E. A., Wu, T. T., Reid-Miller, M., Perry, H. M., and Gottesman, K. S. (1991) *Sequences of Proteins of Immunological Interest*, US Dept. of Health and Human Services, US Government Printing Office, Washington, DC, pp. 2134–2143.
9. Dziegiel, M., Nielsen, L. K., Andersen, P. S., Blancher, A., Dickmeiss, E., and Engberg, J. (1995) Phage display used for gene cloning of human recombinant antobody against the erythrocyte surface antigen, rhesus D. *J. Immunol. Methods* **182** (in press).
10. Orum, H., Nielsen, H., and Engberg, J. (1991) Spliceosomal small nuclear RNAs of Tetrahymena thermophila and some possible snRNA-snRNA base-pairing interactions. *J. Mol. Biol.* **222**, 219–232.
11. Plückthun, A. and Skerra, A. (1989) Expression of functional antibody F_v and Fab fragments in *Escherichia coli*. *Methods Enzymol.* **178**, 497–515.
12. Miller, J. H. (1972) *Experiments in Molecular Genetics*. Cold Spring Harbor Laboratory, Cold Spring Harbor, NY.

CHAPTER 25

Selection of Human Immunoglobulin Light Chains from a Phage-Display Library

Sonia Tyutyulkova, Qing-Sheng Gao, and Sudhir Paul

1. Introduction

Asthma is associated with increased catalytic autoantibodies to vasoactive intestinal peptide (VIP), a bronchodilator and anti-inflammatory neuropeptide found in nerve endings supplying airway smooth muscle and epithelial structures (1). Asthmatic airways obtained at autopsy are deficient in VIP (2), raising the possibility that efficient catalytic hydrolysis of VIP by autoantibodies synthesized locally in the airways or derived by transudation from systemic circulation may be a pathogenetic factor in asthma. With the aim of investigating the possible cause–effect relationship between autoantibodies to VIP and asthma, we have cloned catalytic antibody light (L) chains from the immune repertoire of an exercise-induced asthma patient. We chose to work with the L chains for the following reasons. First, L chains retain the ability to recognize VIP and appear to turn over more rapidly than intact antibodies. Faster catalysis observed with L chains may arise from diminished affinity for the substrate ground state and a more flexible active site than the intact antibody-combining site. Second, F_v species from combinatorial libraries of heavy (H)- and L-chain-variable regions are not likely to reflect the composition of antibodies found in vivo, in that the probability of pairing of the natural H- and L-chain partners in these libraries is low (3). Third, free L chains are found in circulation in vivo (4). Glutathione

From: *Methods in Molecular Biology, Vol. 51: Antibody Engineering Protocols*
Edited by: S. Paul Humana Press Inc., Totowa, NJ

levels are increased in the asthmatic airway *(5)*. A reducing environment may lead to increased levels of L chains by cleavage of disulfide links. We anticipate that availability of recombinant human L chains that catalyze the hydrolysis of VIP will permit direct examination of their disease-causing potential, for example, by examination of airway abnormalities in transgenic mice overexpressing the L chains.

There are other good reasons for constructing human L-chain libraries and selecting individual proteins displaying the desired activities from these libraries. Intracellular catalytic hydrolysis of antigens by L chains within B-lymphocytes could be a factor in antigen presentation and recruitment of T-helper cells. In some forms of amyloidosis and multiple myeloma, the L chains tend to aggregate and form amyloid deposits *(6)*. An immunoregulatory role for free L chains in isotype switching has been proposed *(7)*. Finally, activation of the alternate complement pathway by L chains has been demonstrated *(8)*. The application of phage-display techniques to select antigen-specific L chains described here should facilitate mechanistic studies of these issues.

2. Materials

2.1. Reagents

1. Ampli*Taq* DNA Polymerase (Perkin-Elmer Cetus, Norwalk, CT).
2. Isopropyl-β-D-thiogalactopyranoside (IPTG), ChromaSpin 1000 columns (Clontech, Palo Alto, CA).
3. Low-melting-point agarose, diethylpyrocarbonate (DEPC), phenylmethylsulfonylfluoride (PMSF), *o*-phenylendiamine, chloroform, Triton-100 (Sigma, St. Louis, MO).
4. Lymphoprep (Nyegaard & Co, Norway).
5. RNasin ribonuclease inhibitor (Promega, Madison, WI).
6. *Sfi*I and *Not*I restriction enzymes (New England BioLabs, Beverly, MA).
7. SuperScript RNase H⁻ reverse transcriptase, T4 DNA ligase, DNA ladders (100 bp, 1 kb), DNA quantitation standards, SOC medium, and 2TY (Gibco BRL, Grand Island, NY).

2.2. Buffers and Media

1. TE buffer: 10 mM Tris-HCl, pH 8.0, 1 mM EDTA.
2. PEG/NaCl: 20% polyethylene glycol 8000 (Sigma), 2.5M NaCl.
3. 50X Tris-acetate (TAE) electrophoresis buffer: 242 g Tris-base, 57.1 mL glacial acetic acid, and 100 mL 0.5M EDTA, pH 8.0/1 L dH$_2$O.
4. PBS buffer, pH 7.4: 8 g NaCl, 0.2 g KCl, 1.44 g Na$_2$HPO$_4$, 0.24 g KH$_2$PO$_4$/ 1 L dH$_2$O.

5. 2TY agar plates: Add 15 g bacto-agar to 1 L of 2TY medium, and autoclave for 20 min at 15 lb/s in.^{2} on liquid cycle.
6. TY top agar: add 7 g bacto-agar to 1 L TY medium and autoclave.
7. M9 minimal medium (Difco, Detroit, MI), and GeneClean II Kit (BIO 101, Vista, CA).
8. Bacto-agar (Difco).

2.3. Vectors and *E. coli* Strains

1. Phagemid vector pCANTAB5*his*$_6$ (Cambridge Antibody Technology, Cambridgeshire, UK). A similar vector (without polyhistidine tail) is available from Pharmacia Biotechnology LKB (Recombinant Phage Antibody System).
2. Helper phage VCSM13 (Stratagene, La Jolla, CA).
3. TG1: K12Δ*(lac-pro), supE, thi, hsdD5/F' traD36, proAB, lacI*^{q}, *lacZ* ΔM15 (Cambridge Antibodies Tech).
4. HB2151nal^r: K12Δ*(lac-pro), ara, nal*^{r}*, thi/F', proAB, lacI*^{q}, *lacZ* ΔM15 (Cambridge Antibodies Tech).

2.4. Equipment

1. DNA Thermal Cycler 480 (Perkin-Elmer Cetus).
2. *E. coli* Gene Pulser, ELISA Microplate Reader Model 3550 (Bio-Rad, Hercules, CA).
3. High-performance liquid-chromatography system (ISCO, Lincoln, NE).
4. γ Counter Cobra II and liquid scintillation counter 1600 TR (Packard Instrument, Meriden, CT).

2.5. PCR Primers (see Notes 1 and 2)

PCR primers were synthesized and HPLC-purified by National Biosciences (Plymouth, MN). All primers were made 50 μ*M* in distilled H_2O and kept at –20°C.

2.5.1. Primers for Amplification and Sequencing of cDNA Inserts in pCANTAB5*his*$_6$

LMB3 5'-CAGGAAACAGCTATGAC-3' (primer upstream from the leader sequence)

fd-SEQ1 5'-GAATTTTCTGTATGAGG-3' (primer in the 5' region of gene 3)

2.5.2. Primers for Amplification of Human L Chains

Back (5') primers contain an *Sfi*I restriction site and FOR (3') primers contain an *Not*I restriction site (underlined). The 5' overhang facilitates restriction digestion. Nucleotides 31–50 in the BACK primers correspond to amino acid residues 1–8, and nucleotides 16–39 in the FOR primers, to residues 207–214.

1. κBACK1 (Amplifies κ1 and κ4 V-gene families)
   5'-GTC CTC GCA ACT GC<u>G GCC CAG CCG GCC</u> ATG GCC GAC ATC (C/G)(A/T)G ATG ACC CAG TCT CC-3'

2. κBACK2 (Amplifies κ5 V-gene family)
   5' GTC CTC GCA ACT GC<u>G GCC CAG CCG GCC</u> ATG GCC GAA ACG ACA CTC ACG CAG TCT CC 3'

3. κBACK3 (Amplifies κ2, κ3, and κ6 V-gene families)
   5' GTC CTC GCA ACT GC<u>G GCC CAG CCG GCC</u> ATG GCC GA(A/ T) (A/G)TT GTG (A/C/T)TG AC(G/T) CAG TCT CC 3'

4. λBACK1 (Amplifies λ1, λ2, and λ5 V-gene families)
   5' GTC CTC GCA ACT GC<u>G GCC CAG CCG GCC</u> ATG GCC CAG (G/T)CT G(C/T)(C/G) (C/T)T(C/G) AC(G/T) CAG CC(G/T) (C/G/T)C 3'

5. λBACK2 (amplifies λ3 V-gene family)
   5' GTC CTC GCA ACT GC<u>G GCC CAG CCG GCC</u> ATG GCC TC(C/ T) T(A/C)T G(A/T)G CTG ACT CAG (C/G)(A/C)(A/C) CC 3'

6. λBACK3 (amplifies λ4 and λ6 families)
   5' GTC CTC GCA ACT GC<u>G GCC CAG CCG GCC</u> ATG GCC (A/ C)A(C/T) (G/T)TT AT(A/G) CTG ACT CA(A/G) CC(C/G) C(A/C) 3'

7. κFOR (3' primer for amplification of κ chains)
   5'-CCA TCC T<u>GC GGC CGC</u> ACA CTC TCC CCT GTT GAA GCT CTT-3'

8. λFOR (3' primer for amplification of λ chains)
   5' CCA TCC T<u>GC GGC CGC</u> ACA TTC TGT AGG GGG CAC TGT CTT 3'

3. Methods

3.1. Total RNA Preparation

Human peripheral blood lymphocytes (PBLs) are used as a source for the cDNA library. PBLs are isolated from blood by density-gradient separation on Lymphoprep *(9)*. Total RNA is prepared from 3×10^8 cells using a single-step guanidinium method (*see* Gao et al., Chapter 19).

3.2. cDNA Synthesis (see Notes 3 and 4)

For the generation of cDNA, set up two separate first-strand cDNA reactions using κFOR and λFOR primers.

1. Mix in a microfuge tube:
   a. Total RNA (approx 5 μg)   3   μL
   b. 3'-Primer (κFOR or λFOR), 25 pmol   0.5 μL
   c. DEPC-treated water   16.5 μL

2. Incubate for 10 min at 70°C. Chill on ice.
3. To the mix of step 1, add the following:
    a. dH$_2$O   9.5 µL
    b. 5X Reverse transcriptase buffer   10 µL
    c. 0.1M dithiotreitol (DTT)   5 µL
    d. 0.01M deoxynucleotide triphosphates dNTPs   2.5 µL
    e. RNase inhibitor   2 µL

    DTT, dNTPs, and reverse transcriptase buffer are supplied with the SuperScript Reverse Transcriptase.
4. Place the tube at 42°C for 1 min. Add 1 µL (200 U) GIBCO BRL Super-Script RNase H$^-$ Reverse Transcriptase.
5. Incubate at 42°C for 1 h.
6. Heat to 95°C for 5 min. Then store at –80°C.

3.3. PCR Amplification (see Notes 5 and 6 and Fig. 1)

Set up six separate reactions, each with a 5' κBACK or λBACK primer combined with a 3' κFOR or λFOR primer, respectively. Reaction volume is 50 µL. Use 0.5-mL thin-wall microcentrifuge tubes (Perkin-Elmer Cetus).

1. In six separate tubes add:
    a. BACK primer   0.5 µL (25 pmol)
    b. FOR primer   0.5 µL (25 pmol)
    c. cDNA (from Section 3.2.)   5   µL
2. Set up the following master mix (make enough for 6 reactions):
    a. dH$_2$O   36.5 µL
    b. 10 mM dNTPs   0.5 µL
    c. 100 mM MgCl$_2$ 1.5 µL
    d. 10X PCR buffer   5   µL

    Reaction buffer (supplied with the enzyme) is 10 mM Tris-HCl, pH 8.3, 50 mM KCl, and 0.001% gelatin.
3. To each of the six tubes from step 1 containing primers and template, add 43.5 µL of the master mix.
4. Heat at 94°C for 5 min. Then, add 0.5 µL (2.5 U) Ampli*Taq* DNA polymerase to each tube, cover with two drops mineral oil, and amplify using 30 cycles. Each cycle consists of: 94°C 1 min and 72°C 2 min. Include a final extension step at 72°C for 5 min.
5. Extract with 100 µL chloroform.
6. Separate the PCR products on a 2% low-melting-point agarose gel (in 1X TAE buffer).
7. Cut bands of the appropriate size with sterile surgical blades. Place the gel piece in a sterile 1.5-mL microfuge tube.

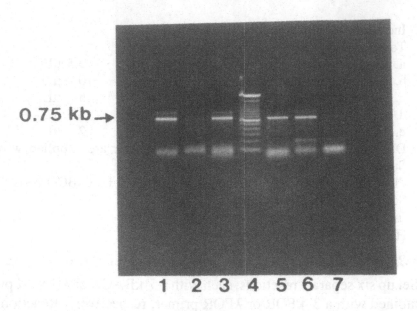

Fig. 1. Ethidium bromide-stained 2% agarose gel electrophoresis of PCR-amplified human κ and λ chains. Amplification done using lane 1, κBACK1 primer; lane 2, κBACK2 primer; lane 3, κBACK3 primer; lane 4, 100-bp DNA ladder; lane 5, λBACK1 primer; lane 6, λBACK2 primer; lane 7, λBACK3 primer. PCR was done using combinations of the indicated κBACK or λBACK primers with the κFOR or the λFOR primer, respectively.

8. Use GeneClean II kit and the protocol supplied by the manufacturer to purify the DNA from the gel. This protocol involves melting the gel with NaI, adsorption of cDNA to glassmilk, and elution in an appropriate volume (20–50 µL) of dH$_2$O.
9. Run 1 µL of the purified sample on a 2% agarose gel containing 0.5 µg/mL ethidium bromide. Run DNA quantitation standards in parallel, and estimate the approximate concentration of the sample by visual comparison with the standards.

3.4. Enzyme Digestion for Cloning into pCANTAB5his$_6$ (see Note 7)

1. Combine PCR products obtained for different families.
2. Digest with *Sfi*I.
   a. 10X NEB buffer 2   20 µL
   b. Acetylated BSA 10 mg/mL   2 µL
   c. *Sfi*I (10 U/µL)   10 µL

d. PCR product   500 ng or greater; sufficient for optimization
of subsequent protocols and library

e. dH$_2$O   to 200 µL

NEB buffer and acetylated BSA are supplied with the enzyme. Incubate overnight at 50°C.

3. Purify *Sfi*I digested PCR product directly from the reaction (without running a gel) using GeneClean II kit. Use the procedure designated as Double GeneClean in the kit.

4. Set up second digestion with *Not*I.

a. 10X NEB buffer for *Not*I   20 µL

b. Acetylated BSA 10 mg/mL   2 µL

c. *Not*I (10 U/µL)   10 µL

d. *Sfi*I digested PCR product   500 ng

e. dH$_2$O   to 200 µL

Incubate overnight at 37°C.

5. Purify using GeneClean II kit, Double GeneClean procedure.

6. Digest pCANTAB5*his*$_6$ in the same way as described above for the PCR products, first with *Sfi*I and then with *Not*I enzyme. After digestion with *Not*I, purify using gel-filtration spin-column chromatography (Clontech ChromaSpin 1000 columns) instead of GeneClean procedure.

3.5. Ligation of Digested PCR Products in pCANTAB5his$_6$

1. Set up a series of pilot reactions (20 µL reaction volume) to determine the optimal ratio of vector:insert DNA. Keep the concentration of the vector constant (50 ng of the double-digested vector) and vary the concentration of the insert DNA.

a. 5X T4 ligase buffer   4 µL

b. pCANTAB5*his*$_6$ (*Sfi*I/*Not*I digested)   50 ng

c. PCR product (*Sfi*I/*Not*I digested, 50 ng/µL)   0.2 µL to 2 µL

d. T4 DNA ligase   2 µL

e. dH$_2$O   to 20 µL

Include a control reaction with vector DNA, but without insert.

2. Incubate overnight at 16°C.

3. Purify the ligation mixture using GeneClean II kit (Double GeneClean procedure), and reconstitute in 10–20 µL dH$_2$O.

3.6. Transformation of E. coli (see Note 8)

1. Prepare electrocompetent cells (TG1 and HB2151).

a. Inoculate 1 L of 2TY medium with 1/100 vol of a fresh overnight culture.

b. Grow cells at 37°C with vigorous shaking to an OD$_{800}$ of approx 0.5–0.7.

c. Centrifuge cells in cold centrifuge bottles at 4000*g* (4°C) for 15 min.

d. Remove the supernatant and resuspend the pellet in a total of 0.5 L ice-cold 10% glycerol.

e. Centrifuge as in step 3, and resuspend the pellet in a total of 0.5 L ice-cold 10% glycerol.

f. Centrifuge as in step 3. Resuspend in a total of 250 mL of ice-cold 10% glycerol.

g. Centrifuge as in step 3. Resuspend in a final volume of 3–4 mL of ice-cold 10% glycerol.

h. Aliquot (100 µL) on ice in sterile microfuge tubes, and store at –80°C. The cell concentration should be about $1-3 \times 10^{10}$ cells/mL. Cells must be kept on ice throughout their preparation.

2. Electroporate 50 µL of electrocompetent cells with 1 µL of the ligation mixtures from Section 3.5. using 0.2-cm cuvets (Bio-Rad) and Gene Pulser set at 25 µF, 2.5 kV, 200 Ω.

3. Immediately add 1 mL of SOC medium, and incubate for 1 h at 37°C.

4. Plate an aliquot of the mixture (0.5 mL) on a 2TY, 100 µg/mL ampicillin, 2% glucose 150×15 mm agar plates, and incubate overnight at 30°C.

5. Count the number of colonies in a 1/4 sector of a plate. Compare the number of colonies observed at different vector:insert ratios. Select the vector:insert ratio giving highest colony number for future ligation reactions.

6. To optimize transformation efficiency, carry out a series of transformations using 50 µL electrocompetent cells and varying amounts of the ligation mixture. Include control reactions with:

a. Closed circular vector DNA.

b. No DNA at all.

c. Unligated *Sfi*I-*Not*I digested vector.

d. *Sfi*I-*Not*I digested vector subjected to ligation in the absence of insert cDNA.

7. The large cDNA library is prepared using optimized ligation and transformation conditions (steps 1–6). Transform 400 µL of electrocompetent cells (0.2-cm cuvets) using appropriately scaled-up ligation mixture and cell number (determined in step 6). Plate aliquots of the transformations on 245×245 mm Nunc plates.

8. Grow overnight at 30°C, flood plates with 5–10 mL 2TY, scrape with a sterile spreader, and transfer into sterile tubes.

9. Freeze aliquots of the cells in 15% glycerol in sterile 2-mL freezing vials (Costar, Cambridge, MA), and store at –80°C.

10. The library size is the total number of colonies that can be grown from the transformation mixture. Because the same L-chain cDNA may be reiterated several times in the library, the library size may not be equivalent to the number of different L-chain cDNA species represented in the library.

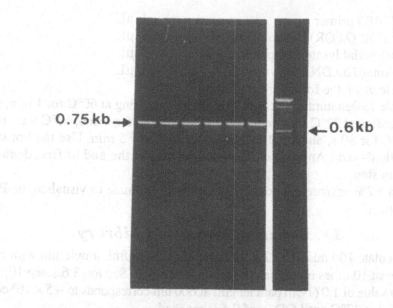

Fig. 2. PCR screening for L-chain inserts in individual bacterial colonies. Lanes 1–6: Lysates of six colonies obtained from the κBACK1/κFOR transformation mixture were amplified using vector-directed LMB3 and insert-directed κFOR primers, and subjected to agarose gel electrophoresis. A 750-bp product is evident. Lane 7, 100-bp DNA ladder.

The diversity of a library can be assessed by sequencing a representative sampling of inserts. If each insert has a unique sequence, the number of L chains in the library approximates the library size.

3.7. Confirmation of Insert Presence by PCR (see Note 9 and Fig. 2)

1. Pick 15 single colonies from the transformation plates using sterile toothpicks.
2. Resuspend colonies in 50 µL 5 mM Tris-HCl, 5 mM EDTA, pH 7.6, and 1% Triton X-100 in 0.5-mL tubes.
3. Heat to 95°C for 10 min in a water bath.
4. Spin for 2 min in a microfuge at 10,000g. Use supernatant as the template source for PCR reaction.
5. Mix in a tube:
   a. dH$_2$O   35.5 µL
   b. 10 mM dNTPs   1   µL
   c. 10X PCR buffer   5   µL
   d. 100 mM MgCl$_2$ 0.75 µL

e. LMB3 primer   1 µL
f. κFOR (λFOR) primer   1 µL
g. Bacterial lysate (template) from step 3   5 µL
h. Ampli*Taq* DNA Polymerase   1 µL

Cycle using the following conditions:

Cycle 1: Denaturation at 94°C for 5 min, annealing at 60°C for 1 min, and extension at 72°C for 1 min. Cycles 2–29: 94°C for 1 min, 60°C for 1 min, 72°C for 30 s, and final extension at 72°C for 5 min. Use the hot start method—add Ampli*Taq* DNA polymerase at the end of first denaturation step.

6. Run a 2% agarose gel containing ethidium bromide to visualize the PCR products.

3.8. Rescue of Phagemid Library

1. Inoculate 100 mL 2TY, 2% glucose, and 100 µg/mL ampicillin with cells at least 10 times more than the total library size (Section 3.6., step 10). An OD value of 1.0 (1-cm path length) at 600 nm corresponds to ~ 5×10^8 cells.
2. Grow at 37°C until OD_{600} of 0.5 is reached.
3. Add 5×10^8 plaque-forming units (PFU)/mL VCSM13 helper phage.
4. Grow at 37°C, 30 min with gentle shaking, and then 30 min with vigorous shaking.
5. Spin the cells for 15 min at 3000g, and resuspend pellet in 500 mL 2TY, 100 µg/mL ampicillin, and 50 µg/mL kanamycin.
6. Incubate overnight at 37°C with vigorous shaking.
7. Spin cells at 3000g for 10 min at 4°C, and use the supernatant containing phage particles in Section 3.9.

3.9. Preparation of Phage Library (see Note 10)

1. Add 1/5 vol PEG/NaCl to the supernatant from step 7, Section 3.8.
2. Mix well and leave on ice for 1 h.
3. Spin at 8000g for 20 min at 4°C.
4. Discard the supernatant, and resuspend the pellet in 1–2 mL of TE buffer.
5. Spin 5 min in a microcentrifuge at maximal speed to remove cell debris.
6. Transfer the supernatant into a new microcentrifuge tube. Repeat the PEG precipitation (steps 1–5).
7. Filter the supernatant through a 0.45-µm filter. Phage preparations may be stored at 4°C for several months or at –80°C for longer periods.
8. Determine concentration of the phage particles photometrically at 269 nm using an absorption coefficient of 3.84 mg^{-1} cm^{-1} *(10)*.
9. Determine the phage titer using TG1 as host bacteria:
   a. Prepare dilutions of phage in 2TY medium.

b. Mix in a tube 10–100 µL of phage solution and 100 µL TG1 host bacteria.
c. Incubate for 10 min at room temperature.
d. Add 3 mL melted TY top agar.
e. Pour on M9 minimal agar plates.
f. Incubate at 37°C.
g. Count plaques, and express data per mL original phage solution.

3.10. Affinity Chromatography for Selection of Binding Clones

Phage particles displaying recombinant antibodies can be isolated by "panning" on antigen-coated plates or by affinity chromatography on immobilized antigen. The protocol we used for selection of VIP-binding clones from a κ L-chain library follows.

1. Incubate 1 mL of immobilized VIP (0.52 mg VIP coupled to CNBr-activated Sepharose 4B; *see* ref. *11* for preparation of the gel) overnight at 4°C with 10^{13} PFU of the phage solution (prepared as in Section 3.9.) in 2% w/v nonfat powder milk in phosphate-buffered saline (PBS) with end-to-end mixing.
2. Pour the gel into a column and wash with (*see* Note 11):
   a. 150 mL PBS.
   b. 25 mL 50 m*M* Tris-HCl, pH 7.5, 0.5*M* NaCl.
   c. 25 mL 50 m*M* Tris-HCl, pH 8.5, 0.5*M* NaCl.
   d. 25 mL 50 m*M* Tris-HCl, pH 9.5, 0.5*M* NaCl.
   e. 25 mL 50 m*M* sodium carbonate/bicarbonate, pH 9.6, 0.5*M* NaCl.
3. Elute the phage particles most strongly bound to the gel with 0.1*M* triethylamine, adjusted to pH 5.5 with HCl.
4. Elute with glycine-HCl buffer, pH 2.7. Neutralize by addition of 1*M* Tris-base.
5. Use phage particles eluted from the column to reinfect logarithmically growing TG1 (for display on the phage surface as a fusion protein) or HB2152 (for expression as soluble fragments) *E. coli* strains (*see* Note 12 for reselection by affinity chromatography).

3.11. Reinfection of E. coli with Eluted Phage

1. Prepare a fresh overnight culture of TG1 or HB2151 *E. coli* (*see* Note 13).
2. Inoculate 10 mL of 2TY with 0.1 mL of the bacterial culture, and grow to OD_{600} 0.8.
3. Add 20 µL of eluate phage particles from the column, and incubate at 37°C for 30 min.
4. Spin the culture at 3000*g* for 15 min at 4°C.

5. Resuspend the cell pellet in 0.5 mL 2TY, and spread on 2TY, 2% glucose, and 100 µg/mL ampicillin agar plate (245 × 245 mm). Incubate overnight at 30°C.
6. Pick single colonies, and grow them for screening as described in Section 3.12.

3.12. Growth of Phagemid Clones in 96-Well Plates

1. Inoculate 150 µL 2TY, 100 µg/mL ampicillin, and 2% glucose with individual TG1 colonies picked with sterile toothpicks in 96-well polystyrene plates (Costar cat # 3595).
2. Grow overnight at 30°C with shaking on a rocker platform.
3. Inoculate 180 µL 2TY, 100 µg/mL ampicillin, 2% glucose, and 5×10^8 PFU/mL VCSM13 helper phage with 20 µL of the overnight culture in 96-well plates, and grow for 2 h at 37°C.
4. Centrifuge plates at 3000g for 15 min.
5. Aspirate the supernatant.
6. Resuspend cell pellet in 200 µL 2TY, 100 µg/mL ampicillin, and 50 µg/mL kanamycin.
7. Grow overnight at 37°C.
8. Centrifuge plates at 3000g for 15 min.
9. Transfer supernatants into new plates. These contain packaged phage particles suitable for binding assays.

3.13. Induction of Soluble L Chains in 96-Well Plates (see Note 15)

1. Inoculate 150 µL 2TY, 2% glucose, and 100 µg/mL ampicillin with single colonies from the reinfection plates (in HB2151), and incubate overnight at 37°C. Use Costar flat-bottom 96-well plates (*see* Note 14).
2. Inoculate 20 µL of the overnight cultures into 180 µL 2TY, 0.1% glucose, 100 µg/mL ampicillin, and grow at 37°C to OD_{600} 0.8. It will take more time to reach this optical density in the plates (compared with the large-scale cultures) because of the poorer aeration.
3. Add isopropyl-β-D-thiogalactopyranoside (IPTG) to 1 mM final concentration, and grow for 24 h at 30°C.
4. Spin the plates at 3000g for 30 min, and transfer the supernatant, containing the secreted antibody fragment, into a new 96-well plate. Use in ELIFA to test binding and expression levels.
5. Keep master plates (from step 1) sealed with Parafilm at 4°C. These can be stored in viable state for 1 wk.

3.14. Screening for L-Chain Expression by Enzyme-Linked Immunoflow Assay (ELIFA)

To screen for expression, use either dot blotting with anti-c-*myc* antibody 9E10 (described by Gao et al., Chapter 19) or ELIFA with antihuman L chains described below.

1. A plate-filtration device from Millipore (part of the Millipore MultiScreen Assay System) and 96-well Millipore MultiScreen-HA 0.45-µm nitrocellulose filtration plates (cat. no. MAHA S45 10 or MAHA N45 10) are used for this assay.
2. Coat the nitrocellulose plates with 50–100 µL/well bacterial supernatants. Incubate for 30 min. Apply vacuum to remove fluid.
3. Block nonspecific binding sites on the nitrocellulose with 200 µL 5% BSA in 50 mM Tris-HCl, pH 8.0, 0.15M NaCl, and 0.05% Tween-20 for 30 min, and apply vacuum.
4. Add antihuman L-chain IgG labeled with horseradish peroxidase (Sigma) diluted in 50 mM Tris-HCl, pH 8.0, 0.15M NaCl, 0.05% Tween-20, and 1% BSA. Incubate for 30 min. Apply vacuum.
5. Wash three times with 200 µL each of PBS and 0.05% Tween-20.
6. Add 100 µL/well developing solution (sodium citrate buffer, pH 5.0, *o*-phenylendiamine 8 mg/10 mL buffer, and 5 µL 30% H_2O_2/10 mL buffer).
7. Develop for an appropriate length of time until yellow color is evident. Stop the reaction with 50 µL 10N H_2SO_4.
8. Transfer supernatants in any clear 96-well plates, and read optical densities at 492 nm using an ELISA reader.

3.15. ELIFA for Screening of the Libraries for Antigen Binding (see Note 16)

1. Use 96-well Millipore MultiScreen-HA 0.45-µm nitrocellulose filtration plates. Coat plates with the antigen. We use 100 µL/well of 100 µg VIP/ mL in 50 mM sodium carbonate/bicarbonate buffer, pH 9.6. Incubate for 30 min at room temperature. Apply vacuum.
2. Block nonspecific binding sites on the nitrocellulose as in step 3, Section 3.14.
3. Add 100–150 µL bacterial supernatants/well. Incubate for 30 min. Apply vacuum.
4. Wash three times with 200 µL/each of PBS and 0.05% Tween-20.
5. Add 100 µL/well antihuman L-chain IgG labeled with peroxidase (diluted in 1% BSA in 50 mM Tris-HCl, pH 8.0, 0.15M NaCl, and 0.05% Tween-20). Incubate for 30 min. Apply vacuum.
6. Wash three times with 200 µL each of PBS containing 0.05% Tween-20.
7. Develop and read color as in steps 6–8, Section 3.14.

4. Notes

1. PCR primers described here are family-specific primers *(12,13)*. We have introduced degeneracies in some of the primers to reduce the number of PCR reactions necessary for library preparation.
2. Codon ACA in κFOR and λFOR primers represent Cys (position 214) in the sense strand. A different codon can be used in this position (e.g., an Ser codon) if dimer formation by S—S linkage is to be avoided.
3. For step 1, use DEPC-treated water *(14)*. It is not necessary to use DEPC water for step 2 of this protocol or any of the subsequent protocols.
4. If a problem is suspected at the reverse-transcriptase step, the efficiency of cDNA synthesis may be tested by monitoring the incorporation of $[\alpha$-$^{32}P]$-dCTP into TCA-precipitable material.
5. Amplification for each family should be carried out in a separate reaction. Combining the primers does not yield satisfactory amplification. Use hot-start PCR method to avoid mispriming.
6. Single bands of the correct size were obtained using the PCR conditions described here (Fig. 1). PCR bands for some families were very faint, since these families are poorly utilized by peripheral blood lymphocytes. If cDNA for the rare families is to be included in the library, larger amounts can be obtained by reamplification using the same conditions as in the original amplification after purification of the PCR product from a gel. PCR conditions for different primer sets should be optimized by varying annealing temperature, extension time, and $MgCl_2$ and dNTPs concentrations.
7. For construction of a fairly large library ($\sim 10^7$ members), the products of at least ten 50-μL PCR reactions from each primer set should be combined. Pooling of different PCR products can be done in the same ratio as the original yield of the products. If PCR products corresponding to rare families are pooled in an increased proportion, the rare families will be overrepresented in the L-chain library.
8. Grow transformed bacteria on agar plates (not in liquid culture) in order to minimize the overgrowth by rapidly proliferating clones, which may alter the representation of different clones in the library. When plating the transformation mixtures, use cell numbers that produce growth of single well-defined colonies. Avoid overcrowding of plates.
9. The presence of inserts can also be determined by comparing the size of the plasmid with a control plasmid without insert. Use the method for rapid disruption of bacterial colonies described in ref. *(15)*.
10. Bacteria used for titering of phage should be plated while the bacterial culture is still in the log-growth phase.
11. The purpose of washing the column with different pH buffers is to elute phage particles with differing affinity for antigen. To determine which of

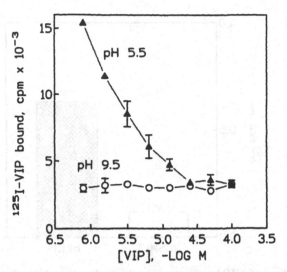

Fig. 3. Saturable ^{125}I-VIP binding by phage particles displaying κ-chains. Particles were recovered from the VIP-Sepharose column in pH 9.5 and 5.5 buffers. Available radioactivity, 35,000 cpm. Assay volume, 150 μL. Phage particle concentration, 250 nM.

the eluate pools should be analyzed further, we screened these for VIP binding by radioimmunoassay. *E. coli* TG1 were reinfected with the eluate pools and grown under identical conditions, the libraries rescued with VCSM13 helper phage, and phage particles were prepared by PEG precipitation (Sections 3.8. and 3.11., respectively). The phage particles were then permitted to bind ^{125}I-VIP as described (*15*) using increasing concentrations of cold VIP as inhibitor. The pH 5.5 eluate pool displayed the lowest IC$_{50}$ for VIP (Fig. 3), suggesting higher-affinity binders. Fifty-six percent of the clones in this pool were subsequently found to be positive for VIP binding.

12. The selected phagemid library can be rescued again with VCSM13 helper phage and phage particles prepared as described in Sections 3.8. and 3.9. for a second round of affinity chromatography. Several rounds of selection, growth, and rescue can be performed until positive clones or clones with the desired characteristics are identified.

13. Use TG1 cells to prepare phage particles for screening and HB2151 cells to prepare soluble L chains for screening. Both TG1 and HB2151 must be grown on minimal medium.

14. Grow clones in 96-well plates with shaking on a rocker platform in a humidified chamber to avoid problems with differential evaporation from border wells.

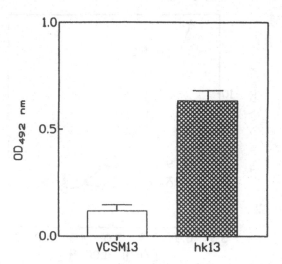

Fig. 4. Binding of VIP by a human κ-chain displayed on phage surface determined by ELISA. The binding of PEG-precipitated phage particles (260 n*M*) to KLH-VIP (10 µg/mL) immobilized on polyvinylchloride 96-well plates is shown. Results are means of three replicates ± SD. VCSM13 helper phage was prepared by PEG precipitation in the same way as hk13 phage particles and used at 260 n*M* in the assay. A peroxidase-labeled anti-M13 antiserum (Recombinant Phage Antibody System Detection Module, Pharmacia) was used to detect phage particles bound to the antigen. Values for binding of the two types of particles to plates coated with KLH alone or BSA alone were essentially identical.

15. To screen the libraries for antigen binding, there are two options: screening for L chains displayed on the phage surface or screening for soluble L chains. In choosing between these options, consider the following:
    a. A great proportion of the expressed gene III protein (up to 90%) will be the wild-type form (as opposed to the fusion protein). As a consequence, L-chain concentrations may not be high enough for detection of binding. To detect binding, it is usually necessary to grow phage particles at a larger scale and concentrate the particles by PEG precipitation prior to assay. This procedure, although possible in 96-well plates, is inconvenient and unsuitable for screening large numbers of clones.
    b. L chains will be displayed on the surface of the phage particles as monomers. At least one L-chain clone displayed on the surface of phage particles was shown to bind VIP (Fig. 4). Masat et al. *(16)* have also recently demonstrated antigen binding by an L-chain monomer. We have successfully used an ELISA with immobilized antigen and anti-fd phage antibody labeled with peroxidase (recombinant phage antibody

system, Detection module, Pharmacia LKB) to confirm antigen binding by selected clones after growing these in large scale and concentrating the particles by PEG precipitation.
  c. Although L chains retain antigen-binding activity, their affinity for the antigen is lower than that of intact antibodies. This imposes restrictions on the choice of the screening assay. In order to increase the apparent affinity of the L chains for the antigen, it is best to use solid-phase assay using antigen immobilized at high densities. This leads to increased avidity, allowing detection of the binding.
16. We used radioimmunoassay for VIP to confirm the data from the initial screening of the library. To demonstrate specific binding of ^{125}I-VIP, 100 μM cold VIP was used as inhibitor in the assay. Displacement of the binding by cold VIP was interpreted to represent specific binding.

References

1. Paul, S. (1994) Catalytic activity of anti-ground state antibodies, antibody subunits and human autoantibodies. *Appl. Biochem. Biotechnol.* **47**, 241–255.
2. Ollerenshaw, S., Jarvis, D., Woolcock, A., Sullivan, C., and Scheibner, T. (1989) Absence of immunoreactive vasoactive intestinal polypeptide in tissue from the lungs of patients with asthma. *N. Engl. J. Med.* **320**, 1244–1248.
3. Gherardi, E. and Milstein, C. (1992) Original and artificial antibodies. *Nature* **357**, 201,202.
4. Berggard, I. and Peterson, P. A. (1969) Polymeric forms of free normal κ and λ chains of human immunoglobulin. *J. Biol. Chem.* **244**, 4299–4307.
5. Smith, L. J., Houston, M., and Anderson, J. (1993) Increased levels of glutathione in bronchoalveolar lavage fluid from patients with asthma. *Am. Rev. Respir. Dis.* **147**, 1461–1464.
6. Stevens, F. J., Solomon, A., and Schiffer, M. (1991) Bence Jones proteins: a powerful tool for the fundamental study of protein chemistry and pathophysiology. *Biochemistry* **30**, 6803–6805.
7. Ioanidis, R. A., Joshua, D. E., Warburton, P. T., Francis, S. E., Brown, R. D., Gibson, J., and Kronenberg, H. (1989) Multiple myeloma: evidence that L chains play an immunoregulatory role in B-cell regulation. *Hematologic Pathol.* **3**, 169–175.
8. Meri, S., Koistinen, V., Miettinen, A., Tornroth, T. G., and Seppala, I. J. T. (1992) Activation of the alternative pathaway of complement by monoclonal lambda L chains in membranoproliferative glomerulonephritis. *J. Exp. Med.* **175**, 939–950.
9. Coligan, J. E., Kruisbeek, A. M., Margulies, D. H., Shevach, E. M., and Strober, W. (1991) *Current Protocols in Immunology*, vol. 2. Wiley, New York.
10. Berkowitz, S. A. and Day, L. A. (1976) Mass, length, composition and structure of the filamentous bacterial virus fd. *J. Mol. Biol.* **102**, 531–547.
11. Paul, S., Volle, D. J., and Sun, M. (1990) Affinity chromatography of catalytic autoantibody to vasoactive intestinal peptide. *J. Immunol.* **145**, 1196–1199.

12. Marks, J. D., Hoogenboom, H. R., Bonnert, T. B., McCafferty, J., Griffiths, A. D., and Winter, G. (1991) By-passing immunization. Human antibodies from V-gene libraries displayed on phage. *J. Mol. Biol.* **222,** 581–597.
13. Marks, J. D., Tristrem, M., Karpas, A., and Winter, G. (1991) Oligonucleotide primers for polymerase chain reaction amplification of human immunoglobulin variable genes and design of family-specific oligonucleotide probes. *Eur. J. Immunol.* **21,** 985–991.
14. Sambrook, J., Fritsch, E. F., and Maniatis, T. (1989) *Molecular Cloning: A Laboratory Manual,* vol. 2. Cold Spring Harbor Laboratory, Cold Spring Harbor, NY.
15. Tyutyulkova, S. and Paul, S. (1994) Selection of functional human immunoglobulin L chains from a phage display library. *Appl. Biochem. Biotechnol.* **47,** 191–198.
16. Masat, L., Wabl, M., and Johnson, J. P. (1994) A simpler sort of antibody. *Proc. Natl. Acad. Sci. USA* **91,** 893–896.

Chapter 26

Purification
of Antibody Light Chains
by Metal Affinity
and Protein L Chromatography

Sonia Tyutyulkova and Sudhir Paul

1. Introduction

Immobilized metal affinity chromatography (IMAC), introduced in 1975 (1), relies on the formation of coordinate bonds between metal ions immobilized on a suitable support and electron donor groups in proteins. A polyhistidine tag (five or six His residues) placed at either the C- or N-terminus of a recombinant protein can form a stable chelate with immobilized transition metals. This allows fractionation of the target protein to 90–95% purity levels in a single chromatographic step (2–4). Metals like Cu^{2+} and Ni^{2+} bind surface-accessible His residues selectively. The high affinity of polyhistidine tags for commercially available metal resins (K_d $10^{-13}M$ or more) allows the use of stringent conditions to remove loosely bound proteins, while retaining the recombinant protein bound to the immobilized metal.

We describe here IMAC for purification of human light (L) chains cloned in pCANTAB5his_6. The recombinant protein contains C-terminal hexahistidine and c-myc tags. The c-myc tag is useful in detection of the recombinant L chain during purification by ELISA. The IMAC procedure yields sufficiently pure L chains for most purposes. Further chromatography on immobilized protein L, a bacterial L chain binding protein (5,6), permits purification of the recombinant protein to apparent homogeneity.

From: *Methods in Molecular Biology, Vol. 51: Antibody Engineering Protocols*
Edited by: S. Paul Humana Press Inc., Totowa, NJ

2. Materials

2.1. Expression of L Chains

1. 2TY medium (Gibco BRL, Grand Island, NY).
2. Phenylmethylsulfonyl fluoride (PMSF; Sigma, St. Louis, MO): 1 mg/mL in isopropanol.
3. Isopropyl-β-D-thiogalactopyranoside (IPTG) (Sigma).
4. Ampicillin (Sigma).
5. Isopropanol (Fisher, Pittsburgh, PA).
6. Orbital shaker (Lab-Line Instruments, Inc., Melrose Park, IL).
7. *E. coli* HB2151nal^r - K12Δ*(lac-pro), ara, nal^r, thi/F', proAB, lacI^q, lacZ ΔM15* (Cambridge Antibodies Technologies).

2.2. Purification of L chains from Medium by Metal Affinity Chromatography (see Notes 1–3)

1. Ni-Nitrilotriacetic acid-Sepharose (NTA) (Qiagen, Chatsworth, CA; 5–10 mg protein binding capacity/mL settled gel).
2. Imidazole (Sigma).
3. β-mercaptoethanol (Sigma).
4. Glycerol (Fisher).
5. SDS-PAGE precast 8–25% polyacrylamide gels (Pharmacia, Piscataway, NJ).
6. Pellicon tangential flow ultrafiltration cassette system with PLGC filter cassette (10-kDa cutoff) (Millipore, Bedford, MA).
7. Phast Electrophoresis System (Pharmacia).
8. Frac-100 fraction collector (Pharmacia).
9. High-performance liquid chromatography system (ISCO, Lincoln, NE).
10. Buffer A: 50 m*M* Tris-HCl, pH 7.2, 0.5*M* NaCl, 0.025% Tween-20, 10% glycerol, 5 m*M* β-mercaptoethanol, 0.02% NaN$_3$.
11. Buffer B: 50 m*M* Tris-HCl, pH 7.2, 0.5*M* NaCl, 1*M* imidazole, 0.02% NaN$_3$.

2.3. Protein L Affinity Chromatography

1. Protein L: Generously provided by L. Björck, Department of Medical and Physiological Chemistry, University of Lund, Sweden.
2. CNBr-activated Sepharose 4B (Pharmacia).
3. Buffer C: 50 m*M* Tris-HCl, pH 8.0, 0.15*M* NaCl, 0.02% NaN$_3$.
4. Buffer D: 50 m*M* glycine-HCl, pH 2.8.

2.4. ELISA for c-myc Tag

1. Anti-c-*myc* antibody: Ascites fluid obtained by growth of cell line 9E10 (ATCC) in pristane-treated mice.

2. c-*myc* peptide standard: AEEQKLISEEDLLRKRREQLKHKLEQLRNSCA (Oncogene Science, Manhasset, NY).
3. Antimouse immunoglobulins (Fc-specific) labeled with peroxidase (Sigma).
4. *o*-Phenylenediamine (Sigma) and hydrogen peroxide.
5. Bovine serum albumin (BSA) (Sigma).
6. Multiscreen Vacuum Manifold (Millipore).
7. Multiscreen 96-well plates fitted with Immobilon P high-protein-binding hydrophobic PVDF filters (cat. # MAIP N45 10, Millipore).
8. ELISA Microplate Reader Model 3550 (Bio-Rad, Hercules, CA).
9. PBS, pH 7.4: 8 g NaCl, 0.2 g KCl, 1.44 g Na_2HPO_4, 0.24 g KH_2PO_4/L water.
10. Wash buffer: 0.05% Tween-20 in PBS.
11. Blocking buffer: 5% BSA in wash buffer.
12. Antibody buffer: 1% BSA in wash buffer.
13. Citrate buffer, pH 5.0: 48.5 mL $0.1M$ citric acid mixed with 51.5 mL $0.2M$ Na_2HPO_4.
14. Developing solution: 4 mg *o*-phenylenediamine and 5 µL 30% hydrogen peroxide in 10 mL citrate buffer. Prepare fresh before use.

3. Methods

3.1. Expression of L Chains

1. Inoculate 10 mL of a fresh overnight culture of the clone selected for purification (in *E. coli* HB2151) in 1 L of 2TY, 0.1% glucose, and 100 µg/mL ampicillin medium. To ensure good aeration, we grow the bacteria in 150–200 mL portions in 1-L flasks.
2. Grow cultures in a bacterial platform shaker at 37°C until OD_{600} is 0.8.
3. Add IPTG to a final concentration of 1 mM.
4. Grow overnight at 30°C with shaking.
5. Centrifuge at 4000g at 4°C. To the supernatant, add PMSF to 5 µg/mL, and use for purification of L chains (*see* Note 4).

3.2. Immobilized Metal Ion Chromatography of L Chains (see Figs. 1 and 2)

1. Concentrate the culture medium from step 5, Section 3.1 to 200 mL using a Pellicon ultrafiltration system (10 kDa cutoff) at 4°C. This step takes about 2 h.
2. Dialyze concentrated medium against 16 L buffer A.
3. Equilibrate 25 mL Ni-NTA gel by washing with 150 mL buffer A.
4. Mix dialyzed supernatant with the equilibrated Ni-NTA gel. Incubate for 1 h at 4°C with end-to-end mixing.
5. Pack the gel into a column, and wash extensively with buffer A at a flow rate of 4 mL/min until A_{280} baseline returns to zero.

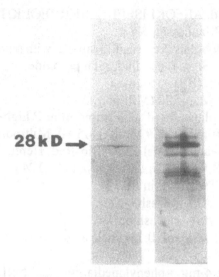

$28\,kD \longrightarrow$

Fig. 1. Silver-stained SDS-polyacrylamide gel showing recombinant human L chain (28-kDa band) fractionated on an Ni-NTA-Sepharose column (right lane) and protein L–Sepharose (left lane). Samples (4 µL) were electrophoresed on an 8–25% gradient gel.

6. Elute bound proteins with a gradient of 0–100% buffer B for 50 min, and then with 100% B for 10 min at a flow rate of 2 mL/min. Collect 2-mL fractions (*see* Note 5).
7. Perform ELISA using anti-c-*myc* 9E10 antibody (*see* Section 3.4.) to determine the elution position of the L chain.
8. Dialyze the c-*myc* stainable fractions for 24 h against a suitable buffer (e.g., PBS, 50 m*M* phosphate buffer or 50 m*M* Tris-HCl, pH 7.4) containing 0.025% Tween-20.
9. Run SDS-PAGE gels to determine the level of purity.

3.3. Protein L Affinity Chromatography

3.3.1. Coupling of Protein L to CNBr-Activated Sepharose 4B

1. Swell 1 g of CNBr-activated Sepharose 4B in 1 m*M* HCl for 15 min at room temperature.
2. Wash the gel with 600 mL 1 m*M* HCl on a sintered glass filter.
3. Transfer the gel into coupling buffer (0.1*M* NaHCO$_3$, pH 8.3) in a 15-mL tube and mix with 1–5 mg protein L in 2 mL coupling buffer.
4. Incubate overnight at 4°C with end-to-end mixing.
5. Centrifuge at 1000*g*. Measure A$_{280}$ of the supernatant to calculate the coupling efficiency ([protein bound to the gel/total amount of protein used] × 100).

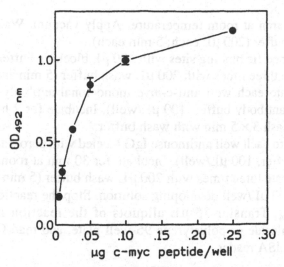

Fig. 2. Reactivity of c-*myc* standard peptide with anti-c-*myc* antibody 9E10 in ELISA.

6. Saturate the remaining NH_2-reactive sites on the gel with 0.2M glycine, pH 8.0, for 2 h at room temperature with end-to-end mixing.
7. Wash the gel five times with coupling buffer containing 0.5M NaCl and then five times with 0.1M sodium acetate buffer, pH 4.0, containing 0.5M NaCl. Store in buffer C at 4°C.

3.3.2. Protein L Purification of L Chains (see Note 6)

1. Pack the protein L-Sepharose (3 mL settled gel) in a column, and equilibrate with 10 vol of buffer C. Monitor effluent absorbance at 280 nm.
2. Load the sample (1 mg protein in buffer C) at a flow rate of 1 mL/min.
3. Wash the gel with buffer C until a stable baseline is reached.
4. Elute bound L chains with buffer D, and immediately neutralize with 1M Tris-base. Collect 1-min fractions (1 mL each).
5. Test fractions by ELISA using anti-c-*myc* antibody (*see* Section 3.4.).
6. Test the purity of c-*myc*-stainable fractions by SDS-PAGE electrophoresis.

3.4. ELISA with Anti-c-myc 9E10 Antibody (see Notes 7 and 8)

1. Place a Multiscreen Immobilon P plate in the Multiscreen Vacuum Manifold. Dispense 50 µL 70% ethanol into each well. Wait for 1 min. Remove the ethanol by applying vacuum, and wash each well with MilliQ water (500 µL). The membrane should be wet when step 2 is performed.
2. Load 50–100 µL sample or c-*myc* peptide standard per well (2.5 µg/mL to 0.05 µg/mL) in PBS or 50 mM Tris-HCl, pH 8.0, and 0.1M glycine. Incu-

bate for 30 min at room temperature. Apply vacuum. Wash three times with wash buffer (200 µL each; 5 min each).

3. Block nonspecific binding sites with 200 µL blocking buffer for 30 min at 37°C. Wash three times with 200 µL wash buffer (5 min each).

4. Dispense into each well anti-c-*myc* monoclonal antibody (MAb) 9E10 (1:2000 in antibody buffer, 100 µL/well). Incubate for 2 h at room temperature. Wash 3 × 5 min with wash buffer.

5. Dispense into each well antimouse IgG labeled with peroxidase (1:2000 in antibody buffer, 100 µL/well). Incubate for 30 min at room temperature. Wash the plate three times with 200 µL wash buffer (5 min each).

6. Dispense 100 µL/well developing solution. Stop the reaction with 50 µL 10N H_2SO_4. Transfer 75-µL aliquots of the reaction mixtures to a polyvinylchloride or polystyrene 96-well plate, and read OD at 492 nm using an ELISA reader.

4. Notes

1. Ni-NTA gel is composed of NTA (nitrilo-triacetic acid) charged with Ni^{2+} and attached to Sepharose CL-6B. It has five open coordination sites on the immobilized Ni^{2+}. IMAC can also be performed using Fast Flow Chelating Sepharose (Pharmacia), which uses iminodiacetic acid as the Ni^{2+} chelator and has six open coordination sites available for protein binding.

2. Since metal chelating gels are positively charged, IMAC is usually performed at high ionic strength to avoid ion-exchange effects. This may also enhance the binding strength of chelated proteins owing to an increased contribution of the hydrophobic effect *(5)*.

3. β-mercaptoethanol is included in the initial steps of the purification in the dialysis and IMAC wash buffer to prevent disulfide bonding of L chains with other proteins. Glycerol and nonionic detergent (Tween-20) present in the IMAC buffer increase the stringency of Ni^{2+}–protein chelation and reduce copurification of irrelevant proteins.

4. Expression levels in culture medium for human L chains range from 0.1 to 1 mg/L. We have observed improved expression levels with low-expressing clones by use of low-density cultures during IPTG induction (initial OD_{600}, 0.4). Sometimes, the expression levels are higher in the periplasmic extract (*see* Gao and Paul, Chapter 19, this vol.).

5. Imidazole absorbs UV light (A_{280} of 1M imidazole is approx 1.0 at 1-cm path length), but protein elution can be monitored because A_{280} increases sharply and then stabilizes at the baseline level of imidazole absorbance. β-lactamase has approximately the same mol wt (30 kDa) as the L chain and coelutes with the latter protein in the early portion of the protein peak. The descending portion of the A_{280} peak contains about 90% pure L chain (Fig. 1).

6. Protein L binds human light of families κI, κIII, and κIV *(7)*.
7. The recombinant L chain contains a 10 amino acid c-*myc* tag recognized by anti-c-*myc* antibody 9E10 at their C-terminus. The c-*myc* peptide used as standard in ELISA is composed of 32 amino acids. The c-*myc* standard peptide and the L chains may not behave identically in the assay. Nevertheless, the ELISA is a useful predictor of relative L-chain concentrations in similarly prepared samples.
8. The assay can detect 0.05 μg/mL c-*myc* standard peptide. Apparent L-chain expression levels in unfractionated culture medium and periplasmic extracts is sometimes misleadingly low, possibly because of protein–protein aggregation or presence of inhibitory substances in crude samples.

References

1. Porath, J., Carlsson, J., Olsson, I., and Belfrage, G. (1975) Metal chelate affinity chromatography, a new approach to protein fractionation. *Nature* **258,** 598,599.
2. Bush, G. L., Tassin, A. M., Friden, H., and Meyer, D. I. (1991) Secretion in yeast. Purification and *in vitro* translocation of chemical amounts of prepro-factor. *J. Biol. Chem.* **266,** 13,811–13,814.
3. Janknecht, R., de Martynoff, G., Lou, G., Hipskind, R. A., Nordheim, A., and Stunnenberg, H. G. (1991) Rapid and efficient purification of native histidine-tagged protein expressed by recombinant vaccinia virus. *Proc. Natl. Acad. Sci. USA* **88,** 8972–8976.
4. Van Dyke, M. W., Sirito, M., and Sawadogo, M. (1992) Single-step purification of bacterially expressed polypeptides containing an oligo-histidine domain. *Gene* **111,** 99–104.
5. Scopes, R. K. (1994) *Protein Purification. Principles and Practices,* 3rd ed. Springer-Verlag, New York.
6. Nilson, B. N. K., Logdberg, L., Kastern, W., Bjorck, L., and Akerstrom, B. (1993) Purification of antibodies using protein L-binding framework structures in the light chain variable domain. *J. Immunol. Methods* **164,** 33–40.
7. Nilson, B. H. K., Solomon, A., Bjorck, L., and Akerstrom, B. (1992) Protein L from Peptostreptococcus magnus binds to the kappa light chain variable domain. *J. Biol. Chem.* **267,** 2234–2239.

CHAPTER 27

Rapid Purification
of Recombinant Antibody Fragments
for Catalysis Screening

Han Huang, Brian Fichter,
Robert Dannenbring, and Sudhir Paul

1. Introduction

A subpopulation of antibodies with high affinity for the substrate ground state is also capable of chemical catalysis *(1)*. However, high turnover by catalysts is dependent on efficient binding to the transition state, not the ground state. Direct screening for catalysis may permit isolation of more efficient antibody catalysts, since this approach obviates the requirement for strong binding to substrate ground states (or presumed transition state analogs). To this end, we have developed methods to purify recombinant antibody fragments rapidly, followed by measurement of their catalytic activity using peptide-methylcoumarinamide conjugates or radiolabeled peptides as substrates.

The procedure is conducted in 96-well plates, permitting purification and assay of large numbers of candidate catalysts in parallel, including positive and negative control clones. The purification step is based on the affinity of a hexahistidine tag in the recombinant antibody fragments for immobilized metal. Hydrolysis assays are performed at nanomolar concentrations of purified recombinant proteins. Only efficient catalysts are detected at these protein concentrations, lessening the chance that the catalytic activity is due to contaminants. The selected clones are then purified in larger scales and their activities confirmed and analyzed by conventional means.

From: *Methods in Molecular Biology, Vol. 51: Antibody Engineering Protocols*
Edited by: S. Paul Humana Press Inc., Totowa, NJ

2. Materials

2.1. Expression of Antibody Clones

Materials for expression of recombinant antibodies in medium and periplasmic extracts are described by Tyutyulkova and Paul, and Gao and Paul (Chapters 19 and 25).

2.2. Antibody Purification in 96-Well Plates

1. Ni-nitriloacetic acid (NTA)-Sepharose (Qiagen, Chatsworth, CA).
2. Millipore (Bedford, MA) Multi-screen apparatus.
3. Filtration plates fitted with 0.65 μm hydrophilic low protein binding filter (Millipore MADV S65 10).
4. Collection plates: Tissue culture treated, low protein binding (Costar 3595, Cambridge, MA).
5. Equilibration buffer: 50 mM sodium phosphate, pH 7.0, 0.5M sodium chloride, 0.025% Tween-20, 0.02% sodium azide, 1 mM imidazole.
6. Wash buffer: 50 mM sodium phosphate, pH 7.0, 0.025% Tween-20, 0.02% sodium azide.
7. Wash buffer 2: 50 mM sodium formate, pH 5.0, 0.025% Tween-20, 0.02% sodium azide.
8. Elution buffer 1: 50 mM sodium formate, pH 3.8, 0.025% Tween-20, 0.02% sodium azide.
9. Elution buffer 2: 100 mM glycine, pH 2.7, 0.025% Tween-20, 0.02% sodium azide.

2.3. Antibody Purification on Spin Columns

1. Ni-NTA spin columns for histidine-protein purification (Qiagen 31315). A silica matrix is used in these columns to impart pressure resistance.
2. Eppendorf (Westbury, NY) 5415C bench-top centrifuge.
3. Buffers described in Section 2.2.

3. Methods

3.1. Expression of Antibody Clones (see Note 1)

1. Transform *Escherichia coli* HB2151 cells with the antibody cDNA library cloned in pCANTABShis_6 (Chapter 25).
2. Grow bacteria on nutrient agar.
3. Pick individual colonies with toothpicks and dip into 200 μL 2YT medium containing 100 μg/mL ampicillin and 0.1% glucose in 96-well plates.
4. Grow the cells at 37°C for 3 h with shaking.
5. Add IPTG to 1 mM to induce recombinant antibody expression. Shake the plates at 30°C for 18 h.

6. Centrifuge plates at 1600*g* for 30 min at 4°C. Transfer 200 μL of supernatants into 96-well filtration plates for antibody purification (Section 3.2.,
   step 3).

3.2. Antibody Purification
in 96-Well Plates (see Notes 2–4)

1. Dispense 100 μL of settled Ni-NTA gel (200 μL slurry) into each well
   of a 96-well filtration plate. Apply suction using a Millipore Multi-screen
   apparatus.
2. Equilibrate the gel by passage of 2-mL equilibration buffer.
3. Dispense 200 μL culture supernatant into each well. Filter the samples at a
   flow rate of <100 μL/min by applying gentle suction.
4. Wash the gel with 2 mL wash buffer 1 (10 × 0.2 mL).
5. Wash the gel with 250 μL of wash buffer 2.
6. Elute antibodies with 250 μL elution buffer 1 into a 96-well catch plate.
7. Elute remaining strongly bound antibodies with 250 μL of elution buffer 2
   into wells containing 20 μL 1*M* Tris-HCl, pH 9.0.

3.3. Antibody Purification
on Spin Columns (see Notes 4 and 5)

1. Equilibrate spin columns with 2 mL (4 × 500 μL) of equilibration buffer.
   Centrifuge at 325*g* to permit passage of fluid through the column.
2. Pass 3-mL culture supernatant or periplasmic extract (6 × 500 μL) through
   the columns.
3. Pass 2-mL (4 × 500 μL) of wash buffer 1 and then 500 μL wash buffer 2
   through the column.
4. Elute bound antibodies with 500 μL of elution buffer 1 and 500 μL of
   elution buffer 2 in separate collection tubes. Perform the second elution in
   tubes containing 40 μL 1*M* Tris-HCl, pH 9.0.

4. Notes

1. Bacterial clones to be screened are grown under identical conditions and
   overgrowth is avoided to minimize well-to-well variations in the level of
   proteases released by the cells.
2. Rapid flow rates in the binding reaction (step 3) can lead to loss of recombinant antibodies in the flow-through. Regulate the flow rate by adjusting
   the positions of the sliding and rotating vacuum control knobs in the Millipore Multi-screen apparatus.
3. The recovery of recombinant antibodies in the eluates can be monitored by
   a dot-blot assay for c-*myc* (Chapter 19). The antibodies are generally
   present in both eluates (pH 3.8 and pH 2.7), with greater recovery obtained

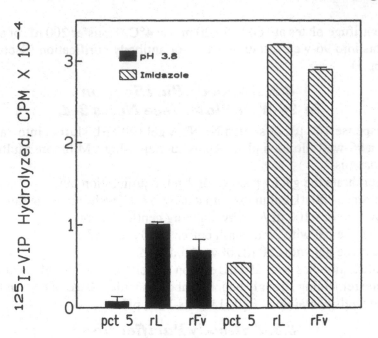

Fig. 1. ^{125}I-VIP hydrolysis by recombinant anti-VIP L chain (rL: clone mk18) and a single chain F_v (rF_v). Values are means of triplicates ±SD observed using 50 μL pH 3.8 or imidazole eluates. The VIP hydrolysis assay was conducted as in Huang et al. (Chapter 28). pct5 denotes eluates from bacterial cultures harboring the control vector without antibody insert.

in the pH 2.7 eluate. Histidine imidazoles are protonated in low pH buffers and cannot coordinate immobilized metal, resulting in release of the recombinant antibody from the matrix. Elution can also be done using 100–250 mM imidazole. The imidazole must be removed by dialysis prior to catalysis assays, since this compound may accelerate acyl-transfer reactions.

4. The proteolytic activity of recombinant antibodies can be assayed using radiolabeled polypeptides or fluorigenic peptide substrates (Chapters 28 and 29). Figure 1 shows the levels of radiolabeled VIP hydrolyzed by eluates containing an anti-VIP recombinant light chain and an anti-VIP F_v, and control eluates prepared from bacteria transformed with vector without antibody inserts.

5. The spin-column procedure can be used to purify comparatively large quantities of recombinant antibodies. Purities of the antibodies are generally

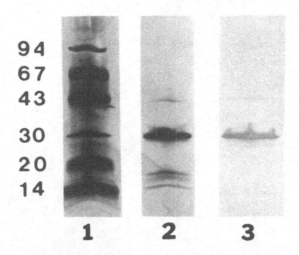

Fig. 2. Silver stained SDS-polyacrylamide gels (8–25%) showing recombinant F_v (lane 2) recombinant L chain (lane 3) in the pH 2.7 eluates from spin columns. Lane 1 shows marker proteins.

>95%. Figure 2 shows silver-stained SDS-polyacrylamide gels with overloaded antibody fragments, corresponding to the bands at approx 27 kDa.

Reference

1. Paul, S., Sun, M., Mody, R., Eklund, S. H., Beach, C. M., Massey, R. J., and Hamel, F. (1991) Cleavage of vasoactive intestinal peptide at multiple sites by autoantibodies. *J. Biol. Chem.* **266,** 16,128–16,134.

CHAPTER 28

Assay of Radiolabeled VIP Binding and Hydrolysis by Antibodies

Han Huang and Sudhir Paul

1. Introduction

High-specific-activity radiolabeled polypeptide probes permit sensitive detection of antigen–antibody interactions. In the case of small polypeptides labeled with ^{125}I, various iodinated forms can be separated by reversed-phase HPLC and resolved peaks characterized by protein chemistry methods. We describe here methods for preparation and purification of vasoactive intestinal (VIP) labeled at Tyr[10] with ^{125}I, and the use of (Tyr[10]-^{125}I)VIP to characterize antibody binding and enzymatic activities.

2. Materials

2.1. Iodination and Purification of ^{125}I-VIP

1. Sodium [125]iodide (Amersham); 17.4 mCi/µg iodine in dilute sodium hydroxide solution.
2. Synthetic VIP (His-Ser-Asp-Ala-Val-Phe-Thr-Asp-Asn-Tyr-Thr-Arg-Leu-Arg-Lys-Gln-Met-Ala-Val-Lys-Lys-Tyr-Leu-Asn-Ser-Ile-Leu-Asn-NH$_2$): Dissolve VIP at 1 mM in 0.1N acetic acid, and store in aliquots at −80°C. The peptide can be purchased from Peninsula Laboratories or Bachem California, or if routine use is anticipated, it can be synthesized at a more reasonable cost by protein synthesis core facilities available at most universities.
3. 0.5M sodium phosphate buffer, pH 7.4.
4. 1 mg/mL chloramine-T in water.
5. 5 mg/mL sodium metabisulfite in water.

From: *Methods in Molecular Biology, Vol. 51: Antibody Engineering Protocols*
Edited by: S. Paul Humana Press Inc., Totowa, NJ

6. Seppak C18 cartridges (Waters, Milford, MA).
7. Glass conical vials for iodination.
8. Reversed-phase HPLC system equipped with a C18 column (e.g., NovaPak C18, 5 μm; Waters) capable of generating binary gradients. We use an Isco HPLC System with two Model 2350 pumps, ChemResearch software, and an S500 Linear multiwavelength absorbance monitor. A flowthrough radioisotope detector (Beckman T-170) is useful for on-line monitoring of effluent radioactivity.
9. Solvent A for HPLC: 0.1% trifluoroacetic (TFA) acid in water.
10. Solvent B for HPLC: 0.1% TFA and 80% acetonitrile in water.
11. γ-Spectrometer (Packard Model 1600, 80% efficiency).
12. SpeedVac centrifuge system (Savant).

2.2. VIP Binding Assay

1. Binding assay buffer: 7.7 mM sodium phosphate, 0.65% sodium chloride, 0.05% sodium azide, 0.005% protamine sulfate, 0.005% bacitracin, 0.5% bovine serum albumin (BSA) (RIA grade, Sigma, St. Louis, MO), 0.025% Tween-20, 25 mM EDTA, pH 7.4.
2. 4 mg/mL γ-globulins (Sigma).
3. 12% polyethylene glycol-6000 (PEG) in water.

2.3. VIP Hydrolysis

1. Hydrolysis assay buffer: 50 mM Tris-HCl, 100 mM glycine, pH 7.7, at 37°C, 0.025% Tween-20.
2. (Tyr^{10}-^{125}I)VIP in hydrolysis assay buffer containing 0.4% BSA.
3. 12.1% trichloroacetic acid (w/v; TCA) in water.

3. Methods
3.1. Preparation and Purification of (Tyr^{10}-^{125}I)VIP

1. Mix 10 μL 0.5M sodium phosphate, pH 7.4, 3 μL 1 mM VIP (10 μg peptide) and 20 μL ^{125}I (2 mCi) in the iodination vial.
2. While slowly vortexing the mixture, add 10 μL of a freshly prepared 1 mg/mL chloramine-T solution. Vortex slowly for 30 s (*see* Note 1).
3. Terminate the reaction by addition of 20 μL 5 mg/mL sodium metabisulphite.
4. Pre-equilibrate a C18 Seppak cartridge with 10 mL solvent B followed by 10 mL solvent A. Transfer the contents of the iodination vial to the barrel of a syringe connected to the Seppak cartridge, wash the vial with 0.5 mL solvent A, and transfer to the syringe barrel. Push the liquid through the cartridge slowly (the flow rate should be <1 mL/min to permit peptide binding). Collect the unbound material.

5. Wash the cartridge with 10 mL solvent A. Collect about 2.5 mL each of the effluent in four tubes.

6. Elute bound peptide with 3 mL solvent B into a glass tube. Count 1-μL aliquots of the solvent B eluate and unbound material from steps 4 and 5. Approximately 50–75% of the initial radioactivity elutes in the solvent B eluate, representing peptide-bound radioactivity.

7. Dry the eluate using a SpeedVac centrifuge equipped with a chemical trap. Redissolve the radiolabeled peptide in 500 μL 75% solvent A/25% solvent B.

8. Fractionate the peptide on a NovaPak C18 column using a gradient of solvent B in solvent A (0–5 min, 25% solvent B; 5–15 min, 25–30% solvent B; 15–95 min, 30–50% solvent B; 95–105 min, 50–100% solvent B) at a flow rate of 0.5 mL/min. Monitor optical density at 214 nm (0.05 AUFS) and radioactivity at full-scale setting of 100 K cpm (detector shielded with one lead disk supplied by the manufacturer). Count 1-μL aliquots of fractions (0.5 mL each) in a γ-counter.

9. The first major peak of radioactivity eluting at 34.6% acetonitrile (Fig. 1) is composed of (Tyr^{10}-^{125}I)VIP (*see* Note 2). Pool fractions corresponding to this peak. The yield of radioactivity in this peak is generally >200 × 10^6 dpm.

10. Mix an equivalent volume of 0.5% BSA in 0.2*M* acetic acid with the radiolabeled peptide pool. Store aliquots of the preparation at –80°C (*see* Note 3).

3.2. VIP Binding Assay

1. Mix 50 μL (Tyr^{10}-^{125}I)VIP (about 30,000 cpm), 100 μL antibody sample and 50 μL unlabeled VIP or buffer in 12 × 75 mm polystyrene tubes. The reaction volume is 200 μL. Unlabeled VIP can be included at varying concentrations up to 100 μ*M* to determine competitive inhibition characteristics and binding affinity. Tubes containing excess unlabeled VIP yield nonsaturable ("nonspecific") binding values.

2. Mix by vortexing, and incubate at 4°C for 16–24 h.

3. Add 25 μL 4 mg/mL γ-globulins to each tube. Mix and then add 1 mL polyethylene glycol to precipitate antigen–antibody complexes (*see* Note 4).

4. Mix well, incubate at room temperature for 5 min, and centrifuge at 3000*g* for 30 mm at 4°C.

5. Aspirate the supernatant with a Pasteur pipet attached to a vacuum source via a collection trap. Suction levels afforded by ordinary laboratory water pumps are sufficient.

6. Determine radioactivity in the pellets using a γ-counter. Counting times permitting registration of ~5000 counts by the instrument are usually suf-

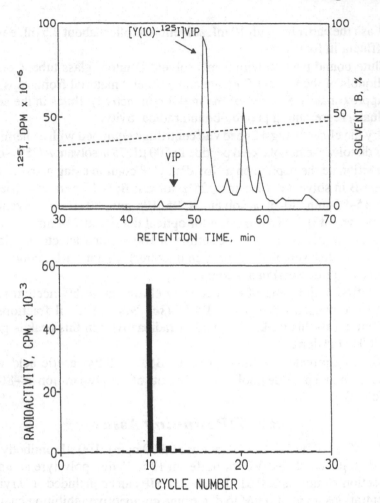

Fig. 1. Preparation of [Tyr^{10}-^{125}I]VIP. *Top:* Synthetic VIP labeled with ^{125}I using chloramine-T was separated on a C-18 Novapak (Waters) column using a gradient of 0.1% TFA in water (solvent A) and 0.1% TFA in 80% acetonitrile and water (solvent B, dotted line) for elution. *Bottom:* An aliquot of the radioactive peak at retention time 51.1 min was subjected to N-terminal amino acid sequencing, and ^{125}I in the effluent from individual cycles was measured.

ficient. Compute saturable binding as: $(cpm_{Tot}-cpm_{VIP,ex})$. Convert binding values into mass units according to:

$$[(cpm_{Tot} - cpm_{VIP,ex})/(cpm \text{ available radioactivity} - cpm_{VIP,ex})]$$
$$\times (\text{molarity of unlabeled VIP} + \text{molarity of radioactive VIP}) \qquad (1)$$

where $cpm_{VIP, ex}$ refers to binding at excess (saturating) concentrations of VIP and cpm_{Tot} refers to total binding without unlabeled VIP or at lower concentrations of the peptide. Antibody binding affinity and capacity can be computed with EBDA and LIGAND programs (*see* Note 5).

3.3. VIP Hydrolysis Assay

1. Mix 50 µL $(Tyr^{10}\text{-}^{125}I)$VIP (about 100,000 cpm) with 50 µL antibody sample and 100 µL hydrolysis assay buffer in 12 × 75 mm polystyrene tubes. Use 50 µL assay buffer instead of antibody sample in control tubes. Mix and incubate at 37°C for 3–24 h with slow shaking in a water bath (*see* Note 6).
2. Add 1 mL 12.1% cold TCA. Vortex and centrifuge at 3000 g for 20 min at 4°C.
3. Aspirate the supernatants and count the pellets using a γ-counter.
4. Compute percent hydrolysis of VIP as:

$$[(cpm_{buffer} - cpm_{antibody})/cpm_{buffer}] \times 100 \qquad (2)$$

where cpm_{buffer} and $cpm_{antibody}$ refer to radioactivity in the absence and presence of antibody, respectively. Reaction kinetics can be studied by obtaining initial rate data at several peptide concentrations and analysis with programs such as EnzFitter (*see* Note 7).

4. Notes

1. There are two Tyr residues available for iodination in VIP (positions 10 and 22). Prolonged oxidation with chloramine-T leads to formation of heavily iodinated peptide variants that are monoiodinated or di-iodinated at either or both Tyr residues.
2. Figure 1 shows the elution profile of the iodination mixture. N-terminal radiosequencing of the first major peak of radioactivity using an automated liquid-phase sequencer with on-line phenylthiohydantoin (PTH) amino acid detection yielded most of the radioactivity in the tenth cycle. A small proportion of the radioactivity was also present in cycle 11, presumably representing residual material from the preceding cycle (1). The radioactivity from both cycles coeluted from a reversed-phase HPLC column with a PTH derivative of authentic ^{127}monoiodotyrosine. These observations indicated that this peak of radioactivity is composed of $(Tyr^{10}\text{-}^{125}I)$VIP. The later eluting radioactive peaks in Fig. 1 yielded radioactivity only in cycle 22 or in cycles 10 as well as 22. The specific activity of the $(Tyr^{10}\text{-}^{125}I)$VIP prepared in this way is 2000 Ci/mmol.
3. Freshly purified $(Tyr^{10}\text{-}^{125}I)$VIP can be essentially completely precipitated with 10% trichloracetic acid or excess anti-VIP antibody. The radiolabeled peptide should be used for immunoassays within 2 mo of preparation.

Approximately 70–80% of the peptide is TCA-precipitable after storage for this length of time. Storage of the peptide without BSA leads to fairly rapid breakdown, assayed by TCA precipitation and reversed-phase HPLC *(2)*.

4. Complexes of VIP with intact IgG (molecular mass 150 kDa) are essentially completely precipitated at a concentration of 10% PEG *(3)*. Increased concentration of PEG (20% w/v) permits precipitation of VIP–light chain complexes and VIP–scF$_v$ complexes *(4)*. Dextran-coated charcoal can also be used to discriminate between bound and free VIP *(5)*. Free peptide is adsorbed by the charcoal, leaving complexes of the peptide in the supernatant. Covalent crosslinking of VIP through Lys side chains using crosslinkers like dithio(bis)succinimidylpropionate, followed by SDS-electrophoresis and autoradiography, permits direct visualization of VIP complexes with larger proteins *(6)*.

5. These programs can be obtained from Elsevier-Biosoft or from the National Institutes of Health, USA (D. Rodbard). The analysis assumes equivalence of antibody interactions with radiolabeled and unlabeled VIP. Binding affinities can also be computed using increasing concentrations of radiolabeled peptide alone (instead of mixtures of radiolabeled and unlabeled peptides). Estimates of binding constants can be obtained by constructions of Scatchard plots (bound peptide vs bound/free peptide). Manual estimates of affinity are subject to significant errors.

6. About 80–90% of the peptide remains TCA-precipitable after incubation for 6 h at 37°C in the absence of BSA and catalysts. Longer incubations should be performed in the presence of 0.1% BSA in the diluent to minimize spontaneous hydrolysis of the peptide *(1)*. Estimates of peptide breakdown by this method correlate very well with those obtained using reversed-phase HPLC to separate intact and degraded peptide (2).

7. The substrate can be radioactive VIP alone at increasing concentrations or a mixture of radioactive VIP with increasing concentrations of unlabeled VIP. In the latter case, the values of cpm hydrolysis decrease with increasing concentrations of unlabeled VIP. The cpm hydrolysis data can be converted into mass units as in Section 3.2.

References

1. Mody, R. K., Tramontano, A., and Paul, S. (1994) Spontaneous hydrolysis of VIP in neutral aqueous solution. *Int. J. Pept. Protein Res.* **44,** 441–447.
2. Paul, S., Sun, M., Mody, B., Eklund, S. H., Beach, C. M., Massey, R. J., and Hamel, F. (1991) Cleavage of vasoactive intestinal peptide at multiple sites by autoantibodies. *J. Biol. Chem.* **266,** 16,128–16,134.

3. Paul, S., Said, S. I., Thompson, A. B., Volle, D. J., Agrawal, D. K., Foda, H., and de la Rocha, S. (1989) Characterization of autoantibodies to vasoactive intestinal peptide in asthma. *J. Neuroimmunol.* **23,** 133–142.
4. Sun, M., Li, L., Gao, Q.-S., and Paul, S. (1994) Antigen recognition by an antibody light chain. *J. Biol. Chem.* **269,** 734–738.
5. Brugger, C., Stallwood, D., and Paul, S. (1991) Isolation of a low molecular mass vasoactive intestinal peptide binding protein. *J. Biol. Chem.* **266,** 18,358–18,362.
6. Stallwood, D., Brugger, C., Baggenstoss, B., Stemmer, P., Shiraga, H., Landers, D., and Paul, S. (1992) Identity of a membrane-bound vasoactive intestinal peptide-binding protein with calmodulin. *J. Biol. Chem.* **267,** 19,617–19,621.

CHAPTER 29

Methods of Measuring Thyroglobulin and Peptide-Methylcoumarinamide Hydrolysis by Autoantibodies

Lan Li, Ravishankar Kalaga, Srinivas Kaveri, and Sudhir Paul

1. Introduction

Polyclonal antibodies often serve as the starting point for interesting studies of new antibody functions and their links with immunoregulation and autoimmune disease. For example, the catalytic activity of naturally formed antibodies was first discovered using human autoantibody mixtures (1,2). Thyroglobulin (Tg), a large water-soluble glycoprotein (mass approx 660 kDa) is a classical target for autoimmune responses. Thyroglobulin is stored in the thyroid colloid and can constitute up to 70% of the total protein in this gland. The protein is iodinated within the thyroid by peroxidase-catalyzed reactions and proteolytic processing of the iodinated Tg leads to formation of the thyroid hormones T_3 and T_4. Autoantibodies to Tg are found in >80% of patients with Hashimoto's thyroiditis, a disease characterized by thyroid damage and hyperthyroidism. Here, we describe a method to measure the catalytic breakdown of Tg by autoantibody fractions. Since Tg contains several repeat domains and antigenic epitopes (3,4), the hydrolytic specificity of the antibodies was determined using a panel of commercially available peptide-methylcoumarinamide (peptide-MCA) substrates. Cleavage of the amide bond linking an amino acid and the coumarin moiety in these substrates serves as a convenient surrogate for peptide bond hydrolysis.

From: *Methods in Molecular Biology, Vol. 51: Antibody Engineering Protocols*
Edited by: S. Paul Humana Press Inc., Totowa, NJ

The peptide-MCA substrates have previously been used to assay the activity of endopeptidases and exopeptidases *(5)*.

2. Materials

1. Thyroglobulin (UCB, Braine L'Alleud, Belgium, or Chemicon, Temecula, CA). Reconstituted in 30 mM sodium phosphate buffer, pH 7.4.
2. 0.5M sodium phosphate buffer, pH 7.4.
3. Chloramine T: 1 mg/mL in water. Prepare fresh before use.
4. Tg-specific autoantibody: This can be purified from patients with Hashimoto's thyroiditis by protein G-Sepharose chromatography followed by Tg-Sepharose chromatography *(6)*. Store antibodies in buffer A.
5. Sodium meta-bisulfite: 2.5 mg/mL in water.
6. Econo-Pac 10DG columns (Bio-Rad, Hercules, CA).
7. Superose-6 gel filtration column (Pharmacia, Piscataway, NJ).
8. Na^{125}I in 0.1N NaOH (Amersham, Arlington Heights, VA).
9. SDS-polyacrylamide gels (4–15%) and Pharmacia Phast System.
10. Nonreducing electrophoresis sample buffer (2X): 2.5 mL 0.5M Tris-HCl, pH 6.8, 4 mL 10% (w/v) SDS, 0.5 mL 0.1% Bromophenol blue, 2 mL glycerol, and distilled water to 10 mL.
11. High molecular weight marker calibration kit (Pharmacia).
12. Kodak XAR5 X-ray film for autoradiography.
13. UMAX Data Scanning System (UC630) equipped with Image 1.43a processing and analysis software (courtesy of W. Rasband, NIH Research Services Branch) and Adobe Photoshop.
14. Buffer A: 50 mM Tris-HCl, 100 mM glycine, 0.025% Tween-20, 0.02% sodium azide, pH 7.7 at 37°C.
15. Buffer B: 0.1% bovine serum albumin (BSA) in Buffer A.
16. Buffer C: 0.5M sodium chloride in Buffer A.
17. Buffer D: 0.01% BSA in Buffer A.
18. Peptidyl-MCA conjugates (Peptides International, Louisville, KY or Sigma, St. Louis, MO). Dissolve in dimethyl-sulfoxide at a concentration of 10 mM and store in aliquots at –80°C.
19. Perkin-Elmer LS-50 fluorimeter with plate reader.
20. 96-well Microfluor W plates (Dynatech, Chantilly, VA).

3. Methods

3.1. Radioiodination
of Thyroglobulin (see Notes 1 and 2)

1. Mix 5 μg Tg (5 μL), 30 μL 0.5M sodium phosphate, pH 7.4, and 0.5 mCi (5 μL) Na^{125}I in a conical glass reaction vial. While gently vortexing this solution, add 20 μL (20 μg) chloramine T. Continue vortexing for 1 min.

2. Terminate the reaction by addition of 100 µL of sodium meta-bisulfite (250 µg). Then add 2 mL buffer B to the reaction vial.
3. Equilibrate an Econo-Pac 10DG column with 5 bed vol of buffer B. Apply the reaction mixture from step 1 on the column. Run the sample completely into the column. Elute with 10 mL buffer A by gravity flow. Collect 1-mL fractions (*see* Note 1).
4. Count 1-µL aliquots from each fraction in a γ-counter. Pool the protein-bound radioactivity eluting at the column void volume. Concentrate the pool to <1 mL using a Centricon-10 ultrafilter device.
5. Apply the sample from step 4 to a Superose-6 column equilibrated with buffer C. Elute at a flow rate of 0.5 mL/min. Count 1-µL aliquots of the fractions (0.5 mL each).
6. To 5-µL aliquots of radioactive fractions, add an equal volume of 2X electrophoresis buffer. Analyze fractions by SDS-polyacrylamide gel electrophoresis.
7. Air dry the gels and expose to an X-ray film. Pool fractions containing a single 330 kDa ^{125}I-Tg band (*see* Note 2).
8. Desalt ^{125}I-Tg solution on an Econo-Pac 10DG column in Buffer D as in step 3.
9. Store ^{125}I-Tg in aliquots of $5–10 \times 10^6$ CPM at –80°C.

3.2. ^{125}I-Tg Hydrolysis (see Notes 3 and 4)

1. Incubate ~10,000 CPM ^{125}I-Tg (~3.9 nM Tg) with anti-Tg or control antibodies in 20 µL Buffer A for 3–16 h at 38°C.
2. Add 20 µL 2X electrophoresis sample buffer. Electrophorese on 4–15% SDS-polyacrylamide gels.
3. Perform autoradiography. Hydrolysis of ^{125}I-Tg is indicated by a reduction in the intensity of the 330 kDa Tg monomer band and appearance of new bands corresponding to lower-sized products.
4. Estimate the intensity of the Tg band by computer-assisted image densitometry. Calculate % hydrolysis as: (band area in diluent – band area in antibody) × 100 / (band area in diluent).

3.3. Peptidyl-MCA Cleavage (see Notes 5–7)

1. Mix the peptide-MCA substrate with antibody in a reaction volume of 60 µL in a 96-well plate.
2. Incubate the plate at 37°C in a humidified chamber.
3. Read fluorescence at desired time intervals (excitation, 370 nm; emission, 460 nm).
4. Correct data for background fluorescence observed in control substrate wells incubated in diluent without antibody. Calculate product concentration by comparison with fluorescence yield obtained with standard aminomethylcoumarin (*see* Note 7).

4. Notes

1. Econo-column fractionation immediately after iodination removes unreacted radioiodine. Subsequent resolutive chromatography on Superose-6 is necessary to remove thyroglobulin fragments generated during iodination reaction. Clean interpretations of the hydrolysis experiments are largely dependent on availability of ^{125}I-Tg displaying a single 330 kDa band in electrophoresis gels. BSA present in the Econo-column buffer minimizes adsorption of Tg by the column. High salt buffer (0.5M sodium chloride) is used in the Superose-6 buffer for the same reason. ^{125}I-Tg stored at −80°C is stable for about 4 wk.

2. Commercially available Tg preparations yield a single-protein band at 330 kDa in nonreducing SDS-polyacrylamide gels. Additional bands are present in some preparations in reducing gels, presumably because cleaved polypeptide fragments are still linked via disulfide bonds.

3. Controls can include antibodies immunoadsorbed with immobilized anti-human antibodies or the flow-through antibodies from the Tg-Sepharose column. The latter are depleted of Tg-reactive antibodies and should display essentially no reaction with substrate.

4. Reaction kinetics can be examined by measuring hydrolysis of a fixed concentration of ^{125}I-Tg mixed with increasing concentrations of Tg. For this purpose, select an antibody concentration and incubation time resulting in less than 30% substrate hydrolysis. The K_m values for natural antibodies with Tg-hydrolyzing activities is in the nM range *(7)*.

5. Several types of peptide-MCA conjugates are available commercially. Anti-Tg antibodies display preferential cleavage at Arg-MCA and Lys-MCA bonds. Examination of specificity can include substrates containing MCA conjugated to basic, acidic, uncharged, or aromatic residues.

6. Repetitive readings at several time points can be obtained to study reaction kinetics. Background fluorescence of peptide-MCA substrates is generally less than 20 fluorescence units.

7. A standard curve is constructed at several concentrations of aminomethylcoumarin (0.5 μM–10 μM/60 μL) and values of product concentration are read off this curve.

References

1. Paul, S., Volle, D. J., Beach, C. M., Johnson, D. R., Powell, M. J., and Massey, R. J. (1989) Catalytic hydrolysis of vasoactive intestinal peptide by human autoantibody. *Science* **244**, 1158–1162.
2. Shuster, A. M., Gololobov, G. V., Kvashuk, O. A., Bogomolova, A. E., Smirnov, I. V., and Gabibov, A. G. (1992) DNA hydrolyzing autoantibodies. *Science* **256**, 665–667.

3. Mercken, L., Simons, M. J., Swillens, S., Massaer, M., and Vassart, G. (1985) Primary structure of bovine thyroglobulin deduced from the sequence of its 8,431-base complementary DNA. *Nature* **316,** 647–651.
4. Dong, Q., Ludgate, M., and Vassart, G. (1989) Towards an antigenic map of human thyroglobulin: identification of ten epitope-bearing sequences within the primary structure of thyroglobulin. *J. Endocrinol.* **122,** 169–176.
5. Sarath, G., De La Motte, R. S., and Wagner, F. W. (1989) Protease assay methods, in *Proteolytic Enzymes: A Practical Approach* (Beynon, R. J. and Bond, J. S., eds.), IRL, Oxford, UK, pp. 25–55.
6. Dietrich, G. and Kazatchkine, M. D. (1990) Normal immunoglobulin G (IgG) for therapeutic use (intravenous Ig) contain cross-reactive idiotype of human anti-thyroglobulin autoantibodies. *J. Clin. Invest.* **85,** 620–625.
7. Li, L., Kaveri, S., Tyutyulkova, S., Kazatchkine, M., and Paul, S. (1995) Catalytic activity of anti-thyroglobulin antibodies. *J. Immunol.* **154,** 3328–3332.

CHAPTER 30

Radiolabeling of Antibodies for Therapy and Diagnosis

Janina Baranowska-Kortylewicz, Glenn V. Dalrymple, Syed M. Quadri, and Katherine A. Harrison

1. Introduction

Radioimmunotherapeutic and radioimmunodiagnostic procedures have been the subjects of nearly 200 clinical trials since 1978. Applications range from diagnosis of tumor deposits to systemic radiation therapy. Originally, murine IgG was the most common antibody form used clinically. Later the antibody fragments, Fab and F(ab')$_2$, were extensively investigated as the alternative radioisotope carriers displaying more favorable pharmacokinetics. Future clinical applications will include products of molecular engineering, such as single-chain antigen-binding proteins, "humanized" (also known as "chimeric") antibodies, human antibodies, and bifunctional antibodies. Selection of antibodies for clinical trials is an extensive and detailed process. The factors to be considered include characterization of the antibody with regard to its interactions with the antigen(s) of interest, nonspecific binding to nontarget tissues, and in vivo pharmacokinetics. In addition, the biological consequences of chemical modifications made during production of the radiolabeled material must be assessed. Ideally, the choice of the radioisotope and radiolabeling methods is individually tailored for each antibody to yield products that display minimally impaired biological properties for any given application. Only seldom can such a detailed approach be afforded. Thus, prior experiences with antibodies and radioisotopes described in the literature are useful in designing the experi-

From: Methods in Molecular Biology, Vol. 51: Antibody Engineering Protocols
Edited by: S. Paul Humana Press Inc., Totowa, NJ

Table 1
Selected Radionuclides Used for Labeling of Antibodies

Isotope	Half-life	Decay	Application	Comments
^{211}At	7.2 h	α	Therapy	Not available commercially
^{212}Bi	1.0 h	$\alpha,\beta-$	Therapy	Short half-life
^{18}F	1.8 h	$\beta+$	Diagnosis (PET)	Short half-life
^{123}I	13.1 h	EC, γ	Diagnosis (SPECT)	Auger electrons, short half-life
^{124}I	4.2 d	$\beta+$ (23%)	Diagnosis (PET)	Not available commercially
^{125}I	60.0 d	EC, X-rays	Therapy	Auger electrons
^{131}I	8.05 d	$\beta-$, γ	Therapy, diagnosis	Optimal half-life
^{111}In	2.8 d	EC, γ	Diagnosis	Optimal imaging characteristics
^{99m}Tc	6.0 h	IT, γ	Diagnosis	From generator, short half-life
^{90}Y	2.7 d	$\beta-$	Therapy	Pure $\beta-$ decay

mental strategies. For each of the commonly used radioisotopes, there are several well-tested methods. A brief overview of available methodologies and specific procedures for radiolabeling with radiometals is given in the following sections.

1.1. Selection of Radioisotope

The choice of the radionuclide for antibody labeling depends first on the intended use, i.e., diagnosis vs systemic radiation therapy. Some clinically useful radioisotopes for labeling of antibodies are listed in Table 1. The half-life of the radionuclide should match pharmacokinetics of the antibody. For example, if the optimum tumor uptake and tumor-to-blood ratios are observed 3 d after the administration of the radiolabeled protein, then radioisotopes with half-lives of a few hours are not very useful.

The emissions from radionuclides used for most imaging methods should be in the form of photons in the energy range of 120–200 keV. Only positron emission tomography (PET) requires the presence of particulate emission (positrons), and the imaging involves photons produced by the annihilation of positrons and electrons. Ideally, the radioisotope selected for immunoscintigraphy should produce only γ radiation. Iodine-123, indium-111, and technetium-99m have excellent energies for γ camera imaging and external counting. Iodine-131 is a versatile radioisotope frequently used for both imaging and therapy, because its half-life is compatible with pharmacokinetics of many antibodies. The time required for antibody to equilibrate in tissues and to give the maximum tumor-to-nontarget ratio should always be given the major consideration when selecting a radiosotope.

Typical radionuclides used for systemic radiation therapy emit α or β particles (^{90}Y, ^{131}I, ^{211}At, ^{32}P), but there is an increasing interest in the use of Auger-electron-emitting radionuclides, particularly iodine-123 and iodine-125. To date, most of the clinical Phase I and II trials have used ^{131}I-labeled antibodies *(1–5)*. This selection is related in part to the simplicity of chemical methods used to label the antibody, a favorable half-life of this isotope, the availability of gamma photons for imaging, and in part to the energy of β particles. However, the use of ^{131}I-labeled antibodies presents a difficult health-physics problem associated with the radiation dose from the γ photons. Frequently an extended hospital admission is required. Other problems include the disposal of ^{131}I released from the patient during hospitalization. The energy of β particles of ^{131}I is too low for optimum therapy of many tumors. Consequently, ^{90}Y is replacing ^{131}I in some radioimmunotherapy applications. This radionuclide (^{90}Y) is a pure β-emitter; the β energy is 2.29 MeV as contrasted to 0.606 MeV (89%) for ^{131}I.

For practical reasons, if the same antibody is considered for diagnosis and therapy, the radiolabeling method should be applicable to both radio-isotopes. A good example is the use of ^{111}In-labeled antibodies for imaging and ^{90}Y-labeled antibodies for therapy. The chemistry of both metals is similar, and a single modification of an antibody with diethylenetriamine-pentaacetic acid (DTPA) services both labeling protocols. A final and very practical reason for choosing the radioisotope is its availability (*see* Table 1).

1.2. Radiolabeling with Halogens

The chemistry involved in the radioiodination of proteins is well established and has been used for decades. Most of the methods rely on the electrophilic substitution in the presence of oxidants (chloramine-T, iodogen). A brief summary of the most commonly used methods and conditions is listed in Table 2. After direct radioiodination, the radiolabel is covalently bound to a tyrosine residue. Proteins are subject to in vivo dehalogenation. This loss of radiolabel causes considerable problems owing to the radiation dose received by the thyroid, stomach, and bladder *(5–7)*. A number of indirect radioiodination methods have been introduced to circumvent this problem. Several extensive reviews on the radioiodination of proteins have been published *(8,9)*.

Table 2
Commonly Used Methods for Radioiodination of Proteins

Oxidant	Description of method
Iodogen	Precoat a radiolabeling tube with iodogen (100 µg/tube), add 0.1–1 mL of 1 mg/mL solution of antibody in PBS, add 5 mCi of sodium radiodide, react at room temperature for 10 min, stop the reaction with 100 µL of 1 mg/mL sodium metabisulfite in PBS, and purify on a Sephadex G-25 column
Chloramine-T	Add 5 mCi of sodium radioiodide to an antibody solution (1 mg/mL, from 0.1–1 mL), mix gently, add 10 µg of chloramine-T dissolved in water at 1 mg/mL, react at room temperature for 1–2 min, stop the reaction with 100 µL of 1 mg/mL sodium metabisulfite in PBS, and purify on a Sephadex G-25 column

1.3. Radiolabeling with Metal (III) Cations

In contrast to radioiodination, the direct labeling of antibodies with metals, such as ^{111}In and ^{90}Y, is not feasible. The antibody must first be modified with an appropriate chelating agent. Among the many methods developed and reported in the literature for coupling of the chelator DTPA to antibodies, the bicyclic anhydride of DTPA has proven to be the most successful *(10)*. The anhydride is available commercially, it is stable at room temperature as long as it is moisture-free, the conjugation protocol is simple and efficient, and antibodies appear to retain their immunoreactivity when one or two DTPA molecules are conjugated to one molecule of protein. The excessive accumulation and retention of radiometals in the liver and bone have prompted development of various derivatives of DTPA and other chelating agents that produce metal complexes with superior in vivo stability. One derivative with reportedly improved in vivo properties is 1-(4'-isothiocyanatobenzyl)DPTA-(ITC-Bz-DTPA). Its reaction with the amino group of lysine residues produces thiourea linkages with proteins *(11)*. Regardless of the chelating agent used, once the antibody–DTPA conjugate is purified, radiolabeling protocols are virtually identical for several metal (III) cations (*see* Sections 3.3. and 3.4.). The apparent simplicity of antibody labeling with radiometals is somewhat deceptive. The method requires a strict control of the DTPA-to-protein ratio (the radioimmunoreactivity decreases rapidly with the increasing number of DTPA molecules conjugated to the same antibody). Because practically any metal can produce a complex with DTPA, every procedure must be conducted with metal-free reagents in metal-free containers. The purity of the radioisotope is also critical. Even seemingly minute contamination with other metals can have detrimental effects on the radiolabeling of antibodies. The protocols described below assume that a high chemical purity is maintained at all stages of conjugate preparation and radiolabeling.

1.4. Recent Clinical Experience

To date, 16 patients with advanced Hodgkin's disease were enrolled in a Phase I clinical trial involving ^{111}In-Bz-DTPA-labeled and ^{90}Y-Bz-DTPA-labeled rabbit antiferritin antibody for diagnosis and therapy, respectively. Figure 1 shows a ^{111}In-Bz-DTPA-antiferritin study of a 28-yr-old man with advanced, recurrent Hodgkin's disease (Stage 3A). He had prior chemotherapy, bone marrow, and stem-cell transplants. Four days prior to imaging, the patient had been injected with 5 mCi ^{111}In-Bz-DTPA-labeled antiferritin (specific activity 3.21 mCi/mg antibody). Note the uptake of antiferritin in tumor deposits in the left supraclavicular region and pulmonary hila (indicated with T). Physiologic uptake in the liver (L) and spleen (S) is also noted. Eight days after the injection of ^{111}In-labeled antiferritin, the patient was injected with the therapeutic dose of 24.2 mCi ^{90}Y-Bz-DTPA-antiferritin (specific activity 13.5 mCi/mg antibody; the dose of 0.19 mCi/kg; four patients participated at each dose level). Since ^{90}Y is a pure β-emitter, direct imaging is not possible. Imaging of photons emitted as a consequence of Bremstrahlung is possible (not shown), but has poor resolution. A follow-up ^{67}Ga study 5 wk after treatment with ^{90}Y antiferritin showed improvement of the supraclavicular mass.

2. Materials
2.1. Preparation of Immunoconjugates

1. Antibodies (*see* Note 1): (a) 5 mg antibody/1 mL (*33 μM*) of 0.05*M* sodium carbonate buffer (pH 8.3) or 0.05*M* HEPES buffer (pH 8.3) for the reaction with ITC-Bz-DTPA, (b) 5 mg antibody/1 mL (*33 μM*) of 0.1*M* sodium carbonate buffer (pH 8.3) or 0.1*M* sodium borate buffer (pH 8.3) for the reaction with the cyclic anhydride of DTPA.
2. ITC-Bz-DTPA.
3. DPTA anhydride (cyclic anhydride of DTPA).
4. Anhydrous dimethylsulfoxide (DMSO).
5. Phosphate-buffered saline (PBS) 0.05*M*, pH 7.2.
6. Sodium citrate buffer, 0.06*M*, pH 5.5.

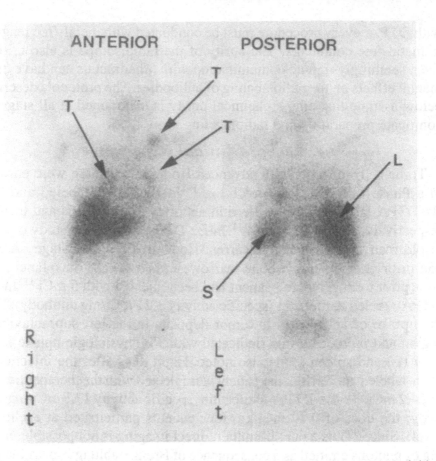

Fig. 1. Radioimmunoscintigraphic image of patient with advanced Hodgkin's disease obtained 4 d after diagnostic dose of ^{111}In-DTPA-Bz-antiferritin. T, tumor; L, liver; S, spleen.

7. Sodium acetate buffer, $0.6M$, pH 5.3.
8. Sodium acetate buffer, $2M$, pH 6.0.
9. Equipment: ultrafiltration devices (Amicon, Inc. Beverly, MA) or size-exclusion columns for purification of immunoconjugates.

2.2. Radiolabeling

1. Immunoconjugates: A conjugate of DTPA and antibody prepared in a reaction with cyclic anhydride of DTPA (DTPA-Ab) or in a reaction with isothiocyanatobenzyl-DTPA (Ab-Bz-DTPA). The conjugate is dissolved at 10 mg/mL in $0.05M$ PBS, pH 7.2.
2. Radioisotopes: [^{90}Y]yttrium chloride (Westinghouse Hanford Co., Richland, WA); [^{111}In]indium chloride (DuPont NEN, Boston, MA).

3. PBS.
4. Sodium acetate buffer, 2*M*, pH 6.0.
5. Sodium acetate buffer, 0.6*M*, pH 5.3.
6. Sodium citrate buffer, 0.06*M*, pH 5.5.
7. Equipment: lead vial and syringe shields; Lucite or other plastic vial and syringe shields; lead or leaded glass and Lucite or other plastic tabletop shields; forceps for remote handling of vials; γ-counter, scintillation counter, dose calibrators (Capintec, Inc, Ramsey, NJ); survey meters (Ludlum Measurements, Inc. Sweetwater, TX), lead-lined waste containers.

2.3. Purification and Quality Control of Radiolabeled Antibodies

1. PBS.
2. 5% human serum albumin.
3. 0.9% saline.
4. NH$_4$OH/CH$_3$OH (1:4, v/v).
5. Chromatography supplies: Sephadex G-l00 and G-50; instant thin-layer chromatography plates (ITLC; Gelman Sciences, Ann Arbor, MI); thin-layer chromatography plates (TLC); size-exclusion HPLC columns.

3. Methods
3.1. Preparation of Antibodies for Labeling

Purification of antibodies from serum, tissue-culture supernatants, or ascites has been described in a number of publications and reviews. Good sources for a comprehensive review of methods and procedures are: *Immunochemical Protocols (12)* and *Antibodies: A Laboratory Manual (13)*. The storage of antibodies prior to labeling does not differ from the usual storage, i.e., the pH of the antibody solution should be neutral. PBS is the most commonly used solution for storing purified antibodies, and the protein concentration of stock solutions are up to 10 mg/mL (*see* Note 2). Usually, the antibody solution is dispensed in convenient volumes (single-use portions) and stored at –20°C.

3.2. Preparation of Immunoconjugates
3.2.1. Attachment of DTPA via ITC-Bz-DTPA

1. Prepare an antibody solution at 5 mg/mL (33 μ*M*) or greater in either sodium carbonate buffer (0.05*M*, pH 8.3) or HEPES buffer (0.05*M*, pH 8.3). The exchange from the storage buffer, usually PBS, to the reaction buffer can be accomplished either by dialysis or ultrafiltration. Regardless of the procedure of choice, use only metal-free buffers.

2. Just prior to conjugation, prepare a 5 m*M* aqueous solution of ITC-Bz-DTPA. Use only freshly prepared solutions.
3. To a 1-mL aliquot of the antibody solution (5 mg/mL in 0.05*M* sodium carbonate buffer, pH 8.3), add 35 µL of ITC-Bz-DTPA solution. This gives a molar ratio of protein to chelating agent of about 1:5. With the usual yield of conjugation of about 40%, this ratio of reagents will provide antibody carrying on average two or less molecules of DTPA. If the reaction is run in the HEPES buffer, it is advisable to add 30 µL of 1.5*M* aqueous solution of triethylamine, pH 8.0, as a catalyst. This addition is not necessary when using carbonate buffer.
4. Allow the reaction to proceed for 2 h at room temperature.
5. Reserve a 10-µL aliquot of the reaction mixture in a metal-free tube for further testing (*see* step 9 in this section).
6. Transfer the reaction mixture into an ultrafiltration device to remove unreacted ITC-Bz-DTPA and to exchange buffer for PBS (in our hands, a Centricon-30 concentrator performs well with only minimal protein losses). After three 1-mL filtrations with PBS, 99+% of the free ligand is removed from the mixture (*see* Note 3). During the fourth and final buffer exchange, concentrate the protein sample to about 10 mg/mL or greater (0.5 mL).
7. Determine the protein content either be measuring the absorbance at 280 nm or using any of the commercial protein assay kits, taking care that the appropriate IgG standard is employed.
8. Transfer the immunoconjugate solution (Ab-Bz-DTPA) into a metal-free vial for radiolabeling, or freeze at –20°C for storage until ready to use.
9. To a tube containing the 10-µL aliquot of the crude reaction mixture (step 5 above), add 5 µL of citrate buffer (0.06*M*, pH 5.5) and 5 µL of acetate buffer (0.6*M*, pH 5.3), and perform labeling as described below (Section 3.5.1.) to determine the number of DTPA residues per antibody molecule.

3.2.2. Attachment of DTPA via Cyclic Anhydride of DTPA

1. Prepare an antibody solution at 5 mg/mL (33 µ*M*) or greater in either sodium carbonate buffer (0.1*M*, pH 8.3) or sodium borate buffer (0.1*M*, pH 8.3). The exchange from the storage buffer, usually PBS, to the reaction buffer can be accomplished either by dialysis or ultrafiltration. Regardless of the procedure of choice, use only metal-free buffers.
2. Dissolve cyclic anhydride of DTPA in anhydrous dimethyl sulfoxide (10 mg/mL; 28 m*M*). Use immediately.
3. To achieve the final substitution ratio of two DTPA residues per one antibody molecule, add 5 molar equivalents of the cyclic anhydride (6 µL) to 1 mL of the antibody solution (5 mg/mL).

4. Allow the reaction to proceed for 2 h at room temperature.
5. Reserve a 10-µL aliquot of this reaction mixture in a metal-free tube for further testing (follow directions from Section 3.2.1., step 9, and then proceed with procedures described in Section 3.5.1.).
6. Transfer the reaction mixture into an ultrafiltration device to remove unreacted DTPA and its anhydride, and to exchange buffer for PBS (in our hands, a Centricon-30 concentrator performs well with only minimal protein losses). After three 1-mL filtrations with PBS, 99+% of the free ligand is removed from the mixture (*see* Note 3). During the fourth and final buffer exchange, concentrate the protein sample to about 10 mg/mL or greater (0.5 mL).
7. Determine the protein content either by measuring the absorbance at 280 nm or using any of the commercial protein assay kits, taking care that the appropriate IgG standard is employed.
8. Transfer the immunoconjugate solution (DTPA-Ab) into a metal-free vial for radiolabeling or freeze at –20°C for storage until ready to use.

3.3. Radiolabeling with Yttrium-90

1. Thaw an appropriate volume of the immunoconjugate, and allow it to warm up to room temperature (*see* Notes 4 and 5).
2. To the reaction vial containing 2 mg of DTPA-Bz-Ab in 200 µL of PBS, add an equal volume (200 µL) of 2M sodium acetate buffer, pH 6.0.
3. Place the reaction mixture in a Plexiglass™ shielding container.
4. With a metal-free pipet tip, transfer the desired amount of the ^{90}YCl$_3$ solution, i.e., 50 mCi in 10 µL of 0.1M HCl, into the reaction vial (*see* Note 6). Gently shake the vial to mix its content. Withdraw about 1 µL of the reaction mixture, and check its pH using a pH paper. The pH should be about 6 or slightly less. If the pH is higher, add an additional volume, usually 50 µL are sufficient, of 2M sodium acetate buffer.
5. Allow the reaction to proceed at room temperature for 1.5 h (*see* Note 7).
6. To terminate the reaction, add 50 µL of 0.01M solution of DTPA in water, pH 6.5. Allow the mixture to equilibrate for about 5 min, and apply to the top of the Sephadex G-100 column (30 × 1.5 cm) through the intracath as shown in Fig. 2 (*see* Note 8). In cases where the sterile and pyrogen-free product is required for human use, do not prerun the Sephadex column with BSA.
7. After the reaction mixture has run into the column packing, gently apply 1 mL of PBS through the intracath to rinse the tubing and sides of the column. Allow PBS to run into the beads. Remove the intracath, and switch the valve to the PBS reservoir. Adjust the solvent flow rate to about 1 mL/min.
8. Collect 10 mL (the void volume equivalent; *see* Note 9) of the eluant into the waste vial (fraction 1). Switch the valve to start collection of the prod-

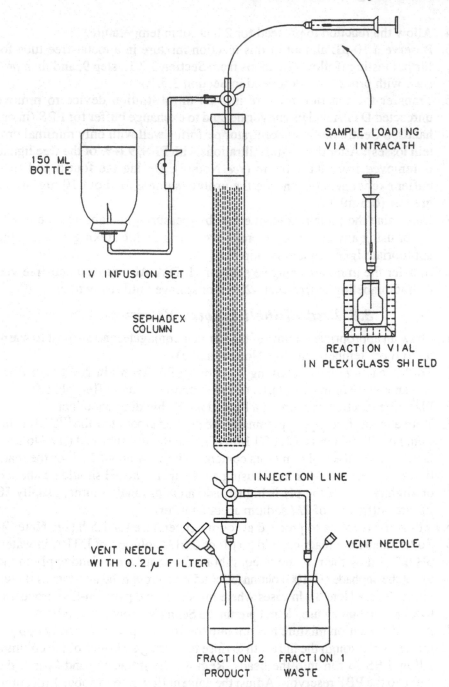

Fig. 2. Representative setup for purification of radiometal-labeled proteins (for ^{111}In-labeled antibodies use lead shields).

uct (fraction 2; 6 mL). Close the valve, and replace the fraction 2 vial with a new collection vial, switch the valve, and continue to collect the eluate (6 mL). If the on-line radioactivity detector is available, collect the entire radioactive protein peak into a single vial.

9. Measure the radioactivity collected with the protein fraction (*see* Note 10). For columns pretreated with BSA, the recovery is about 80%; for columns without BSA prerun, the usual yield is 50–60%, depending on the quantity of antibody used in radiolabeling. The losses are particularly substantial when the total protein content is <200 µg. In these instances, it is advisable to consider a smaller column. A convenient disposable column can be prepared in a 10-mL syringe barrel (*see* Note 11).

10. Determine protein content in fractions 2 and 3 either by measuring the absorbance at 280 nm or using any of the commercial protein assay kits, taking care that the appropriate IgG standard is employed.

11. Calculate the specific activity as a ratio of µCi ^{90}Y to µg protein. Under the conditions described in this protocol, the specific activity is between 10 and 15 µCi/µg.

12. Reserve aliquots of fractions 2 and 3 for quality-control testing as described in Section 3.5.2.

3.4. Radiolabeling with Indium-111

1. Thaw an appropriate volume of the immunoconjugate, and allow it to warm up to room temperature.

2. To the reaction vial containing 1 mg of DTPA-Ab in 100 µL of PBS, add 50 µL of 0.6M sodium acetate buffer (pH 5.3) and 50 µL of 0.06M sodium citrate buffer (pH 5.5).

3. Place the reaction mixture in a lead-shielded container.

4. With a metal-free pipet tip, transfer the desired amount of the ^{111}InCl$_3$ solution, i.e., 8 mCi in 40 µL of 0.1M HCl, into the reaction vial. Gently shake the vial to mix its contents. Withdraw about 1 µL of the reaction mixture, and check its pH using a pH paper. The pH should be about 5.5 or slightly less. If the pH is higher, add an additional volume of 0.6M sodium acetate buffer. Usually 20 µL are sufficient.

5. Allow the reaction to proceed at room temperature for 1 h (*see* Note 12).

6. To terminate the reaction, add 50 µL of 0.01M solution of DTPA in water, pH 6.5. Allow the mixture to equilibrate for about 5 min and apply to the top of the Sephadex G-100 column (15 × 1 cm) through the intracath as shown in Fig. 2. In cases where the sterile and pyrogen-free product is required for human use, do not prerun the Sephadex column with BSA.

7. After the reaction mixture has run into column packing, gently apply the 1 mL of PBS through the intracath to rinse the tubing and sides of the col-

umn. Allow PBS to run into the beads. Remove the intracath, and switch the valve to the PBS reservoir. Adjust the solvent flow rate to about 1 mL/min.

8. Collect 5 mL (the void volume equivalent) of the eluant into the waste vial (fraction 1). Switch the valve to start collection of the product (fraction 2; 3 mL). Close the valve or replace the waste vial (fraction 1) with a new collection vial. Switch the valve and continue to collect the eluate (fraction 3; 3 mL). If the on-line radioactivity detector is available, collect the entire radioactive protein peak into a single vial.

9. Measure the radioactivity collected with the protein fraction (*see* Notes 8 and 10). For columns pretreated with BSA, the recovery is about 80%; for columns without BSA prerun, the usual yield is 50–60%, depending on the quantity of antibody used in radiolabeling. The losses are particularly substantial when the total protein content is <200 μg. In these instances, it is advisable to consider a smaller column. A convenient disposable column can be prepared in a 5-mL syringe barrel.

10. Determine protein content in fraction 2 either by measuring the absorbance at 280 nm or using any of the commercial protein assay kits, taking care that the appropriate IgG standard is employed.

11. Calculate the specific activity as a ratio of μCi ^{111}In to μg protein. Under the conditions described in this protocol, the usual specific activity is about 4–6 μCi/μg.

3.5. Quality Controls

3.5.1. Determination of the Number of DTPA Residues Conjugated to an Antibody Molecule

1. To a vial containing 10 μL of the crude reaction mixture described in Section 3.2.1., step 9, containing 3.2×10^{-4} μmol of Ab and 1.6×10^{-3} μmol total DTPA, add 1 μCi (2.1×10^{-8} μmol) of ^{111}InCl$_3$ and 4 μL of nonradioactive InCl$_3$ solution (1 mM in 0.01M HCl).

2. Allow the reaction to proceed at room temperature for 60 min.

3. Prepare three 10-cm long ITLC plates by placing 2 μL of the labeling mixture about 1 cm from the bottom of each plate, air-drying, and eluting in 0.9% saline.

4. Determine the radioactivity associated with the protein (at the origin) and unreacted DTPA (the upper part of the plate) either by counting 0.5-cm sections of the plate in a γ-counter or using any of the commercial radioactivity scanners. Figure 3 shows a typical radioactivity scan.

5. Calculate the number of DTPA residues per protein by multiplying the fraction of counts associated with the origin (protein-bound radioactivity) by the total DTPA-to-antibody ratio used in a conjugation reaction. For example, if 5 molar equivalent of DTPA are reacted with 1 molar equiva-

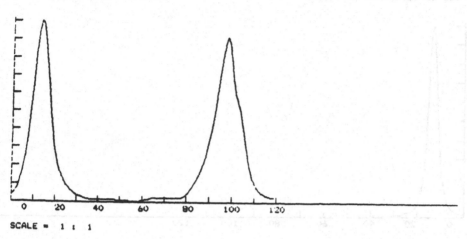

FULL SCALE COUNTS = 60119

SCALE = 1 : 1

```
ZONE #  1    X ⌄  10 - 20

ORIGIN      1       SOLVENT FRONT    100

  SONC #   BEGIN      END     PEAK      AREA    RANK    %ROI    %TOTAL      RF
       1       0        31      13     659511      2   46.270   44.456     .121
       2      78       115      97     765845      1   53.730   51.624     .970


COUNTS IN REGIONS    1425356
TOTAL COUNTS         1483511
```

Fig. 3. Typical radioactivity scan of the crude reaction mixture from conjugation of DTPA anhydride to antibody at 10:1 molar ratio; ITLC plate was eluted with 0.9% saline and scanned using Vista-100 radioactivity counter.

lent of antibody and the fraction of counts associated with protein is 0.4, then the number of DTPA residues bound per molecule of antibody is 2.

3.5.2. Determination of the Radiochemical Purity of Radiolabeled Antibody

The quickest and most convenient method used in the determination of the radiochemical purity of the radiolabeled antibody is ITLC.

1. Dilute the sample to be tested with PBS to a concentration of about 2 μCi/ μL, and divide it into two 100-μL portions.
2. To one of the 100-μL aliquots, add 10 μL of 0.01M DTPA, pH 6.5. Apply each sample to a separate ITLC plate, and allow to dry.

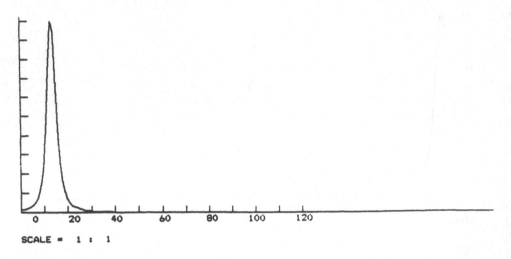

FULL SCALE COUNTS =   6671

SCALE = 1 : 1

ZONE # 1   X = 10 - 20

ORIGIN   0   SOLVENT FRONT   200

SQNC #	BEGIN	END	PEAK	AREA	RANK	%ROI	%TOTAL	RF
1	3	23	13	37826	1	100	94.617	.∨o5

COUNTS IN REGIONS   37826
TOTAL COUNTS   39978

Fig. 4. Typical radioactivity scan of ITLC plate for radiometal-labeled antibody-DTPA conjugate, in this case ^{90}Y-DTPA-Bz-antiferritin, after purification on a Sephadex column.

3. Elute both plates with 0.9% saline or 0.06M acetate buffer.
4. After the solvent front is about 1 cm from the top, remove the plates from the developing chamber (a glass jar with a reasonably tight cover is sufficient), allow to air-dry, and either scan for radioactivity (Fig. 4) or cut into 0.5-cm pieces and determine their radioactive content in a γ-counter (*see* Note 13).
5. Calculate the radiochemical purity by dividing the radioactivity associated with the origin by the total radioactivity on the plate.
6. Analyze both test samples (with and without DTPA) at 24-h intervals for 5–7 d to establish the stability of radiolabeled immunoconjugate (*see* Note 14). For most clinical applications, the release criteria for radiochemical purity is set at 95% or more of the radiolabel bound to protein.

3.5.3. Determination of the Immunoreactive Fraction

Most of radiolabeling methods can be damaging to the biological properties of antibodies. Any loss of immunoreactivity can have a detrimental effect on the in vivo behavior of the antibody. In preparation for a clinical trial, it is particularly important to measure and document the binding properties of radioimmunoconjugates. Binding assays vary with each antibody. Therefore, a specific recommendation is not made here. The FDA is a good source for any information about quality-control requirements for antibodies to be used in the clinic (*see* Note 15).

4. Notes

1. The amounts of protein and molar ratios are based on the use of IgG-size antibodies. Revise these figures when using antibody fragments or IgM-size proteins.
2. Caution: Buffers and vials for storage of antibodies prior to labeling with radiometals, such as ^{90}Y or ^{111}In, should be metal-free.
3. The removal of the excess unreacted DTPA can also be accomplished on a size-exclusion column (15 × 1 cm) taking care that only metal-free buffers and pipet tips are used. Satisfactory results are also obtained with dialysis.
4. Before using radioactive isotopes, consult your Radiation Safety Office for proper procedures for handling and disposal of radioactive materials.
5. Specific activity of no-carrier-added ^{90}Y is about 48.9 Ci/µmol. To label each DTPA molecule in 0.1 mg of a 1:1 DTPA-Ab conjugate, as much as 32.6 mCi of ^{90}Y are required. However, the yield of labeling is considerably improved when about a threefold molar excess of conjugated DTPA over radiometal is employed, i.e., for 0.1 mg of the 1:1 DTPA-Ab conjugate, use 10 mCi or less of ^{90}YCl$_3$. The above-described procedure has been successfully employed in labeling with up to 100 mCi ^{90}Y. When using smaller quantities of the radioisotope, adjust the amount of the antibody–DTPA conjugate keeping the concentration of the protein at about 5–10 µg/µL.
6. Most suppliers provide ^{90}YCl$_3$ in 0.1M HCl but the concentration in mCi/µL varies. Therefore, the volume of HCl added to the reaction mixture may change from the volume indicated above. As a general rule, avoid dilute radioisotope solution.
7. It is advisable to check the reaction progress at 60 min using ITLC.
8. Determine the radioactivity left behind in the reaction vial. Use this residual sample to determine the radiochemical yield. Dilute the residual sample with PBS to about 2 µCi/µL. Place 1 µL of this solution about 1 cm from the bottom of the ITLC plate. Proceed as described in Section 3.5.2.

9. Determine the void volume with Blue Dextran. In our hands, this size column has a void volume of 10–11 mL.
10. Preparations to be used in a clinical trial are dispensed by a radiopharmacist into a syringe according to a strictly-defined protocol. At this time, a 0.05-mL sample is removed for quality-control tests and verification of the isotope identity required by the FDA on all clinical-grade preparations. To avoid radiolysis of protein at high specific activities, 5% human serum albumin is added to a final concentration of 1%. A sample (0.5–1.0 mL) is taken for sterility and pyrogen testing. The dose to be administered to the patient is stored in a syringe equipped with a shielded syringe holder until the results of pyrogen tests are available.
11. Measure the radioactivity left in the loading syringe with tubing, on the 0.2-µm filter and outflow tubing, and on the column. This information is needed to keep track of the radioactivity distribution and for the radioactive waste disposal records.
12. It is advisable to check the reaction progress at 45 min using ITLC.
13. In a routine protocol employed in our laboratories, each final radiolabeled antibody preparation is also analyzed on a size-exclusion HPLC column (Biosil SEC250, Bio-Rad Laboratories, Richmond, CA) with a dual detection (radioactivity and UV absorbance). In addition to HPLC and ITLC testing, we use TLC methods to verify the quality of each preparation. The plates are silica gel, and the solvent is a 4:1 (v/v) mixture of 95% ethanol and concentrated ammonia. Selected radioimmunoconjugate preparations are also tested on nonreducing SDS-PAGE gels (5–15% gradient).
14. Each radioimmunoconjugate to be used in vivo undergoes extensive stability testing in human blood and serum, and murine liver homogenate to determine the rate of degradation and to identify metabolites.
15. Each lot of antibody produced must pass release tests prior to use for human studies. After radiolabeling, the radioimmunoconjugate must be tested to show that the protein retains its immunoreactivity, the labeling method has not introduced impurities, and the fraction of an unbound radioisotope, if any, conforms with the release criteria.

References

1. Press, O. W., Eary, J., Badger, C. C., Appelbaum, F. R., Wiseman, G., Martin, P. J., and Bernstein, I. D. (1993) High-dose radioimmunotherapy of lymphomas. *Cancer Treat. Res.* **68,** 13–22.
2. Press, O. W., Eary, J. F., Appelbaum, F. R., Martin, P. J., Badger, C. C., Nelp, W. B., Glenn, S., Butchko, G., Fisher, D., and Porter, B. (1993) Radiolabeled-antibody therapy of B-cell lymphoma with autologous bone marrow transplant. *N. Engl. J. Med.* **329,** 1219–1224.

3. Czuczman, M. S., Straus, D. J., Divgi, C. R., Graham, M., Garin-Chesa, P., Finn, R., Myers, J., Old, L. J., Larson, S. M., and Scheinberg, D. A. (1993) Phase I dose-escalation trial of iodine-131-labeled monoclonal antibody OKB7 in patients with non-Hodgkin's lymphoma. *J. Clin. Oncol.* **11,** 2021–2029.

4. Finkler, N. J., Muto, M. G., Kassis, A. I., Weadock, K., Tumeh, S. S., Zurawski, V. R., Jr., and Knapp, R. C. (1989) Intraperitoneal radiolabeled OC125 in patients with advanced ovarian cancer. *Gynecol. Oncol.* **34,** 339–344.

5. Muto, M. G., Finkler, N. J., Kassis, A. I., Howes, A. E., Anderson, L. L., Lau, C. C., Zurawski, V. R., Jr., Weadock, K., Tumeh, S. S., and Lavin, P. (1992) Intraperitoneal radioimmunotherapy of refractory ovarian carcinoma utilizing iodine-131-labeled monoclonal antibody OC125. *Gynecol-Oncol.* **45,** 265–272.

6. Vriesendorp, H. M., Herpst, J. M., Germack, M. A., Klein, J. L., Leichner, P. K., Loudenslager, D. M., and Order, S. E. (1991) Phase I-II studies of yttrium-labeled antiferritin treatment for end-stage Hodgkin's disease, including Radiation Therapy Oncology Group 87-01. *J. Clin. Oncol.* **9,** 918–928.

7. Crowther, M. E., Ward, B. G., Granowska, M., Mather, S., Britton, K. E., Shepherd, J. H., and Slevin, M. L. (1989) Therapeutic considerations in the use of intraperitoneal radiolabelled monoclonal antibodies in ovarian carcinoma. *Nucl. Med. Commun.* **10,** 149–159.

8. Wilbur, D. S. (1992) Radiohalogenation of proteins: an overview of radionuclides, labeling methods, and reagents for conjugate labeling. *Bioconjugate Chem.* **3,** 433–470.

9. Fritzberg, A. R., Berninger, R. W., Hadley, S. W., and Wester, D. W. (1988) Approaches to radiolabeling of antibodies for diagnosis and therapy of cancer. *Pharm. Res.* **5,** 325–334.

10. Hnatowich, D. J., Layne, W. W., Childs, R. L., Lanteigne, D., Davis, M. A., Griffin, T. W., and Doherty, P. W (1983) Radioactive labeling of antibody: a simple and efficient method. *Science* **220,** 613–615.

11. Brechbiel, M. W., Gansow, O. A., Atcher, R. W., Schlom, J., Esteban, J., Simpson, D. E., and Colcher, D. (1986) Synthesis of 1-(*p*-isothiocyanatobenzyl) derivatives of DTPA and EDTA. Antibody labeling and tumor-imaging studies. *Inorg. Chem.* **25,** 2772–2781.

12. Manson, M. M. (ed.) (1992) *Methods in Molecular Biology*, vol. 10, *Immunochemical Protocols*. Humana Press, Totowa, N.J.

13. Harlow, E. and Lane, D. (1988) *Antibodies: A Laboratory Manual*. Cold Spring Harbor Laboratory, Cold Spring Harbor, NY, pp. 283–319.

Index

A

AbM, 28–41
Acetylcholine antibodies, 159
Acetylcholinesterase, 205–207, 211
  activity, inhibition by F(ab)$_2$, 216
  antibody, 211–221
Active site, 377
Active site titration, 220, 221
Adjuvants, 124, 130, 193
Affinity,
  of antibody, 375
  estimation, 94, 96, 97
  immunoblotting, 156–159, 165–169
  maturation, in vitro, 329
  for metals, 395
Aggregation, noncovalent, 112
Aligned matches, 2, 61
Alkaline phosphatase, 266
  coupling to antibody, 175
Allotype, 151
Amber mutation, 294
Amino acid sequence alignment, 1, 28, 29
Aminopterin, 126
Ampicillin resistance, 277
Amyloid fibril, 53, 70
Anti-idiotypic antibody, 173, 177, 183–199
  catalytic activity of, 207, 208, 211–221, 223
  monoclonal, 193
  opioid mimicry, 183
  polyclonal, 192
  purification of, 189–191, 193–195
  screening for, 217

Anti-morphine activity, 191
Antibody,
  affinity, 142, 143, 149
  analysis by isoelectric focusing, 153–155, 167, 168
  anti-idiotypic, 173, 177, 183–199
  avidity, 143, 149
  biotinylation of, 195
  capture, 244, 248
  catalysis, contaminants, 403
  catalysis, theoretical and practical limitations of, 238
  catalytic, 203–208, 211, 223, 234, 239, 295, 303, 377, 417
  clonality, 151–160
  clones, expression of, 404
  combining sites, concentration of, 315
  to DNA, 265
  humanized, 73, 251
  immobilized, 244
  as internal images, 174, 183, 211
  labeling with radioisotopes, 177, 178, 423–438
  microheterogeneity, 153, 158
  mutants of, 266, 276, 294, 298, 319, 326, 330
  phage display, and chaperonins, 343
  preparation, for radiolabeling, 429
  production, large-scale, 127, 128
  purification, 114, 136, 215, 274, 291, 302, 307, 395, 403
    in 96-well plates, 404, 405
    on spin columns, 404, 405
  specificity search, 3, 14

subunits, reduced and alkylated,
111–121
to transition state analogs, 237
valency, 143
Antigen, coating of nitrocellulose, 167
Antigen–antibody binding,
solid phase, 147–149
liquid phase, 144–147
Antigenic clusters, 177
Antigenic epitopes, 140–142
Ascites production, 127, 135, 136,
214, 215
Asthma,
catalytic antibodies in, 207
VIP autoantibody in, 377
Atropine derivatives, 205
Auto-anti-idiotype, 155
Autoantibodies,
catalytic activity of, 121, 207, 208,
223, 224, 281
to DNA, 207, 223, 265
to thyroglobulin, 417
to VIP, 121, 207, 281, 377
Autoantibody clonotype, 156
Autoimmune aspects of catalytic
antibodies, 207, 208
Autoimmune disease, 171, 223, 224,
417
Autoimmunity, pathological, 171
Autoradiography, 107–109, 154, 269

B
β-barrel structure, 22
β-sheet structure, 18, 52
B-DNA, 265
B-lymphocyte activation, 104
B-lymphocytes, V-gene expression,
99–109
Bence Jones proteins, crystal struc-
ture, 53–60
Blood group antibodies, 159
Bone marrow transplantation,
antibodies in, 157
Brookhaven Protein Database, 17

C
c-myc, ELISA for, 399
c-myc expression, dot-blots for, 291,
294
c-myc tag, 282, 302, 327
Cα database constraints, 31
C_ε gene, 253
C_κ gene, 253
Canonical loops, 23, 31
Canonical residues, 24
Carbohydrate antibodies, 329
Carrier proteins, 124, 184, 188, 189
Catalysis, screening for, 237, 403
Catalytic activity,
in L-chain, 377
measurement of, 219, 220, 231–
233, 419, 420
Catalytic antibodies, 203–208
acetylcholinesterase, 211–221
anti-idiotypic, 211–221
autoimmune aspects, 207, 208
to DNA, 207, 208, 223, 234
esterolytic, 303
purification of, 229, 230
removal of contaminants, 224
screening strategies, 237–250
to thyroglobulin, 207, 417–420
and transition state analogs, 237, 239
to VIP, 121, 207, 281, 377
Catalytic efficiency, 239
Catalytic specificity, 420
Catalytic triad, 295
catELISA, 245, 249
cDNA,
cloning, 289
insert identification by PCR, 290
preparation, 282, 288, 289
by reverse transcription, 308
synthesis, 380-381
CDR,
classes, 25
combinational search, 4, 14
conserved residues, 60–67
construction, 22, 23

diversification in vitro, 331, 340
germ-line, 60–67
grafting, 269, 270, 278, 340
length of, 23, 24
modeling, 29–37
randomization, 330
remodeling, 32–36
CDRH3,
and antibody specificity, 14
loop, 24
modeling, 33–35, 40
structural diversity, 23
variability of, 3
CDRL1 modeling, 31–33, 36
Chaperonins, 343–351
effect on engineered bacteriophages 347–350
GroES and GroEL, 345, 346
in intracellular expression of antibody, 346, 347
and protein folding, 345
Chemical warfare agents, 205
Chemiluminescence, 156
Chloramine-T, 410, 413
CHO cells, 258
Cholinergic receptor sites, 205
Chromatography, for interaction analysis, 85–88
Clonal selection, 151
Cloning,
of hybridomas, 134, 135, 218
by limiting dilution, 127
of V domains, 273, 274, 284, 300, 343, 371
CNBr coupling, 189, 190
Cofactors, for antibody catalysis, 204
Combinatorial libraries, 329, 343, 355, 377
Combining-site structure, 17–41
Complementarity determining regions, *see* CDR
Complementarity determining loops, 23
Computer simulation of chromatographic data, 88, 96

Conformational searching, 26
CONGEN program, 26, 29, 30
Conjugation to carrier protein, 184, 188, 189
Crystal structure,
alternative conformations, 56
database, 17
effect of solvent, 55, 56
Crystal-packing interactions, 41
Crystallization,
by batch precipitation, 90
buffers and precipitants, 88, 89
by dialysis, 90
methods, 90, 91, 95
by vapor diffusion, 91
Crystallography, 84, 85
Cytocentrifugation, 104

D
D-minigenes, 3, 12
Deletion mutations, 319
Dextran, 142
Disease-associated autoantibodies, 172
Disulfide bonds, intramolecular, 112
DNA antibody, 265, 266
DNA antibody clonotype, 156
DNA hydrolysis by antibodies, 223, 234
Domain shuffling, 337
DTPA, 427, 429, 430

E
E. coli strains, 277
Electroporation,
of bacteria, 290, 314, 369, 370, 384
of SP2/0 cells, 258
yields, 314
ELIFA, 389
ELISA, 126, 147, 175–177, 261
competitive inhibition, 176, 177
screening for anti-idiotypic antibody, 217
screening for catalytic antibodies, 245, 247–250

Energy minimization, 36, 37
Epitope mapping, 94, 96, 171–180
Epitopes, 140–142
  conformational, 141, 172
  linear, 172
  nonrepeating, 141
  repeating, 141, 142
  sequential, 140, 141
Error rate, *Taq* polymerase, 319
Esterolytic sF$_v$, 297
Euglobulin precipitation, 218
Expression of chimeric immunoglobulin genes, 251–262
Expression vector, 254, 258, 266,
  282, 334, 362

F
F episome, 325
F(ab)$_2$,
  immunization with, 216
  preparation of, 215
Fab,
  and chaperonins, 346
  gene-cassette, combinatorial, 355
  libraries, 355–376
  preparation of, 116, 117, 230
  reduction and alkylation, 117
Fd fragments, 119
Feeder suspensions, 126
Filamentous bacteriophages, 343
Flow linear dichroism, 226, 227
Fluorescence yield, 420
Force fields, 26, 30
Framework construction, 22, 29
Framework region and generic drift, 65
Fusion of cells, 125, 126, 133, 134,
  216, 217
F$_v$, single chain, 201, 265, 281, 300,
  312, 337, 341, 346

G
Gapped duplex DNA, 319
Gapped DNA, repolymerization of,
  325

Gene tandem, construction and
  expression, 252–255
Gene3, 282, 334, 392
Geneticin G-418, 255
Germ-line genes, 60–67
  aligned, 61
Glutaraldehyde crosslinking, 156,
  157
gpl20 antibody, 156
GroEL, 345
GroES, 345
Ground state, 403
Growth factors, 126

H
H-chain,
  affinity purification, 118, 119
  and binding specificity, 111
  goldfish, 4
  and L-chain, probability of
    pairing, 377
Halogens, radiolabeling with, 425,
  426
Haptens, 124, 140, 157, 204, 237,
  304
Hashimoto's thyroiditis, 156, 207,
  417
HAT medium, 125, 134
Heat shock proteins, 345
Heavy chain, *see* H-chain
Helper phage, 322, 348, 350, 365,
  372
Hinge region, 18
Histidine tag, 266, 294, 302, 395, 403
HIV antibody, 3, 156
HPLC, size exclusion, 85–89, 92–94
Human Fab fragments, 355
Human Fab libraries, direct cloning
  method, 370
Human immunoglobulin light chains,
  selection of, 377–401
Human lymphocytes, 380
  isolation and culture of, 103, 104
Humanized antibodies, 73, 251

Hybridoma cell lines, 123, 216
  karyotype, 252
Hybridomas, screening for catalytic
  antibodies, 243, 247–249
Hydrophilic residues, 28
Hydrophobic residues, 28, 30
Hypermutability of CDRs, 281
Hypermutation, 330
Hypoxanthine-phosphoribosyl-transferase,
  125

I
Idiotype, 152
  mapping, 173–180
Idiotope–anti-idiotypic network, 155,
  208, 211
Idiotypic cross reactivity, 191
Idiotypic specificity, 191
IgE, chimeric, 251–262
IgG,
  mRNA, GC content, 374
  reduction and alkylation of, 114
  -Sepharose, 274
IgM, purification of, 218, 219
Imidazole, 400
Immobilized metal affinity chroma-
  tography, 291, 292, 303, 313,
  395, 397, 398
Immunization protocols, 123–125,
  130–133, 216
Immunoblotting, 156–159, 168, 169,
  261, 262
Immunoconjugates, 427, 429, 430
Immunogenicity, of antibodies, 251
Immunogens,
  boronic acid, 204
  difluoroketones, 204
Immunoglobulin,
  conjugation to reporter molecules, 193
  fold, 18
  genes, chimeric, 251–262
  genes, expression in mammalian
    cells, 251–262
  superfamily, 52

Immunoreactivity, of radiolabels,
  425, 437
In situ hybridization, 99–109
Indium-111, radiolabeling with, 433,
  434
Infectivity, 345
Inosine, 331, 335, 340
Insecticidal toxins, 205
Insertion mutations, 319
Interfacial surface, 58
Internal image, 174, 183, 211
Intrasplenic injection, 124
Iodine, labeling with, 426
Iodogen, 177
IPTG, 268, 277, 294, 375, 400
Isoelectric focusing, 152–155, 167,
  168, 292
  recycling, 155

J
J_H-C_H locus, 252
J_K-C_K locus, 252

K
Kabat database, 2, 14, 28, 29
Kinetic screening, 242, 243
Klenow fragment, 326
K_m, of antibodies, 281, 295, 420

L
L-chain,
  affinity purification, 118, 119
  anti-ground state, 281
  antigen binding by, 393
  binding of VIP by, 111, 120, 377
  casts, 53, 57, 59
  deposition disease, 53, 70
  dimerization, 68, 74–76, 92
  dimers, structure, 51–78
  expression of, 397
  expression levels, 400
  expression, screening for, 389
  expression in soluble form, 388
  genes, cloning of, 372

κ, 57–60
λ, 53–57
  libraries, 377–393
  pathological aggregation, 53
  preparation without denaturation,
    115–119
  purification of, 395–401
  self-association, 68–73
  VIP hydrolysis by, 120, 121
lac promotor, 293
lacZ promoter, 375
Leader peptide, 276, 282, 294, 301,
    362
Libraries,
  combinatorial, 329, 343, 355, 377
  human, 355, 377
  L-chain, 377–401
  phage display, 338, 343, 355, 377
  superinfection of, 365, 372
  V_H and V_L domains, 266, 300,
    329, 344, 355
Library,
  diversity of, 390
  generation strategy, 337
  screening for antigen binding, 389
  size, 384, 390
Ligase chain reaction, 329
Ligation, 273, 289, 310, 374, 383
Light chain, *see* L-chain
Linkers, 284, 293, 299, 300, 334,
    357

M
Metal cations, radiolabeling with,
    426
Metal coordination sites, 400
Misfolding, 346
Molecular dynamics, 22
Molecular modeling, 17–41
  ab initio, 25, 26
  combined method, 27, 30
  database/knowledge-based
    method, 23

Monoclonal antibody,
  antiphosphonate, 304
  purification of, 114, 136, 215
  subunits, purification of, 114, 115,
    218, 219
Morphine, conjugation to albumin,
    188, 189
Morphine antibodies, 192, 196
Morphine-binding site, 198
Multiple myeloma, 51
Murine monoclonal antibodies, 123–137
Mutagenesis,
  efficiencies, 325
  methods, 319–320
  random, 329–341
  reaction, oligonucleotide-directed,
    324
  site-directed, 269, 270, 276, 319–
    327
  template, uracil-labeled, 319
Mutagenic oligonucleotide(s), 269
  annealing of, 324
Mutant strand, extension and ligation
    of, 324
Mutants,
  libraries of, 329–341
  sequencing, 326
  sequencing and expression of, 339,
    340
Mutation efficiency, 320
Mutation rate, 330
Mutations, types, 319, 320
Myasthenia gravis, antibodies in, 159
Myeloma cell lines, 124
Myeloma proteins, 153

N
Natural autoantibodies, 171
Neuropeptide, 377
Nick translation, 260, 261
Nonspecific binding, 375
Northern hybridization, 259, 260
Nucleic acids, antibodies to, 265, 266
Nucleotide alignment, 2–11

O

Oligonucleotide(s),
-directed mutants, 319
phosphorylation, 323
purification, 332
spiked, 331, 340
synthesis, 334
Oligosaccharide antigens, 142
Opioid(s), 183, 184
ligands, conjugation to
immunogenic proteins,
184, 188, 189
ligands, receptor-binding portions,
184
receptor antibodies, 183, 184, 197,
198
receptor antibodies,
growth-inhibitory effects,
197
receptors, 183, 197, 198
Organophosphate intoxication,
vaccination against, 205
Organophosphorus compounds,
catalytic antibodies to, 205
Overlap extension method, 269
Overlap extension, linkage by, 289
Oximes, 204

P

φ, ψ difference plots, 37, 40
Panning, selection by, 338, 365, 372,
373, 387
Paratopes, 140, 143
Passive immunization, 206
PCR,
amplification of L-chain, 381
amplification of V domains, 272,
273, 288, 289, 308, 309
annealing temperature, 277, 293
assembly, 299
assembly, of Fab libraries, 356,
367
conditions, 390
hot start, 390

linkage by, 309
primers, 270, 284, 330–332
family-specific, 381, 390
for L-chain repertoire cloning,
381
for repertoire cloning, 300,
356–364
for sequencing, 379
specificity of, 312
screening, 385, 392
yield, 374
*pel*B, 301, 362
Peptide methylcoumarinamide, 295,
417, 419, 420
Peptide bond hydrolysis, 418
Periplasmic extract, 291, 311
Peroxon antibody, 206
Phage amplification, 349
Phage display, 338, 339
chaperonin-assisted, 343
of L-chains, 392
libraries, of Fab, 355–376
Phage elution, 387
Phage libraries, 338, 343, 355, 377,
386
Phage selection, 349
Phage titers, improved, 345, 346, 350
Phagemid, 362, 369, 375, 379
library, rescue of, 386, 391
vectors, 282, 283, 294
vectors, use in mutagenesis, 322
Phenylacetate hydrolysis, assay of,
312, 315
Phosphonate haptens, 204
Phosphorothioate nucleotide, 319, 325
Plasma cell dyscrasia, 53
Plasmacytomas, 51, 125
Plasmid construction, 334
Plasmids, 254, 255, 266, 267, 277,
283, 301, 302, 345
Point mutations, 319
Polyclonal antibodies, 112, 139
comparison with monoclonal
antibodies, 139–150

Polyethylene glycol, fusion with, 133, 134
Polymerase errors, 293
Pristane, 5
Promoter,
cytomegalovirus, 256
lac, 293
T7 RNA polymerase, 253, 254
tac, 301
Protease substrates, 281
Protein A, 116, 136, 215, 243, 266
affinity chromatography, 215
Protein G, 114, 136, 243, 244
Protein L chromatography, 395, 398, 401
Proteolytic antibody fragments, antiground-state, 281–295
Puromycin resistance, 255, 256

R
Radiochemical purity, 435
Radioconjugates, 426
Radioimmunoassay, 126, 147, 178, 194
competitive, 178
Radioimmunotherapy, 423, 425
Radioiodination,
methods, 426
of thyroglobulin, 418
Radioisotopes, selection of, 424
Radiolabeled antibodies, clinical experience, 427
Radiolabeled VIP, 406
Radiometal labeled proteins, 432
Radionuclides, characteristics of, 424
Radiosequencing, 412, 413
Raidolabeling, quality controls, 434
Ramachandran plots, 38–40
Random mutants, 320
Recombinant antibodies,
proteolytic activity, 406
rapid purification for catalysis screening, 403–407
Region analysis, 12
Regulatory elements, 251

Renaturation of proteins, 115–120
Replica plating, 268, 269
Restriction sites, 252, 254, 266, 293, 299, 301, 309, 326, 360, 382, 383
in V-genes, 293
Rheumatoid arthritis, 207, 224
RNA,
hybridization, 260
preparation, 282, 287, 288, 308, 356, 365, 370, 380
probes, 105, 106
secondary structure, 374

S
Salmonella O-polysaccharide, 329
scF$_v$, *see* single chain F$_v$
Scleroderma, 207, 224
Secretion signal, 276
Segment swapping, 269, 270, 276
Selection of antibody-producing clones, 126, 127
Selection of clones by affinity chromatography, 387
Self ligation, of vector, 374
SEQHUNT, 1–15
Sequence pattern match, 2, 3
Sequencing of mutants, 325, 326
Sex pili, 375
Side-chain,
construction, 27-28
location of, 27, 30
rotamer libraries, 27
Single chain F$_v$, 265–278, 281
anti-ground state, 281
catalytic, 281, 201, 312
cDNA preparation, 288, 289
and chaperonins, 346
dimerization, 341
expression, 274, 275, 302
large-scale purification, 311
libraries, 266, 300, 337
PCR cloning of, 288, 289, 298, 299

purification, 274, 302
screening for, 268, 269, 275, 310
-VIP complexes, precipitation of, 414
Single-stranded phagemid DNA, preparation of, 322
Single-stranded template DNA, 322
removal of, 324
Site-directed mutagenesis, 319–327
Size-exclusion chromatography, 72, 92, 93
and affinity estimation, 94, 96, 97
and epitope mapping, 94, 96
and heterologous interaction, 93
Solvent accessible residues, 292
Solvent shielding, 28
Soman antibody, 206
Stop codon, 364
Substrate,
affinity for, 377
antibody binding to, 281
chromogenic, 242
fluorigenic, 242
peptides, 295
phenylacetate, 303
Supercoiled DNA, cleavage of, 226, 231, 234
Surface plasmon resonance, 334, 339–341
Synthetic antibody genes, 329–341, 343
Synthetic antibody libraries, 329, 343
Systemic lupus erythematosus,
anti-DNA antibodies in, 207, 224, 265
catalytic antibodies in, 207, 208, 224

T

T5 exonuclease, 326
T7 lysozyme, 276
T7 RNA polymerase promoter, 253, 266, 276
T7 DNA polymerase, 326

tac promotor 301, 314
Taq polymerase, 272, 288
Tetrahedral haptens, 204, 304
Thin layer chromatography, 196
Thrombin, 266
Thyroglobulin, 171
antibodies, 171–180
antibody clonotype, 156
hydrolysis, 417–419
Thyroid hormones, 417
TLC, 14
Topoisomerase I, anti-idiotypic antibodies to, 207
Transudation, 377
Transfection, 258, 259
Transformation, 273, 277, 310
Transformation efficiency, 344, 383, 384
Transition state, 203, 204, 237, 403
Transition-state analogs, 237–242, 304
competitive binding to, 242
ELISA for, 245, 247–250

V

V domain cloning, 273, 274
V gene expression, 99
V gene synthesis, by ligase chain reaction, 336
V_H cDNA preparation, 288, 289
V_H domain libraries, 266, 300
V_H gene fragments, cloning of, 371
V_H gene-family usage, 107, 108
V_H library randomization, 337
V_H probes, 104–106
V_k exon, 253
V_L cDNA preparation, 288, 289
V_L dimerization and *lacZ* activation, 75
V_L domain libraries, 266, 300
V_L library randomization, 337
V_L–V_H domain orientation, 334
V_L–V_L contacts, 55, 73
Variable domain, structure of, 2, 3

Vasoactive intestinal polypeptide, *see*
  VIP
VIP, 207, 281, 295
  assay for binding, 409–413
  assay for hydrolysis, 410
  autoantibodies to, 121, 207, 281,
    377
  binding, radioimmunoassay for,
    391, 393
  deficiency of, 377
  hydrolysis of, 295
  immobilized, 387

iodination and purification of, 410
TCA precipitation, 413

W
Western blotting, 119, 120, 149, 155,
  156, 292

Y
Yttrium-90, radiolabeling with, 431

Z
Z-DNA, 265, 269

Methods in Molecular Biology™ Series

Methods in Molecular Biology™ manuals are available at all medical bookstores. You may also order copies directly from Humana by filling in and mailing or faxing this form to: Humana Press, 999 Riverview Drive, Suite 208, Totowa, NJ 07512 USA, Phone: 201-256-1699/Fax: 201-256-8341.

☐ 55. **Plant Cell Electroporation and Electrofusion Protocols**, edited by *Jac A. Nickoloff, 1995* • 0-89603-328-7 • Comb $49.50 (T)

☐ 54. **YAC Protocols**, edited by *David Markie, 1995* • 0-89603-313-9 • Comb $69.50 (T)

☐ 53. **Yeast Protocols:** *Methods in Cell and Molecular Biology,* edited by *Ivor H. Evans, 1995* • 0-89603-319-8 • Comb $69.50 (T)

☐ 52. **Capillary Electrophoresis:** *Principles, Instrumentation, and Applications,* edited by *Kevin D. Altria, 1995* • 0-89603-315-5 • Comb $64.50 (T)

☐ 51. **Antibody Engineering Protocols**, edited by *Sudhir Paul, 1995* • 0-89603-275-2 • Comb $69.50

☐ 50. **Species Diagnostics Protocols:** *PCR and Other Nucleic Acid Methods,* edited by *Justin P. Clapp, 1995* • 0-89603-323-6 • Comb $69.50 (T)

☐ 49. **Plant Gene Transfer and Expression Protocols**, edited by *Heddwyn Jones, 1995* • 0-89603-321-X • Comb $69.50 (T)

☐ 48. **Animal Cell Electroporation and Electrofusion Protocols**, edited by *Jac A. Nickoloff, 1995* • 0-89603-304-X • Comb $64.50 (T)

☐ 47. **Electroporation Protocols for Microorganisms**, edited by *Jac A. Nickoloff, 1995* • 0-89603-310-4 • Comb $69.50

☐ 46. **Diagnostic Bacteriology Protocols**, edited by *Jenny Howard and David M. Whitcombe, 1995* • 0-89603-297-3 • Comb $69.50

☐ 45. **Monoclonal Antibody Protocols**, edited by *William C. Davis, 1995* • 0-89603-308-2 • Comb $64.50

☐ 44. **Agrobacterium Protocols**, edited by *Kevan M. A. Gartland and Michael R. Davey, 1995* • 0-89603-302-3 • Comb $69.50

☐ 43. **In Vitro Toxicity Testing Protocols**, edited by *Sheila O'Hare and Chris K. Atterwill, 1995* • 0-89603-282-5 • Comb $69.50

☐ 42. **ELISA:** *Theory and Practice,* by *John R. Crowther, 1995* • 0-89603-279-5 • Comb $59.50

☐ 41. **Signal Transduction Protocols**, edited by *David A. Kendall and Stephen J. Hill, 1995* • 0-89603-298-1 • Comb $64.50

☐ 40. **Protein Stability and Folding:** *Theory and Practice,* edited by *Bret A. Shirley, 1995* • 0-89603-301-5 • Comb $69.50

☐ 39. **Baculovirus Expression Protocols**, edited by *Christopher D. Richardson, 1995* • 0-89603-272-8 • Comb $64.50

☐ 38. **Cryopreservation and Freeze-Drying Protocols**, edited by *John G. Day and Mark R. McLellan, 1995* • 0-89603-296-5 • Comb $79.50

☐ 37. **In Vitro Transcription and Translation Protocols**, edited by *Martin J. Tymms, 1995* • 0-89603-288-4 • Comb $69.50

☐ 36. **Peptide Analysis Protocols**, edited by *Ben M. Dunn and Michael W. Pennington, 1994* • 0-89603-274-4 • Comb $64.50

☐ 35. **Peptide Synthesis Protocols**, edited by *Michael W. Pennington and Ben M. Dunn, 1994* • 0-89603-273-6 • Comb $64.50

☐ 34. **Immunocytochemical Methods and Protocols**, edited by *Lorette C. Javois, 1994* • 0-89603-285-X • Comb $64.50

☐ 33. **In Situ Hybridization Protocols**, edited by *K. H. Andy Choo, 1994* • 0-89603-280-9 • Comb $69.50

☐ 32. **Basic Protein and Peptide Protocols**, edited by *John M. Walker, 1994* • 0-89603-269-8 • Comb $59.50 • 0-89603-268-X • Hardcover $89.50

☐ 31. **Protocols for Gene Analysis**, edited by *Adrian J. Harwood, 1994* • 0-89603-258-2 • Comb $69.50

☐ 30. **DNA–Protein Interactions**, edited by *G. Geoff Kneale, 1994* • 0-89603-256-6 • Paper $64.50

☐ 29. **Chromosome Analysis Protocols**, edited by *John R. Gosden, 1994* • 0-89603-243-4 • Comb $69.50 • 0-89603-289-2 • Hardcover $94.50

☐ 28. **Protocols for Nucleic Acid Analysis by Nonradioactive Probes**, edited by *Peter G. Isaac, 1994* • 0-89603-254-X • Comb $59.50

☐ 27. **Biomembrane Protocols:** *II. Architecture and Function,* edited by *John M. Graham and Joan A. Higgins, 1994* • 0-89603-250-7 • Comb $64.50

☐ 26. **Protocols for Oligonucleotide Conjugates:** *Synthesis and Analytical Techniques,* edited by *Sudhir Agrawal, 1994* • 0-89603-252-3 • Comb $64.50

☐ 25. **Computer Analysis of Sequence Data:** *Part II,* edited by *Annette M. Griffin and Hugh G. Griffin, 1994* • 0-89603-276-0 • Comb $59.50

☐ 24. **Computer Analysis of Sequence Data:** *Part I,* edited by *Annette M. Griffin and Hugh G. Griffin, 1994* • 0-89603-246-9 • Comb $59.50

☐ 23. **DNA Sequencing Protocols**, edited by *Hugh G. Griffin and Annette M. Griffin, 1993* • 0-89603-248-5 • Comb $59.50

☐ 22. **Microscopy, Optical Spectroscopy, and Macroscopic Techniques**, edited by *Christopher Jones, Barbara Mulloy, and Adrian H. Thomas, 1993* • 0-89603-232-9 • Comb $69.50

☐ 21. **Protocols in Molecular Parasitology**, edited by *John E. Hyde, 1993* • 0-89603-239-6 • Comb $69.50

☐ 20. **Protocols for Oligonucleotides and Analogs:** *Synthesis and Properties,* edited by *Sudhir Agrawal, 1993* • 0-89603-247-7 • Comb $69.50 • 0-89603-281-7 • Hardcover $89.50

☐ 19. **Biomembrane Protocols:** *I. Isolation and Analysis,* edited by *John M. Graham and Joan A. Higgins, 1993* • 0-89603-236-1 • Comb $64.50

☐ 18. **Transgenesis Techniques:** *Principles and Protocols,* edited by *David Murphy and David A. Carter, 1993* • 0-89603-245-0 • Comb $69.50

☐ 17. **Spectroscopic Methods and Analyses:** *NMR, Mass Spectrometry, and Metalloprotein Techniques,* edited by *Christopher Jones, Barbara Mulloy, and Adrian H. Thomas, 1993* • 0-89603-215-9 • Comb $69.50

☐ 16. **Enzymes of Molecular Biology**, edited by *Michael M. Burrell, 1993* • 0-89603-322-8 • Paper $59.50

☐ 15. **PCR Protocols:** *Current Methods and Applications,* edited by *Bruce A. White, 1993* • 0-89603-244-2 • Paper $54.50

☐ 14. **Glycoprotein Analysis in Biomedicine**, edited by *Elizabeth F. Hounsell, 1993* • 0-89603-226-4 • Comb $64.50

☐ 13. **Protocols in Molecular Neurobiology**, edited by *Alan Longstaff and Patricia Revest, 1992* • 0-89603-199-3 • Comb $59.50

☐ 12. **Pulsed-Field Gel Electrophoresis:** *Protocols, Methods, and Theories,* edited by *Margit Burmeister and Levy Ulanovsky, 1992* • 0-89603-229-9 • Hardcover $69.50

☐ 11. **Practical Protein Chromatography**, edited by *Andrew Kenney and Susan Fowell, 1992* • 0-89603-213-2 • Hardcover $59.50

☐ 10. **Immunochemical Protocols**, edited by *Margaret M. Manson, 1992* • 0-89603-204-3 • Comb $69.50

☐ 9. **Protocols in Human Molecular Genetics**, edited by *Christopher G. Mathew, 1991* • 0-89603-205-1 • Hardcover $69.50

☐ 8. **Practical Molecular Virology:** *Viral Vectors for Gene Expression,* edited by *Mary K. L. Collins, 1991* • 0-89603-191-8 • Paper $54.50

☐ 7. **Gene Transfer and Expression Protocols**, edited by *Edward J. Murray, 1991* • 0-89603-178-0 • Hardcover $79.50

☐ 6. **Plant Cell and Tissue Culture**, edited by *Jeffrey W. Pollard and John M. Walker, 1990* • 0-89603-161-6 • Comb $69.50

☐ 5. **Animal Cell Culture**, edited by *Jeffrey W. Pollard and John M. Walker, 1990* • 0-89603-150-0 • Comb $69.50

Name _____

Department _____

Institution _____

Address _____

City/State/Zip _____

Country _____

Phone # _____ Fax # _____

"T" denotes a tentative price. Prices listed are Humana Press prices, current as of June 1995, and do not reflect the prices at which books will be sold to you by suppliers other than Humana Press. All prices subject to change without notice.

UK, Europe, Middle East, and Africa: Order directly from Chapman & Hall by faxing to: +44-171-522-9623.

Postage & Handling: *USA Prepaid (UPS):* Add $4.00 for the first book and $1.00 for each additional book. *Outside USA* (Surface): Add $5.00 for the first book and $1.50 for each additional book.

☐ **My check for $_____ is enclosed**
   (Drawn on US funds from a US bank).

☐ **Visa**   ☐ **MasterCard**   ☐ **American Express**

Card # _____

Exp. date _____

Signature _____